Problem-based Psychiatry

Problem-based Psychiatry

DAVID MEAGHER MD, PhD, MSc (Clinical Teaching), MRCPsych

Foundation Chair, Head of Teaching & Research in Psychiatry, School of Medicine, University of Limerick. Consultant Psychiatrist, Mid-West Mental Health Service

HENRY O'CONNELL MRCPsych, MCPsychl, MSc, MD

Consultant Psychiatrist, Laois Offaly Mental Health Service and Adjunct Associate Clinical Professor, University of Limerick School of Medicine

JOHN McFARLAND MD

Senior Lecturer, School of Medicine, University of Limerick, Consultant Psychiatrist, Mid-West Mental Health Service. Dean for Postgraduate Training in Psychiatry, UL-Midwest Deanery of the College of Psychiatrists for Ireland

NOREEN MOLONEY MSc, MRCPsych, MCPsychl

Senior Registrar, Mid-West Mental Health Service

The late **MAEVE LEONARD, MD, MRCPsych**

Former Clinical Tutor (Psychiatry), School of Medicine, University of Limerick

For additional online content, visit StudentConsult.com

ELSEVIER

Content Strategist: Jeremy Bowes
Content Development Specialist: Veronika Watkins
Project Manager: Anne Collett
Design: Ryan Cook
Illustration Manager: Paula Catalano

Printed in the UK

Last digit is the print number: 9 8 7 6 5 4 3 2 1

Working together to grow libraries in developing countries

www.elsevier.com • www.bookaid.org

CONTENTS

PREFACE

This textbook has been developed as a practical resource to support students through their educational attachments in psychiatry during medical school training. The four-year graduate entry programme at the University of Limerick was established in 2007 and emphasizes problem-based learning techniques throughout. The chapters of this book have been developed by the teaching faculty in collaboration with our medical students over the lifetime of our school through an iterative process using feedback from students. This has allowed us to road test the material to ensure that it is stimulating and that the content emphasizes practical information that supports students as they engage with the complex world of clinical psychiatry. Each chapter represents a protected teaching session that is facilitated by the teacher (typically a member of our clinical faculty) in highly interactive small-group settings.

The material has also been used in the clinical induction programme for our basic specialist trainees and is designed to support education that is vertically integrated. The material considers clinical challenges from a multidisciplinary perspective and is therefore also suited for blended learning scenarios. Each case is designed to bring the learner on a journey that consists of situations where key knowledge about the topic being studied is considered in the context of a clinical conundrum. While the scientific basis of psychiatry is emphasized, our extended faculty of clinicians have contributed to ensure the authenticity of the case histories and to keep each case firmly grounded in the challenges of real-world practice. In addition, we have maintained careful attention to the recognized learning objectives for psychiatry teaching as suggested by internationally recognized regulatory bodies, which have helped to ensure coverage across the clinical spectrum.

The cases are designed to facilitate a learning journey, wherein the students consider questions that relate to an evolving clinical scenario. The students are provided with the material prior to the protected teaching sessions, and thus, teaching time is focused upon exploring student understanding of the material and exercising this new information to promote deeper learning, while also allowing flexibility around time allocation to aspects that students find most challenging to understand and digest. For the teacher-facilitator, the material is structured to promote student engagement, while allowing time for the teachers to observe the learners and encourage participation across the members of the small-group. Over the years, both students and teachers have repeatedly reported their enjoyment and enthusiasm for this approach to formal teaching sessions. In particular, teachers have remarked how they find the sessions more powerful because they have much less speaking to do during sessions and can thus better observe and facilitate the students.

Finally, we would like to thank our students for their help in developing the content of this book and for helping us to make it as student-friendly as possible. We have also benefitted immeasurably from the wisdom of our clinical colleagues who have embraced the teaching programme with great vigour, generously giving their time and now enjoying the dividend of our former students joining our clinical faculty as many have undertaken careers in psychiatry. We have patiently developed this educational material and, inevitably, this journey has spanned almost a decade—a period during which one of the principal authors, Dr Maeve Leonard, died. Maeve contributed crucially to the original chapters of the book, and we hope that the final product does justice to her dedication, generosity and kindness.

Ar dheis Dé go raibh a h'anam.
David Meagher, John McFarland, Noreen Moloney, Henry O'Connell.
Graduate Entry Medical School
University of Limerick
December 2020.

ACKNOWLEDGEMENTS

The author team would like to acknowledge and offer their grateful thanks to the following contributors, whose input and support were invaluable in producing the chapters in this book:

Dimitrios Adamis MD, MRCPsych, Consultant Psychiatrist, Sligo Mental Health Services

Zahoor Ahmad MBBS, MRCPsych, Consultant Psychiatrist, Kildare/West Wicklow Mental Health Service

Fahad Awan FCPS, MRCPsych, Consultant Psychiatrist, Mid-West Mental Health Service

Dario Bagaric MD, PhD, Consultant Psychiatrist, Mid-West Mental Health Service

Ahmad Bashir MCPsychI, Senior Registrar, Mid-West Mental Health Service

Diarmuid Boyle MCPsychI, MRCPsych, Senior Registrar, Mid-West Mental Health Service

Gurjot Brar MRCPsych, MCPsychI, Clinical Tutor, School of Medicine, University of Limerick

Richard Cahill MB, MRCPsych, Consultant Psychiatrist, Laois Offaly Mental Health Service

Aisling Campbell MRCPsych, MMedSC, Consultant Psychiatrist and Head of Department of Psychiatry, University College Cork

Aidan Collins MB, DPM, Consultant Psychiatrist, St Vincent's Hospital, Dublin

Catherine Corby MRCPsych, MSc, Consultant in Liaison Psychiatry, University Hospital, Limerick and Honorary Senior Lecturer at University of Limerick

Walter Cullen MD, MICGP, MRCGP, General Practitioner and Professor of Urban General Practice, UCD School of Medicine

Cara Daly MRCPsych, Senior Registrar, Carlow/Kilkenny/South Tipperary Mental Health Service

James Daly MMedSc, MRCPsych, Consultant Psychiatrist, Laois Offaly Mental Health Service and Adjunct Senior Clinical Lecturer, University of Limerick School of Medicine

Rachel Davis MRCPsych, Consultant Psychiatrist (Child and Adolescent Psychiatry), Mid-West Mental Health Service

Patrick Devitt MD, MRCPsych, Consultant Psychiatrist Adjunct Senior Lecturer in Psychiatry, University of Limerick School of Medicine

Eoin Devereux PhD, Professor of Sociology, University of Limerick, Adjunct Professor in Contemporary Culture at the University of Jyvaskyla, Finland

Patrick G. Doyle MRCPsych, Consultant Psychiatrist (Retired), Mid-West Mental Health Service

Colum Dunne PhD, Director of Research, School of Medicine, University of Limerick

Aslam Malik Elahi MRCPsych, Consultant Psychiatrist, Kildare West Wicklow Mental Health Service

Darran Flynn MRCPsych, Consultant Psychiatrist, Waterford Mental Health Service

Eithne Foley MRCPsych, MA, CBT, Consultant Child and Adolescent Psychiatrist, Mid-West Mental Health Service

Maurice Gervin MRCPsych, MD, Consultant Psychiatrist and Executive Clinical Director, Laois Offaly Mental Health Service

Kevin Glynn BA, MSc, BMBS, MRCPsych, Senior Registrar in Old Age Psychiatry, St James's Hospital Dublin

Gautam Gulati MD, FRCPI, FRCPsych, Consultant Psychiatrist, Adjunct Associate Clinical Professor, School of Medicine, University of Limerick

Zafrullah Hamzah MRCPsych, Consultant Psychiatrist, Mid-West Mental Health Service

Noel Hannan MRCPsych, Consultant Psychiatrist (Intellectual Disability), St Raphaels, Cellbridge, Co Kildare

David Hickey MB, Registrar in Psychiatry, Mid-West Mental Health Service

Ed Holland MB, BSc, DCH, MRCPsych, Consultant Psychiatrist, Laois Offaly Mental Health Service and Adjunct Senior Clinical Lecturer, University of Limerick School of Medicine

H El Sheikh Idris MRCPsych, MRCPI, DPM, DCP, DMMD, Consultant Psychiatrist, Laois Offaly Mental Health Service

Muhammad Javed MRCPsych, MCPsychI, FRCPC, Consultant Psychiatrist, Waterford Mental Health Service

Michael Jennings, Principal Social Worker (Retired), Mid-West Mental Health Service

Brendan Kelly MD, PhD, FRCPsych, FRCPI, FTCD, Professor of Psychiatry, Trinity College Dublin, Consultant Psychiatrist, Tallaght Hospital, Dublin

Mary Kelly MRCPsych, Consultant Psychiatrist (Intellectual Disability), Mid-West Mental Health Service

Peter Kirwan MRCPsych, Consultant Psychiatrist (Retired), Mid-West Mental Health Service

Erik Kolchus MRCPsych, Consultant Psychiatrist (Psychiatry of Later Life), Mid-West Mental Health Service

Kevin Lally MSc, MRCPsych, MCPsychI, Senior Registrar, Mid-West Mental Health Service

Niamh Liddy MSc, Clin Pharm, MRCPsych, MCPsychI, Senior Registrar, Mid-West Mental Health Service

Mas Mohamad Mahady MRCPI, MRCPsych, Consultant Psychiatrist (Perinatal Psychiatry), Mid-West Mental Health Service

Professor Geraldine McCarthy MRCPsych, Consultant Psychiatrist (Psychiatry of Later Life), Sligo Mental Health Service and Associate Professor of Psychiatry, NUIG School of Medicine

Deirdre McGrath MD, MMEd, FRCP, FRCPI, Head of School, University of Limerick School of Medicine

Helena McKeague FFARCSI, Senior Lecturer in Medical Education (Problem Based Learning), School of Medicine, University of Limerick

Frank McKenna MRCPsych, MCPsychI, Senior Registrar, Cork Mental Health Service

Lisa McLoughlin MRCPsych, Consultant Forensic Psychiatrist, Central Mental Hospital, Dublin

Anna Maria Meaney MD, MRCPsych, Consultant Psychiatrist, Psychiatry of Later Life, Mid-West Mental Health Service

Ian Moloney DCH, DPM, MRCPsych, Consultant Psychiatrist, Laois Offaly Mental Health Service

Faisal Mohd MRCPsych, MCPsychI, Clinical Tutor, School of Medicine, University of Limerick

Maria Moran MRCPsych, Consultant Psychiatrist, Intellectual Disability, Brothers of Charity, Galway

Deirdre Mulryan MRCPsych, Consultant Psychiatrist (Rehabilitation Psychiatry), Galway/ Roscommon / Mayo Mental Health Service

Valerie Murphy MRCPsych, Consultant Psychiatrist (Intellectual Disability), Cork Mental Health Service

Owen Mulligan MD, MRCPsych, Consultant Psychiatrist, General Adult Psychiatry, Sligo-Leitrim Mental Health Service

Declan Murray MD, MRCPsych, Consultant Psychiatrist, Adjunct Senior Lecturer in Psychiatry, University of Limerick School of Medicine

Ayesha Nazir MRCPsych, Consultant Psychiatrist, Longford Westmeath Mental Health Service

Mary B. O'Brien MSc, MRCPsych, Consultant Psychiatrist, Laois Offaly Mental Health Service

Muireann O'Donnell MSc Occ Health, DRCOG, MRCPsych, MCPsychI, Registrar, Mid-West Mental Health Service

Antonia O'Keefe MRCPsych, MCPsychI, Senior Registrar Child and Adolescent Psychiatry, Mid-West Mental Health Service

Seamus O'Flaithbheartaigh, Consultant Psychiatrist, Rehabilitation and Recovery Psychiatry, Mid-West Mental Health Service

Susan O'Hanrahan MRCPsych, Consultant Psychiatrist (Child and Adolescent Psychiatry), Mid-West Mental Health Service

Donal O'Hanlon MRCPsych, Consultant Psychiatrist and Clinical Director, Kildare West Wicklow Mental Health Service

Roisin O'Sullivan MRCPsych, MCPsychI, Consultant Psychiatrist (Liaison Psychiatry for Later Life), Tallaght University Hospital, Dublin

Vishnu Pradeep MRCPsych, MCPsychI, Senior Registrar, Mid-West Mental Health Service

Gerry Rafferty MRCPsych, MCPsychI, Registrar, South Tipperary Mental Health Service

Muhammad Ammad Rauf MRCPsych, Consultant Psychiatrist, Laois Offaly Mental Health Service

Paul Reynolds MRCPsych, Consultant Psychiatrist, (Psychiatry of Later Life), Mid-West Mental Health Service

Tom Reynolds MRCPsych, Consultant Psychiatrist, (Psychiatry of Later Life), Mid-West Mental Health Service

Mark Roe MRCPsych, MPhil, PhD, Consultant Psychiatrist, Laois Offaly and Longford Westmeath Mental Health Service

Marcel Steenkist RANP, MA, GradDip, MSc, Psychotherapist, Laois Offaly Mental Health Service

Narayanan Subramanian, Consultant Psychiatrist, Mid-West Mental Health Service

Sheila Tighe MSc(Pharm), MD, MRCPsych, Consultant Psychiatrist, Mid-West Mental Health Service

Art illustrations by Claus Castenskiold

(I) Introduction

David Meagher ▦ Helena McKeague ▦ Deirdre McGrath ▦ John McFarland

This textbook is designed to provide a comprehensive and engaging learning resource for those learning and teaching psychiatry and mental health. The case-based narrative style allows for highly accessible and practical content that echoes how the practising clinician applies their knowledge about mental disorders in everyday practice. The informal style encourages students to actively engage with the material before, during and after scheduled teaching sessions, allowing for greater digestion, analysis and retention of the subject matter, while also promoting life-long learning. The book is primarily designed for medical students and their educators to provide a user-friendly, but comprehensive, resource to support the psychiatry programme. The chapters can readily be adapted to provide a framework to engage other groups—postgraduate trainees in psychiatry, nurses and allied healthcare professionals—that want to engage with practical, clinically orientated learning in psychiatry.

The stimulus for this case-based textbook was our experience at the University of Limerick (UL) Medical School. In the early years of the programme, we used a hybrid curriculum that integrated traditional lecture-based methods and problem-based learning (PBL). However, over time, the interactive case-based approach occluded the need for lectures as our students consistently indicated that they found these sessions more stimulating and useful. Not surprisingly, our final year students reported that the year was particularly intense with a significant cognitive load, and that receiving knowledge in a way that facilitated retention and allowed information to be readily contextualized in terms of its real-world application was most helpful. The effectiveness of this case-based material is evidenced by repeatedly high student satisfaction and enjoyment ratings, and by the number of our students who ultimately choose psychiatry as a career. Indeed, more than a dozen of the authors of chapters in this book are graduates of our programme now engaged in postgraduate training in psychiatry.

To ensure adequate coverage of all knowledge, skills and attitudes relevant to clinical psychiatry, we have developed the material alongside a careful review of recognized learning objectives for psychiatry teaching. This identified that combining learning outcomes that are recommended by three bodies—(1) the Royal College of Psychiatrists (RCP), (2) the Association of Directors of Medical Student Education in Psychiatry (ADMSEP) and (3) the Australian Medical Council (AMC)— allowed for a comprehensive list of desired outcomes for medical student training in psychiatry. Each chapter in the book includes clearly defined learning objectives that can be identified at the beginning of each case and reviewed prior to the conclusion of the teaching session to ensure adequate learning has been achieved.

The consistency in the quality of the individual chapters has been promoted through a process of student feedback, whereby students were asked to anonymously identify elements of the protected teaching programme that they found less useful, including identifying the three 'best' and three 'worst' chapters. We also found that rotating cases across the teaching faculty allowed for feedback from the teachers' perspective.

Design and format

This textbook is designed to take the reader on a journey through each principal learning topic in psychiatry. Each chapter follows the narrative of a named 'patient' through 6–7 'stations', gradually delving more deeply into the subject matter and prompting the student to stop and think about the scenario as it develops, thus promoting better understanding and deep learning. Each chapter provides material suited to a one-hour interactive teaching session. All the chapters have been road-tested by the authors over the past seven years to optimize their suitability for small- and medium-group teaching sessions.

This textbook consists of 26 case-based chapters, each addressing an important area of clinical psychiatry. There are also introductory sections on psychiatric assessment; clinical psychopathology and a section showing the style of the main chapters of the book via 'Martha: Enquiry-based Learning'.

Each chapter of this book has been written by a team of authors that includes at least one of the main textbook authors (all of whom are academic members of the Department of Psychiatry at UL School of Medicine), along with faculty members who deliver the material in protected teaching sessions and other identified experts who are national and international experts outside UL. The book has an Irish origin, but our programme includes a high percentage of students from North America and across Europe. Therefore, this textbook has been written in a way that is easily comprehensible by students and doctors-in-training in all English-speaking countries.

Several of the chapters are used in our UL-College of Psychiatrists of Ireland training programme to support protected teaching sessions. In some cases, students who engaged with the early drafts of this material at the commencement of our UL Medical School programme have progressed to re-engage with it as postgraduate trainees in psychiatry and, most recently, as trainers. Furthermore, the material is orientated to support vertical training over much of the lifetime of medical learning.

'Signposted' Problem-based Learning

Problem- (or case-) based pedagogies have become the preferred approach for learning in many medical schools across the globe, including our programme, where the ethos of student-centred, interactive, inquiry-based methods has formed the mainstay of our curriculum. The early years of the programme embrace a relatively purist approach to PBL, which emphasizes self-directed learning such that by the time the students reach their final year, they have developed the type of critical thinking that allows for a modified approach to the final year. This ensures that the learning objectives and key clinical challenges can be proactively delivered, with class teaching time almost exclusively devoted to small-group discussions of clinically relevant and practical scenarios.

Moreover, we describe the delivery of our teaching sessions as 'signposted' PBL, wherein students are provided with information around each clinical question that arises in each case, which encourages the discussion of both correct and incorrect ideas in a safe environment that can be readily structured to promote participation across the group with elaboration and organization of knowledge to promote deeper learning. This approach is suited to the demands of the final year programme, which needs to cover a considerable amount of material in each discipline of medicine in a short period. In our programme, this typically involves 4–5 cases per week.

How to use this textbook as a student

This book is intended to allow user-friendly engagement with the key learning objectives for over two dozen presentations that are relevant to the practice of clinical psychiatry. The book is designed to be easy to read, with clinical narratives that are intended to stimulate the reader by raising important questions about our understanding and management of mental illness.

A key aspect of the learning process is to proactively embrace the material such that formal teaching sessions can be used to explore issues concerning knowledge, better comprehend the material and promote deeper and enduring learning. In short, students should have already read each chapter before it is formally covered in protected teaching sessions. This requires some discipline to remain ahead of the flow of new material during attachments, but ultimately is a highly efficient means of understanding the material. We have tried to design the book so that it is suitable for an initial casual read (e.g. at the commencement of an attachment), followed by a more formal and detailed read of each session immediately before it is covered in protected teaching, and followed by detailed exploration and knowledge organization during teaching sessions. Our knowledge of what promotes sustained and dynamic retention of knowledge supports this approach as an efficient means of optimally absorbing the material.

As a student, inevitably, one's knowledge of these problems will be tested in terms of confirming knowledge—demonstrating an ability to apply this knowledge in clinical scenarios. It is useful for each chapter to consider the question of *'how might this be tested in an examination?'* and to that end, we suggest that all students try to put themselves into the shoes of an examiner—how can knowledge be reliably tested in a manner that can be applied consistently to a (usually large) group of students who are sitting for an examination? In general, clinical examinations are the component of the exam wherein students of different ability separate out. It should be recognized that some aspects of knowledge are more suited to being tested in a simulated clinical setting, and to that end, we have listed potential objective structured clinical examination (OSCE) stations to facilitate students preparing for the clinical component of the examination, which many report as being the most stressful aspect of the examination process.

We hope that this textbook is both an informative and enjoyable resource to support your educational journey through psychiatry.

How to use this textbook as an educator

The level of detail is designed to enable it to be covered within the typical clinical attachment in psychiatry that students undertake within modern medical curricula, which is typically between four and eight weeks. Each case has undergone rigorous road testing, having been delivered within the time-pressured environment of our six-week long final year clinical attachment in psychiatry. This has helped to optimize the pacing of material so that it can be efficiently covered within the required time frame. Within our programme, we include an initial induction week that focuses on revisiting and developing existing knowledge about clinical psychiatry and preparing students for the subsequent five weeks of clinical attachments, emphasizing history taking and conducting the mental state assessment. The latter part of the induction week includes covering six 'core' cases that orient students to the common and more severe clinical presentations (e.g. acute psychosis, acute mania, depression and anxiety disorders) so that the remaining 20 cases can be covered in the protected teaching sessions during the remaining five weeks of clinical psychiatry attachment. This schedule can be readily adapted as needed. The learning outcomes provided can be constructively aligned with the assessment of knowledge and clinical skills.

Martha's 'case' (see section IV, below) is designed to introduce enquiry-based learning to those who are not familiar with it.

(II) The Psychiatric Assessment

Introduction

History taking and the MSE are the most important diagnostic tools in a psychiatrist's toolkit. Physical examination and clinical investigations are helpful in clarifying a diagnosis in some cases, but most psychiatric diagnoses are syndromal (i.e. they reflect patterns of symptoms) and are not readily identified with specific biological measures. In no other area of medicine is the skill of clinical interviewing so important as in psychiatry, where, in addition, many patients have problems in communicating their difficulties because of their illness (e.g. paranoid patients may find it difficult to share their beliefs and experiences with others). It is frequently necessary to obtain a collateral history from a trusted source to clarify the accuracy of details and to get a sense of a patient's usual or 'baseline' functioning.

For any student of psychiatry, they must recognize that interviewing is a skill that can only be mastered with lots of practice, as a key element is to have a natural flow to the interview. The novice interviewer spends more time thinking up their next question rather than reacting to the specifics of a patient's response, while the seasoned clinician instinctively modifies their questioning according to the assessment as it unfolds. Having a standard structure in your mind is a crucial starting point. In practice, the skilled interviewer will deviate from this, allowing the patient to dictate the direction, but will ultimately make sure that all the different areas are covered.

A full psychiatric assessment includes history taking, MSE, a collateral history, physical examination and appropriate investigations. The case formulation is the final aspect of the complete assessment process and includes a case synopsis, differential diagnosis, a description of likely aetiological factors, a management plan and an assessment of likely prognosis. Moreover, the psychiatric history is intended to answer the question, 'Why is this particular patient sick, in this way, at this time?' It charts the patient's journey to this point in time and therefore has a longitudinal character. The MSE reflects the patient's current psychopathology and is thus much more cross-sectional. This section deals with history taking, MSE and formulation in some depth, while section III explores the key aspects of psychopathology.

The Psychiatric History

- Introductions and Demographics
- Context of the Assessment (venue, how patient arrived at the assessment)
- Presenting Complaint
- History of Presenting Complaint
- Past Psychiatric History
- Past Medical and Surgical History
- Drug History
- Family history
- Substance Misuse
- Personal History
  - Early Life & Development
  - Education
  - Occupational history
  - Relationship history
- Social History
- Forensic History
- Premorbid Personality

Mental Status Examination

- Appearance and Behaviour
- Speech
- Mood and Affect (and risk assessment)
- Thinking
  - Form
  - Content
- Perceptual Disturbances
- Cognition
- Insight

Formulation

- Case Synopsis
- Differential Diagnosis
- Aetiology
- Management Plan
- Prognosis

The psychiatric history

Taking a good psychiatric history requires that the interviewer simultaneously attends to a variety of challenges, including facilitating the patient, observing patient behaviour while closely listening to what is said (and not said!) and how, and finding a balance between allowing the patient to tell their story while also interjecting to clarify particular points of note, as well as steering the conversation through the necessary components of a thorough history. It is important to plan such encounters and to make oneself aware of as much background information as possible as this can minimize any potential misunderstandings while also equipping the interviewer to demonstrate accurate empathy with the patient's perspective. It is important to remember that often patients have already had to explain their difficulties to other people before you engage with them, while some patients will have issues with paranoia and/or irritability. Sometimes, it may be necessary to have several interactions to obtain a full history.

A note on questioning style

Always begin with open questions. This facilitates the patient telling you their story in their own words and will yield more information than a litany of closed questions. Closed questions are appropriate to clarify or establish particular issues. An open question might be 'what are the main problems that you have been having?' or 'what has brought you to see me today?' Use closed questions to clarify specific points, for example, 'have you ever felt that life is not worth living?' or 'have you ever felt like harming yourself?' Leading questions, such as 'do you wake up earlier in the morning now?' should be avoided and a more, non-directive style should be employed, for example, 'can you describe your sleep?' This allows the patient to describe their experience more fully. It also avoids a situation where the patient is trying to give 'the right answer' to please (or sometimes, mislead) the interviewer. The responses to leading questions about auditory hallucinations ('do the voices talk to each other about you?') or thought interferences ('do you have the experience of thoughts being placed into your head?') need to be interpreted carefully to avoid erroneously making a diagnosis of schizophreniform psychosis. Note that there is a marked difference between a patient responding with a simple 'yes' than 'yes, they make remarks about my behaviour'.

It can be useful to consider questioning about risk, for example, as a series of ever-decreasing circles that start very open ('how have you been feeling about yourself?' and 'how do you see the future?') to becoming gradually more narrow in focus ('do you ever feel that life is not worth living or that you would not mind if you suddenly died?', to 'do you ever have thoughts of harming yourself in any way?'), to quite precise questions regarding thoughts of self-harm, self-harm behaviour and planning, and actual suicidal intent.

Conducting an interview is like a dance—sometimes, it is a straightforward process wherein the patient is a willing and capable historian. At other times, it can be a more delicate process. It is important to try to avoid upsetting or annoying the patient, especially when patients are feeling irritable or paranoid. Some patients are frustrated that their beliefs are not being taken seriously enough or are doubted by others. In such cases, the experienced interviewer follows the general rule of patient interviewing 'neither collude nor collide'. This can be best achieved by empathizing with the patients' experience and emotional response rather than necessarily agreeing with delusional or other unusual ideas. Use of phrases, such as 'I'd like to try to understand that some more. Can you explain that in more detail?' or 'that sounds very difficult. How has that affected you?'

Setting the scene

It may sound obvious, but you should begin your interview by introducing yourself and any co-interviewers to the patient. In general, it is best to refer to the patient by title and surname in the first instance. Then, if the patient subsequently invites you to address them by their first name, you should do this. Ensure you know the names and relationships of anyone accompanying the patient and ask the patient if they would like them to remain in the room. Outline the purpose of the interview, explain confidentiality, and roughly how long the interview will take. As a general rule, it is useful to summarize the introductory discussion by saying that 'my task is to make it as easy as possible for you to tell your story and provide the information that can help us to establish how we can best help you'. Assure the patient that they can stop the interview at any time if they so wish, and that you are there to listen to their story and help them with their difficulties. Giving the patient a sense of control in this way helps to establish rapport.

It is useful to establish who the primary help seeker is, for example, a man with alcohol dependence may be presented as 'my wife has threatened that she would leave if I didn't do something about my drinking' or a psychotic person may feel they were 'forced' to come by a parent or general practitioner (GP).

Introductions and demographics

This should include key sociodemographic details, such as name, address, date of birth, contact information, ethnic origin, GP details, next of kin and their contact information.

Presenting complaint

This should briefly encapsulate how the patient presented to you at this particular time, the source of referral and the patient's description of their reason for seeking help and what they perceive as their main current difficulties. This is their subjective account of their 'problem list', and it should include quotes of the patient's responses where possible. Typically, a principal problem list should contain no more than 3–4 'main problems'.

History of presenting complaint

This is a more detailed and specific analysis of the presenting problem and should include details on symptom duration, onset and progression and any identifiable triggers. The frequency of symptoms, and aggravating and alleviating factors, should be explored. One must establish the effect on functioning and the impact on the patient's life. The interviewer should enquire if these symptoms were ever experienced in the past and, if so, what helped at that time. Use patient quotes liberally to represent the patient's subjective account accurately. This can be useful to look back on at subsequent meetings to gauge progress. Moreover, it can be especially useful for other interviewers when assessing the patient subsequently.

It is often useful to ask the patient 'when were you last feeling well/your normal self?' Longstanding difficulties raise the issue of temperament or personality as a factor. For example, a person with persistent low mood dating back to teenage years may have dysthymic disorder with or without a comorbid acute depressive exacerbation.

THE IMPORTANCE OF DETERMINING BASELINE FUNCTIONING

Psychiatric interviewing is not straightforward and establishing what the patient is normally like allows you to determine how unwell they are or how far off baseline they have become. It is important not just to rely on a narrative account, such as 'I was happier,' but to ask the patient for examples of what they used to do that they are not doing now. Collateral history from someone who knows the patient well is also a good way to get a sense of a person's baseline. Moreover, with acute presentations of major disorders, such as psychosis and mania, collateral history is sometimes the principal source of information. When information is gathered from third parties, it should be documented in the psychiatric assessment together with details of the informant.

Past psychiatric history

Obtain a chronological list of previous psychiatric episodes/diagnoses with details of all inpatient, outpatient and GP care. Document whether inpatient care was voluntary or involuntary. Note specific treatments and the efficacy of these, for example, psychological, psychotropic medications and electroconvulsive therapy (ECT). Enquire about episodes of self-harm in the past and any treatment received. It is important here to document the patient's perspective on what they found helpful (or unhelpful) in the past.

Past medical and surgical history

Obtain a chronological list of diagnoses, treatments and consider possible relationships to psychiatric illness. Past medical and surgical history is important in terms of the cause of mental disorders (e.g. hypothyroidism and depressive illness, treatment with drugs, such as steroids and psychosis). It may also impact treatment choices because of cardiac status, pharmacokinetics and drug interactions.

Drug history

List all current medications using generic drug names together with the details on dose and frequency of administration. Note any previous psychotropic medications (and why these were discontinued) and any known drug sensitivities. Note that decisions around the choice of antidepressant and antipsychotic medications are strongly influenced by previous experiences of effectiveness and tolerability.

Family history

Include a family tree of the patient, siblings, parents and offspring documenting any psychiatric illnesses. For deceased relatives, document the age and cause of death. Enquire about a family history of suicide, alcohol and substance misuse. Relationships with family members should be explored and documented in this section. Moreover, it is increasingly recognized in pharmacogenetics that a family history of response to psychotropic medication can guide optimal choice for your patient.

This can be completed as a diagram for visual clarity. The general rules for drawing a family tree are shown in Fig. II.1.

Substance misuse

Ask the patient about their use of alcohol, street drugs, over the counter medications or drugs not prescribed for them. For each drug ask about the age of first use and longitudinal history, including quantity. It is important to try to clarify the recency of use. If appropriate, explore features of dependence.

Personal history
EARLY LIFE AND DEVELOPMENT

Document any known issues during pregnancy, delivery or in the postpartum period. Enquire about the attainment of developmental milestones, noting any delays (e.g. 'Did your mother/parents ever tell you that you had problems with walking or talking?'). Enquire about the family unit and the environment in the early years and any periods of separation or bereavement in childhood.

A simple family tree includes details of parents, siblings and children (and any other family members who have been affected by mental illness

Males are noted as a square ☐, with females as a circle ◯, and unknown or nonbinary gender as a diamond ◇.

Affected members are denoted by shading in the symbol (e.g. ■), deceased members are noted by a line through the symbol (e.g. ⊘)

Marital or other partnership is denoted by a horizontal connecting line between members ☐—◯

An ended relationship (e.g. divorce, legal separation is denoted by a double line ☐—//—◯ separating this horizontal)

Descent is denoted by a vertical line descending between parents, while sibship is denoted by a horizontal line with a descending individual vertical line for each sibling.
Siblings are ordered from left (eldest) to right (youngest).

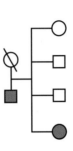

Twins are denoted by a diagonal line with a connector for monozygotic twins

Fig. II.1 The general rules for drawing a family tree.

As a general probe, it is useful to ask 'were you happy as a child?' and 'were you a good mixer? Did you make friends easily?'. It is useful to enquire about the style of parenting they received (e.g. strict, disciplinarian, loving) and any childhood adversity, such as significant losses, physical, emotional or sexual abuse and neglect. Note that there is a need to alert patients that you may be obligated to report disclosed historical child sexual abuse if the abuser is still alive or may pose a risk to others in any way.

EDUCATION

Document the patient's experience in primary and secondary school noting any bullying, conduct or other issues. Note academic performance and document the highest level of education reached. It is useful to explore the degree to which the patient engaged with extracurricular activities, such as sports, music, drama and other clubs, as this gives a sense of their character while growing up.

OCCUPATIONAL HISTORY

Give a chronological list of jobs the patient has held and reasons for leaving jobs and ask the patient to account for periods of unemployment.

RELATIONSHIP HISTORY

Document current and major past relationships, durations of each and reasons for breaking up. If appropriate, enquire about sexual orientation. Ask about children, with whom they reside and the patient's relationship with them. In terms of current relationships, it is important to document the character of the relationship, especially in terms of whether it is close, supportive and confiding in nature as these are key aspects that are linked to vulnerability towards mental ill-health.

Social history

Ask about current accommodation and the patient's current financial situation. In particular, establish if there are any significant debts. Enquire about psychosocial stressors and social supports. Establish the daily activities of the patient and how this compares to previous baseline activities.

Forensic history

Obtain a chronological list of any interactions with law enforcement, any cautions, arrests, convictions and prison sentences. Furthermore, ask about any pending legal proceedings. Enquire about any violent offences or offences involving weapons.

Premorbid personality

Ask the patient what they are like when 'well', and to describe themself as a person—highlighting how others might describe them and enquiring about 'good' and 'bad' points. Specific questioning regarding introversion vs extroversion, obsessionality, perfectionism, moodiness and positivity in perspective, impulsivity (including incidences where this has been an issue) and spiritual/religious beliefs. It is important to realize that the patient's description may be unreliable as it tends to be coloured by their prevailing mental state. It may be more useful to ask how others would describe them or to rely on collateral sources of information. A list of suggested probes to assess premorbid personality are provided in Box II.1.

BOX II.1 ■ Suggested probes to assess premorbid personality

1. Are you outgoing or more of a home body?
2. Do you enjoy socializing, or do you generally prefer your own company?
3. How do you perform in groups – do you like to be at the centre of attention?
4. Do you have any perfectionistic traits?
5. How are you in terms of things like punctuality, order, cleanliness?
6. Do you sometimes spend too long on tasks when it is not necessary?
7. Are you normally a cautious person or do you like to jump straight in?
8. How long do you usually take when deciding about purchasing new items?
9. Have you ever got into trouble because of making rash decisions?
10. Are you generally positive or negative when thinking about everyday life?
11. Would you describe yourself as a glass half-full or half-empty person?
12. Do you suffer from mood swings or periods of persistent pessimism?

The Mental State Examination

The MSE is the process by which we document our observations of the patient's mental state at the time of the interview, including the presence and severity of mental symptoms, which are also known as psychopathological disturbances. It is cross-sectional and, in contrast to the psychiatric history, is objective rather than subjective. It is based upon all observations during the interview process. Much of the information documented under the MSE section is gathered or apparent during the general assessment process (Box II.2); however, usually, these observations are supplemented by clarifying questions towards the end of the interview.

BOX II.2 ■ The Mental State Examination

- Appearance and behaviour
- Speech
- Mood and affect (and risk assessment)
- Thinking (form and content)
- Perceptual disturbances
- Cognition
- Insight

The MSE is one of the key skills of psychiatry, and students must become familiar with the recognized scheme for describing the MSE. This is typically viewed as including seven separate sections (although there are subsections in each of these). It is important to follow the scheme in the correct order, and students may find the use of a mnemonic helpful to pin down the order (i.e. remember ASMTPCI). A widely suggested mnemonic is 'A Smart Medic Takes Particular Care Innately'. Some students find more quirky mnemonics connect better. A favourite in our programme was suggested by Dr Elizabeth Dunbar as 'A Saucy Maid Tickles People Coming In'. Just how and why they are tickled and where it is they are coming in to is uncertain but use whatever works best for you!

Appearance and behaviour

Comment on the apparent age of the patient, physical appearance, demeanour, dress and level of self-care. These should be as objective as possible and neutral in tone (e.g. a person can be unusual in attire but should not be described as foolish or ridiculous—even if you perceive this to be the case!). Remember that it is important to be respectful of patients who present with unusual or odd behaviours, but that the clinician must navigate the territory between objective documentation while not trivializing or ignoring unusual behaviour.

You should note the activity level of the patient during the interview, their spontaneity, level of eye contact, any agitation and general attitude to the interview. Comment on rapport—was the patient guarded or suspicious? Were they socially appropriate, cooperative, distractible, disinhibited or overfamiliar? Did the patient display any abnormal movements?

Rapport is an important aspect of the assessment and should be considered as a two-way process. Sometimes students or training doctors may blame themselves for interviews that do not go well and in which they find it difficult to connect with the patient and form a productive rapport. It is important to note that one of the characteristics of psychosis is that it includes experiences that are generally outside of normal experience and therefore frequently difficult for the assessor to fully empathize with. This is not the fault of the assessor however, merely an objective observation that it was difficult to establish good rapport during this interview and it also is an important factor in explaining circumstances where it is difficult to gather a full history as the patient is guarded or otherwise uncommunicative.

Speech

The patient's volume, tone and rate of speech should be noted. Ascertain whether the patient is a focused and fluent historian or if their speech is rambling, circumstantial or tangential. Take note of a reduced or increased amount of speech or any abnormal breaks in the conversation. Document any word-finding difficulties (such as nominal dysphasia) and document any abnormalities in the content of speech, such as personalized language (e.g. neologisms or metonyms: see section III, below). If you do not note any abnormalities, it is appropriate to comment on the relative negatives in your findings by stating 'speech was normal in flow, form and content'.

Note that speech can be considered the audible expression of thinking, and it can be difficult at times to decide whether phenomena should be described as disturbances of thinking or speech. In general, disorders of speech content relate to the repetition of phrases or use of words in an unusual manner. Other disturbances of content (such as delusions or intrusive thoughts) are typically considered as disturbances to thought content. However, there is considerable flexibility in terms of in which cases these phenomena are reported—it is not unusual, for example, to comment at this point of the MSE that a patient with mania 'has evidence of pressurized speech with a flight of ideas and loosened associations' even though the latter two phenomena are more indicative of thought flow and form.

Mood, affect and risk assessment

It is important to document both the patient's subjective description of mood and your objective sense of their mood state. It is often useful to rate this in terms of score between 0 (unbearably low) to 10 (perfectly fine). At times there can be a disparity between the subjective and objective reporting of mood when a patient equates emotional discomfort (e.g. dysphoria) with depressed mood, which is typically a more pervasive and sustained phenomenon (Box II.3).

Affect is the objective assessment of the patient's expression of their emotions. A description of the patient's affect in terms of range (e.g. flattening refers to the reduced range), appropriateness in expression (e.g. blunting refers to a lack of appropriateness to circumstances) and tone in terms of expression over time (e.g. labile if very changeable).

BOX II.3 ▪ Questions that can be used to explore mood and risk of self-harm

Questions to elicit low mood include the following

- How have you been feeling in your mood?
- Does your mood change over the day?
- Have you been able to enjoy things?
- How have you been feeling about yourself?
- How do you see the future?

Questions to elicit elated mood include the following

- How has your mood been recently?
- How good have you felt?
- Has your mood been changeable?
- How are your levels of confidence?
- Have you been feeling special, important or empowered?
- Does anything upset you?

Questions to elicit thoughts of self-harm include the following

- How have you been feeling about the future?
- Have you ever felt that life is not worth living?
- Have you ever wished that you would not wake up?
- Have you ever thought that people would be better off without you?
- Have you ever thought about harming yourself or ending it all?
- Have you thought about how you might do it?
- Have you made any preparations?
- Have you tried to harm yourself?
- What would stop you doing it?
- Are you considering harming yourself at present?
- What methods have you considered?

Thinking

During the MSE, we aim to get an appreciation of the patient's thinking in terms of: (1) stream (or flow); (2) form (or structure of thoughts, including their organization and how thoughts are connected); (3) content (the themes of thoughts, e.g. delusions, obsessions); and (4) possession of thought (whether the thoughts are 'interfered' with in any way, e.g. thought insertion, withdrawal, broadcasting).

In terms of eliciting abnormal thought content and possession, it is often useful to begin with a question, such as '*is there anything in particular on your mind at the moment?*' or '*has anything been bothering you lately?*' It can be useful to facilitate patients with the comment '*Sometimes when people are unwell or stressed, they have unusual thoughts or experiences...*' Further examples of useful questions are presented in Box II.4 below.

BOX II.4 ■ Questions that can used to explore for abnormalities of thought content and form

- Are you ever worried that people are talking about you, following you or trying to harm you in any way? Who do you think is behind it (e.g. Mafia, MI5, ISIS, aliens) *Persecutory Delusion*
- Have you ever felt you were under the control of some external force or power? *Delusion of Control / Passivity*
- Has anything happened recently that has been very important for you? (e.g. the traffic light changed, and you realized you had been chosen to lead people) *Delusional Perception*
- Did you experience a sense of perplexity where you had some sense of inexplicable change in your environment? You sensed 'Something is not quite right' *Delusional Mood*
- Do you have a sense that people are paying attention to you? Do you ever receive messages from the television/radio/newspaper? *Delusion of Reference*
- Do you feel you have committed a grave sin or crime? Do you deserve to be punished for that? *Delusion of Guilt*
- Do you have any special gifts or power? Are you famous in any way? *Delusion of Grandiosity*
- Do you ever feel you are 'made to' act or feel in a certain way? Do you ever feel that your thought or feelings are outside of your control? *Passivity*
- Do you feel financially secure? Are others trying to take your wealth? *Delusion of Poverty*
- Do you think something terrible has or will happen to you? Do you feel doomed? Do you ever feel part of your body is dead? *Nihilistic Delusion*
- Are you able to think clearly now? Do you think your thoughts are being interfered with in any way?
  1. For example, those thoughts are being put into your head...*insertion*
  2. or taken out...*withdrawal*
  3. or that others can hear your thoughts...*broadcast*
- Do you ever draw a blank in your thoughts? Do your thoughts ever stop suddenly and unexpectedly when your thinking was fine moments before? *Thought Block*

Perception

In this section of the MSE, we are interested in identifying abnormalities that the patient may be experiencing in any sensory modality. For both delusions and hallucinations, it is important to establish the degree of conviction. Useful questions include the following: Is it possible that you are mistaken? Do you think there could be another explanation? Could your mind be playing tricks on you? (See also Box II.5.)

BOX II.5 ■ Questions to elicit perceptual disturbances

Has it ever happened that you have heard a noise (*Elementary*) or a voice when there was nobody around to account for it?
- Just one voice or more? Male/female? Can you identify who they are?
- Do they talk to each other? ... talk directly to you?
- Do they comment on what you are doing?
- Do you think they are coming from your own mind or can you locate where in the room they are coming from? Are you hearing them through you?
- Are they as clear as my voice?
- Can you stop them?
- When do they happen? (going to sleep / waking up)
- Do you feel they are real or could there be another explanation?

Continued on following page

Box II.5   (Continued)
- Has it ever happened that you have **seen** something that others did not appear to see?
- Has it ever happened that you have felt something strange in your body, for example, someone touching you when no one was there? Electricity? Muscles being squeezed? Itching or a sense of there being insects under your skin?
- Has it ever happened that you have **smelled / tasted** something that others did not appear to smell / taste?

Cognition

The assessment of cognition begins as you first observe the patient and then progresses to include eliciting specific aspects of performance, usually with formal testing. Bedside testing of cognition can be supported by cognitive batteries, such as the mini-MSE or the Montreal cognitive assessment test, which have the added advantage of providing scoring systems that are linked to significant impairment. However, both tools are subject to restrictions in their use and assessment of cognition can be readily achieved through a systematic process of observing the patient and conducting some simple tests of each cognitive modality. A scheme for this is provided in Box II.6.

BOX II.6 ■ A scheme for bedside/office-based assessment of cognitive function

This includes commenting on their level of consciousness, orientation, attention, short and long-term memory, executive abilities and visuospatial functioning.
- How alert and aroused are they? What is their level of **awareness** of their environment and capacity to engage in a coherent conversation? (e.g. Can I ask you your name? Where are you from? Why are you in the hospital?)
- Assess **Orientation** to time, place and person (others and themselves). Typical questions include the following: What is your name? Where is this place? Why are you here? Can you tell me what day it is, and the date? What month (year) are we in? What do you think that I do for a living? Who is that person (key nurse) over there?
- Consider their **attention** levels—are they able to focus and sustain the conversation? Formally, test for attention using a simple test, such as the reciting the months of the year forwards (ability to focus attention) and backwards (ability to sustain attention). Generally, people under age 65 years should be able to recite the months backwards to January without error. For those over age 65 years, they should be able to recite the months of the year backwards to July with no more than one omission. Other tests of attention are less preferred as they involve aspects of cognition other than attention (e.g. serial sevens require mathematical ability; spelling 'world' backwards requires literacy) and are thus subject to bias. Counting back from 20 to 1 requires minimal mathematical ability and, is thus, impacted upon mostly by the ability to maintain attention to the task.
- **Short-term memory** can be assessed by asking the patient if they can recall your name (presuming that you have provided this at the beginning of the assessment!). More formally, you can document their ability to recall three words after a delay. This is done by asking them to acknowledge and recite three words (e.g. red, cat, ball), and then asking them to repeat this after five minutes has elapsed. It should be noted if the patient can recall the three words with or without specific cueing (e.g. 'can I give you a clue—it's a colour' or 'it's a type of animal'). Normal performance is to recall all three words. Short-term memory can also be assessed by a name and address (e.g. Mr John Green, 27 Main Street, Clonmel, Co. Tipperary).
- **Long-term or remote memory** can be assessed by asking about verifiable personal details (names of family members, operations they have undergone), which should be available in medical case

Continued on following page

Box II.6 (Continued)

notes and memory for well-known figures (e.g. who was the president before Michael D Higgins? Who was the Irish soccer manager at Italia 90? Who was the American president assassinated in 1963?).

- **Executive function** relates to abilities, such as organization and planning, concept formation and word/idea generation. This can be readily tested by asking the patient to generate as many words as they can beginning with a particular letter in the alphabet (e.g. letter 'F') or animals that you might find in a zoo or types of motor car. It is usual to be able to reach ten words within a minute.
- **Visuospatial function** can be tested by asking the patient to identify the shape of objects in their environment, the relative distance between objects (e.g. which is closer, the television or the window?) and through formal tests, such as the ability to copy overlapping pentagons or insert a particular time into a circular clock. Note that these latter tests are impacted by motor skills.

When impaired performance is evident, it is usual to follow-up with a second test, and if they also perform poorly on this, formal and more detailed testing may be indicated. A patient with normal cognitive function can usually be described as follows: 'Ms Z readily engaged with the interview and was able to converse without any difficulties in terms of attention and concentration. Formal testing indicated that she was orientated to time, place and person, and she was able to recite the months of the year backwards without error. In terms of memory, she had a good short-term recall for three objects and also was able to recount her previous medical history accurately and name our most recent past president. Executive function appeared intact in terms of her ability to explain her story in a logical and sequenced manner and to list more than ten words beginning with 'F' within a minute. She completed the overlapping pentagons test indicating intact visuospatial abilities'. When there are impairments, the description can be amended accordingly.

Insight

There are several facets to 'complete insight', and it is better to avoid terms, such as 'insightless', as there are four principal elements (or levels) to insight that warrant clarification and few patients can be truly considered to be lacking insight. For the psychiatric assessment and future management, it is important to establish these four aspects of insight, namely:

1. Does the patient acknowledge that they have a problem?
2. Do they recognize that they are unwell?
3. Do they recognize their problems/experiences as symptoms, and are these symptoms attributed to psychological/psychiatric illness.
4. Does the patient believe they need help, and are they willing to accept treatment?

Note that insight is a key determinant of the need to consider involuntary treatment. Insight may be present for some symptoms and not for others, e.g. a patient may accept that they have schizophrenia but may not recognize a delusional idea as evidence of illness.

Formulation

A psychiatric formulation should attempt to explain why this patient is unwell, in this way, at this time.

Synopsis

It should begin with a synopsis of 2—3 sentences that include demographic details and salient features of the patient's history, MSE and physical examination.

Differential diagnoses

A discussion of differential diagnoses, with evidence for and against each differential, should be included. The provisional diagnosis should be identified.

Aetiological factors

A discussion of relevant aetiological factors utilizing a biological, psychological and social approach should be included. This should explore predisposing, precipitating and perpetuating factors. It is often helpful to present this as a table, utilizing the framework presented in Table II.1. Of note, there may be substantial overlap in the content of the nine cells here, e.g. family history of mental illness may lead to biological, psychological and social predisposing, precipitating and perpetuating factors. Moreover, some cells may be empty. The purpose of the table is to help to pull together the key elements of the case in a logical way.

TABLE II.1 ■ Biopsychosocial Formulation of Aetiology

	Biological	Psychological	Social
Predisposing factors	e.g. genetic, perinatal, substance misuse	e.g. early life experiences, cognitive style, bereavement	e.g. deprivation
Precipitating factors	e.g. noncompliance, substance misuse	e.g. relationship difficulties, loss	e.g. lack of support, debt
Perpetuating factors	e.g. noncompliance, substance misuse	e.g. cognitive distortions	e.g. social isolation, unemployment, financial problems

Management plan

The proposed management plan should include any relevant investigations and discuss treatment in terms of immediate and longer-term treatments, again using a biological, psychological and social approach.

Prognosis

A patient-specific statement on short- and long-term prognosis should be included highlighting good and poor prognostic indicators and reflect the natural history of the diagnosed disorder, course of illness (acute versus insidious), initial and/or previous response to treatment, level of insight, compliance with treatment, family history of response to treatment, premorbid adjustment and relevant social supports or lack thereof.

(III) Clinical Psychopathology

The purpose of this section is to introduce the reader to concepts that are relevant to understanding how symptoms of disturbed brain function present as mental symptoms. Psychopathology is the study of the symptoms of mental disorders and includes both the subjective account of the patient and descriptions of observed disturbances by the clinician. It involves the dissection and categorization of symptoms so that they can be understood in terms of clinical diagnosis and treatment.

What are the symptoms of disturbed brain function?

Disturbed functioning in the brain can produce a wide range of neurological and psychological symptoms and signs. Psychiatrists are especially interested in eliciting psychological (or mental) symptoms and understanding how they relate to psychiatric illnesses. These can include disturbances to behaviour, speech and language, mood and affective expression, thinking, perception and cognition. In addition, the ability to organize and sequence behaviour and integrate information to respond coherently can be affected by mental disorders. From a practical perspective, an important aspect of serious mental illnesses is that the ability to make rational decisions can be impaired in a way that sometimes require that patients receive help against their will, the so-called involuntary treatment, and which reflects a unique aspect of psychiatric care.

What is meant by the terms 'functional' and 'organic' when applied to mental disorders?

Historically, one of the ways of categorizing mental disorders has been to describe them as 'organic', wherein a reliable and discernible physical insult is identified as causing the disorder versus 'functional', wherein a consistent neuropathophysiological abnormality is not evident. It is important to recognize that this does not mean that symptoms of 'functional' mental disorder are any less 'real' but rather that the neural underpinnings are subtle such that they have not yet been identified in a way that allows for diagnosis by medical science. The biological era that has dominated psychiatry practice over the recent past was expected to unearth the underlying pathophysiology of common functional mental disorders. Although there have been considerable advances in understanding these conditions, disturbances that might allow for reliable diagnostic testing have remained elusive. In practical terms, all presentations of mental disturbances have a potential organic basis that should be ruled out before identifying them as functional. This is important when formulating a differential diagnosis, which should include possible physical causes and functional psychiatric conditions.

What is the difference between 'neurotic' and 'psychotic' symptoms?

Symptoms of mental illness can be divided according to their relationship to normal everyday experience. In psychosis, the person experiences symptoms that are outside the realm of normal experience and impact upon their experience of reality. These symptoms include delusions (abnormal beliefs that are not justified or rational) and hallucinations (perceptual experiences that occur without an external stimulus). It is more difficult for clinicians to empathize with psychotic symptoms as they are typically not based upon a rational interpretation of reality and are outside normal experience.

In contrast, neurotic symptoms include a variety of symptoms that are within normal experience but are excessive. Reality testing and insight are retained. These include anxiety, obsessive–compulsive phenomena and fears about health and wellness. The excessive nature of these experiences is a subjective judgement but closely relates to their functional impact. For example, many people experience intrusive obsessional thoughts that can be associated with compulsive behaviours (e.g. rechecking that the doors are locked and that appliances are unplugged at night). However, when this occurs at an intensity that interferes with one's ability to get to bed at a timely hour, it is considered pathological. Similarly, it is not uncommon to feel anxious in novel social circumstances, but when this anxiety is of an intensity that causes social avoidance that impacts upon one's quality of life, then it can be considered to have a pathological functional impact. The term 'neurotic' is also used, often in an uncomplimentary or pejorative way in everyday language (e.g. he or she is 'so neurotic') and has, thus, been largely retired. Nevertheless, the distinction between neurotic and psychotic symptoms is an important aspect of understanding psychiatric symptoms and diagnoses. In general, illnesses that include psychotic symptoms are more serious and are placed higher on the diagnostic hierarchy.

Do psychotic symptoms differ according to diagnosis?

Psychotic symptoms share the characteristic of being outside normal experience and linked to diminished insight on the part of the person experiencing the symptoms. Beyond that, they have quite different qualities or 'flavours' that allow them to be distinguished as organic versus functional, and affective versus schizophreniform.

In organic psychosis, symptoms are typically quite simple and often relate to the immediate environment. Delusional ideas frequently include themes of paranoia about having things stolen or being poisoned or that their environment is not how it is represented, for example, medications are poisons being used to punish or harm and that the ward is a prison. Hallucinations are often in tactile or visual sensory domains, which are less common in functional psychosis where auditory hallucinations are the most common. Simple auditory hallucinations do occur in organic psychosis (e.g. noises in the background), but second- and third-person 'voices' expressing complex ideas are much more suggestive of functional illness. Delusional ideas in functional psychosis can often include complex and systematized patterns with bizarre or scientifically implausible content.

Psychotic symptoms also have a different character in affective versus schizophreniform presentations. At the core of understanding, this distinction should be made by considering the relationship of the experiences to prevailing mood state, and whether they are mood-congruent (which suggests an affective origin for psychosis) or not. Mood congruence reflects the extent to which the symptoms are in-keeping with or secondary to mood. In psychotic depressive states, delusional ideas typically have themes or nihilism, guilt or imminent death/serious illness and thus reflect a sense of self-reproach and hopelessness or pointlessness. In mania, delusional ideas are typically about empowerment, special abilities or talents, status, fame or wealth and thus reflect the elevation of mood with expansive and unduly positive thinking.

Other psychotic symptoms are not readily linked to mood as they are dominated by themes of persecution or passivity. In psychosis associated with schizophrenia and related disorders (e.g. schizoaffective disorder, delusional disorder), there is often an underlying theme of passivity, i.e. that an external force can influence or control aspects of one's experience that would normally be under one's own control (e.g. thinking, emotions, behaviour). The sufferer is unable to prevent this happening as it is outside their volition and is thus described using the phrase *passivity*. These symptoms are often referred to a 'schizophreniform' and include a variety of experiences that were first described by Kurt Schneider (1959) as symptoms of first-rank that are suggestive of schizophrenia and thus sometimes also referred to as Schneiderian first-rank symptoms. These symptoms include the external influence of thinking (inserting, removing or broadcasting thoughts) and third-person auditory hallucinations where the subject is commented upon or referred to in the third-person (e.g. 'he's trying to fool them that everything is all right') rather than directly addressed as in second person hallucinations (e.g. 'you are evil, you should harm yourself'). See Box III.1 for more details.

BOX III.1 ■ Schneider's first-rank symptoms of schizophrenia

Auditory hallucinations

- A voice or voices repeating the subject's thoughts out loud.
- Voices that are discussing or arguing about the subject and that refer to him/her in the third person.
- Auditory hallucinations taking the form of a commentary on the subject's thoughts or behaviour.

Delusions of thought interference

- Thought insertion where unusual ideas or thoughts are described by the subject as being placed into their mind by an external agency.
- Thought withdrawal where the subject describes that their thoughts are being removed by an external agency.
- Thought broadcasting is the experience that the subject's thinking is no longer confined within his/her own mind but is shared by or is accessible to other people.

Made feelings, impulses or actions

- The experience that actions, sensations, bodily movements or emotions are generated by an outside agency that takes over the will of the subject.

Primary delusional experiences

- Delusional perception—the belief that a normal perception has special significance or meaning. This includes a normal perception (e.g. traffic lights turning green), which is interpreted as meaning that the person is a saint).
- Primary delusions are abnormal beliefs that arise like 'thought bubbles' and that cannot be considered as secondary to other beliefs or the prevailing mood.

True versus 'pseudo' psychosis

Another distinction is between true psychosis and related symptoms that lack the quality of psychosis in terms of their perceptual nature and associated insight. This refers particularly to hallucinations where a true auditory hallucination is perceived like a true perception, i.e. in external space and as real. In contrast, auditory pseudohallucinations are often described as 'voices inside my head' that the person recognizes is not based upon a real external stimulus. Such experiences are often described as being distinguishable from normal experiences by their character (e.g. described as not sounding like a real voice). True hallucinations are perceived as having an external source. Similarly, for thought content, patients can present with abnormal ideas that are similar to delusions but not held with the same intensity, are fleeting and relate to situational factors rather than an internal morbid experience. It is important to recognize that pseudo-psychotic symptoms are not 'false' or unimportant and that, in addition to occurring in vulnerable persons (e.g. emotionally unstable personality or those with dissociative disorder) and/or during periods of marked stress, they also commonly occur in major functional psychotic conditions, such as schizophrenia. These phenomena emphasize the importance of assessing serious mental symptoms in detail that should include their character, how they are experienced, their emotional significance, how they relate to events in the person's life and the conviction with which they are held (e.g. are they acted upon by the person?).

Neurosis and nonpsychotic symptoms

Traditionally, nonpsychotic symptoms of mental illness have been referred to as 'neurotic'. However, this term has been subsumed into the language of everyday life, often with a negative attribution ('you are so neurotic') that it has been largely retired by the psychiatry community. Nevertheless, the concept has some merit as it encapsulates mental disturbances that are often part of the normal experience of everyday life but that are exaggerated or experienced in excessive ways and therefore have a functional impact upon the person. In addition, the person recognizes that they are abnormal and has insight into their nature as evidence of mental distress or illness. Included among these symptoms are intrusive worries and ruminations, obsessional thoughts, compulsive behaviours, intrusive recollections of negative events, somatization and hypochondriacal. Central to this is that these are experiences that we all can recognize and often empathize with (e.g. experiencing stomach cramps when under stress or avoiding walking under a ladder on the street for fear it may bring bad luck). However, with illness, these symptoms become problematic in terms of impaired functioning (e.g. being late for work because of repeatedly checking that all the doors are locked and that appliances are unplugged).

Distinguishing between symptoms that relate to illness versus underlying personality

An important concept in understanding mental symptoms is how they relate to a person's underlying personality and belief systems. We all have beliefs that are shaped by our life experiences, cultural and religious background; that somebody with a different background may perceive as unusual or even abnormal. These ideas are not irrational but can be perceived as outside of normal belief systems for many other humans and are referred to as overvalued ideas.

The ego can be understood as that part of the mind that mediates between the conscious and unconscious. It is responsible for reality testing and gives a sense of personal identity. Overvalued ideas are typically 'ego-syntonic' in that they are consistent with our personal belief system and perceived as our own thoughts. In contrast, ego-dystonic thoughts are not consistent with our belief system and perceived by us as abnormal. Having thoughts about the need for cleanliness or order is a frequent ego-syntonic experience, but where these dominate thinking and cause anxiety if resisted, they become abnormal and are perceived by the person as undesirable and ego-dystonic. Obsessionality is a common (and often useful) personality trait, but having intrusive obsessional thoughts that lead to time-consuming and functionally disabling (compulsive) behaviours that are unwanted by the person are typically attributed to illness rather than a personality trait (e.g. obsessive–compulsive disorder [OCD]). Similarly, experiencing intrusive thoughts regarding behaviours, such as gambling or substance use, are typically viewed as ego-syntonic and not attributed to illness (although this distinction is increasingly challenged).

Another important consideration regarding the nature of mental symptoms is their pattern over time. Personality is a relatively consistent phenomenon that is expressed in traits that are evident across the various domains of our life and that are stable over time. In contrast, most mental illnesses follow a phasic pattern over time with recovery (or relative recovery) between episodes. There is thus a distinction between difficulties that reflect a state or phase than those that persist as traits (i.e. state versus trait). This distinction is complicated by the fact that personality and illness are not mutually exclusive concepts such that persons with obsessional personality are more prone to developing obsessional symptoms when unwell (e.g. as part of depressive illness or OCD). Moreover, in many cases, psychiatric illness can involve persistent residual symptoms that over time share many characteristics of personality traits.

Disturbances to thinking

These can include abnormal content of thoughts or disturbed thought processes (i.e. the construction or mechanics of thinking). It is important to note that our ability to recognize disturbances of thinking is heavily dependent upon speech as this is the principal mechanism by which our thought processes and their content are expressed. As an example, patients with mania frequently present in a highly energized state that includes loud and fast speech with content that can rapidly switch from topic to topic. These phenomena are referred to as 'pressure of speech' and 'flight of ideas', which are considered disturbances of speech and thought-form, respectively. In such cases, patients can often express a variety of grandiose beliefs (e.g. having special abilities or being on an important mission) that reflect delusions, which are disturbances of thought content. Distinguishing between speech, language, thought-form and content could be challenging, and it is not necessary for students to necessarily distinguish the precise focus of the disturbance, but rather note its presence and significance.

Thought content

Disturbances to the content of one's thoughts is a fundamental component of most mental disorders. These disturbances range from thoughts that we all experience daily, and that are associated with psychic discomfort (e.g. anxious ruminations) to thoughts that are grossly bizarre and scientifically implausible (e.g. delusional ideas that one can control the weather through our behaviour). Some disturbances relate very directly to external experiences and specific life events (e.g. intrusive recollections with posttraumatic stress disorder [PTSD]), while others arise as part of an intense internal morbid experience (delusional ideas with emerging schizophrenia).

It is thus important to explore abnormal thought content in terms of its principal theme, the impact upon the person's sense of well-being (safety, mental integrity) and emotional state, the plausibility of the beliefs, their relationship to past experiences, the capacity to resist or exclude the thoughts from one's mind, the conviction with which they are held, any associated actions and the willingness of the person to see the thoughts as reflecting illness.

Ruminations are any recurring thoughts or worries. Ruminating is repetitively going over a thought or a problem without managing to resolve the issue. It is commonly seen in depressive and anxiety disorders but is also part of the normal everyday experience where ruminating is part of the worrying or brooding process.

Obsessions are recurrent, intrusive, unwanted ego-dystonic thoughts, images or urges that are not inherently pleasurable. They are distressing and anxiogenic and are often accompanied by a sense of compulsion. Attempts to resist obsessional thoughts are often associated with worsening anxiety. Themes include hygiene, contamination, safety, symmetry or order, and sometimes religious or bizarre sexual or aggressive themes. Some patients experience a sense of more general '*obsessional angst*' where they obsess about the meaning of things (e.g. life) or experience persistent thoughts about 'what if'. Obsessions are frequently associated with compulsive behaviours ('*compulsions*', e.g. hand washing, checking) that are repetitive, and although goal-directed, they are ultimately without a useful purpose. Obsessional thoughts are common in all humans and often involve an element of magical thinking (e.g. 'if I count to ten repeatedly then my football team will score'), but with OCD, they are recognized as excessive and harm one's functioning.

Intrusive recollections are a specific type of recurring thought that is a feature of PTSD and refer to the person reliving a traumatic event through recurrent and intrusive thoughts or memories about the traumatic event. They are frequently accompanied by distressing nightmares or perceptual experiences, such as flashbacks (or 'daymares') with autonomic arousal. They are frequently triggered by situations that are of emotional significance or have symbolic relevance to the traumatic event (e.g. encountering violence on a television programme that reminds one of an assault).

Overvalued ideas are thoughts that are considered unusual or unreasonable by their intensity or conviction. They are strongly held but not to delusional intensity, in that the person typically has good insight into the fact that they are very personal and that others might not share them or may perceive them as unusual. They are usually understandable in the context of the individual's personality, culture or life experiences. An important distinction from overt psychosis (i.e. delusional ideas) is that insight is maintained as the idea is not unshakeable. Overvalued ideas may be featured in conditions, such as morbid jealousy, hypochondriasis, dysmorphophobia (a belief that one is abnormal in appearance) and anorexia nervosa. Political or religious extremism is sometimes explained in terms of overvalued ideas.

In morbid jealousy, the person has an unjustified belief and excessive concern that their significant other is being unfaithful. This occurs most commonly as an overvalued idea (based upon a vulnerability in terms of personality, alcohol use issues or sexual dysfunction), but on occasions, can reach delusional intensity (so-called 'delusional jealousy'); in such cases, it poses a major risk for being acted upon with violence (including homicide). In such cases, it is important to carefully assess the nature of the beliefs and the extent to which they may be acted upon (e.g. checking personal possessions, movements, phone activity). Of note, infidelity is not an uncommon feature of everyday life such that a key consideration is to what extent the person has justification for their suspicions. In morbid jealousy, the focus is typically more ego-centric and relates to the perceived betrayal by another person, while with infidelity, the focus is often upon how and with whom it is occurring. In short, where such beliefs occur as part of the illness, they principally relate to an internal morbid process rather than actual external evidence. Morbid jealousy is also sometimes referred to as 'Othello syndrome', referring to the character in Shakespeare's play, *Othello*, who murdered his wife as a result of a false belief that she had been unfaithful.

Delusions are often described as fixed, false beliefs that are not understandable in the context of a person's personality or background. They are not reasonable, often illogical and insight is lacking. Classically, fully formed delusions are all of the above, but it should be noted that in the emerging stages (or as the ideas soften as one recovers) delusional ideas may not be held with absolute certainty. In addition, delusions are not necessarily false—the partner of a person who has delusional jealousy might also be unfaithful! Moreover, delusional themes are frequently shaped by one's personality or background and are therefore not entirely independent of these. In the 20th century, religious themes were extremely common in delusions, while in the 21st-century, themes that relate to technology and the internet are very common.

Delusions can involve a variety of different themes that can assist with diagnosis (see Table III.1). Delusions can be classified in terms of whether they are bizarre or non-bizarre (often in terms of whether they have any plausibility). Bizarre delusions are implausible, are not derived from normal life experience and are difficult to understand. For example, a patient may feel that aliens are transmitting messages to the chosen people through a radio transmitter implanted in their brain. A good example of a non-bizarre delusion would be delusions of love or infidelity; while they may be false, they are not beyond the realms of possibility. Bizarre delusions are more indicative of a schizophrenia-spectrum disorder. Delusions could also be primary or secondary. Primary delusions (also called 'autochthonous delusions') cannot be understood because of circumstances or events or are secondary to one's mood state. Conversely, secondary delusions relate to the prevailing mood (grandiose delusions in mania or delusions of guilt in depression) and can also occur as secondary to a primary delusion (e.g. 'I can save people from damnation' may be secondary to a primary delusion that 'I am God's special messenger').

The experience of a primary delusion can have different elements or follow recognized themes that are: (i) delusional mood, which is the vague feeling that 'something is not quite right', but that the nature of what is different is not yet clear; (ii) delusional intuition, which involves the occurrence of sudden, out-of-the-blue delusional ideas; (iii) delusional perception, wherein a normal object or perception is attributed a delusional meaning (e.g. a traffic light changed from green to red, and the person realized that he had been chosen to lead people into the promised land); and (iv) delusional memory, wherein a person remembers an event but belatedly attributes a delusional significance to it. The concept of primary delusions is often debated by psychiatrists. However, ultimately, if a patient experiences delusional ideas without any plausible basis or understandability in terms of other mental phenomena, then they can be considered primary and raise the possibility of a diagnosis of schizophrenia or related conditions.

Some themes for delusional ideas are described in Table III.1.

TABLE III.1 ■ Delusional Themes

Delusional Theme	Example
Delusions of reference	The belief that others are paying undue attention to one by monitoring one's behaviour or communicating abnormal ideas through the television, radio, internet or other means.
Delusions of control/passivity	The belief that an external agent is interfering with one's thoughts, actions or emotions.
Delusions of persecution	The belief that other(s) are attempting to cause one harm or are interfering with one's privacy, reputation or ability to prosper.
Delusions of grandiosity	The belief that one has special abilities, attractiveness, wealth or status.
Delusions of guilt	The belief that one is responsible for bad events or has committed a terrible action.
Delusions of jealousy	The unjustified belief that one's partner is unfaithful.
Hypochondriacal delusions	Delusional belief that one has a specific illness.
Nihilistic delusions (Cotard's syndrome)	The belief that one does not exist, is already dead or putrefying, or that they have lost their blood or body parts/organs.
Erotomania (de Clerambault's syndrome)	Belief (erroneous) that one is in a relationship with another individual (typically outside one's social strata, such as a wealthy or famous person).
Delusional Misidentification Syndromes	
Capgras syndrome	The belief that a spouse or close relative has been replaced by an imposter.
Fregoli delusion	The delusion of doubles where there is a belief that a person, often a stranger, is a familiar person in disguise. Typically the delusional person believes that they are being persecuted by the person they believe is in disguise.
Doppelgänger	The belief that one has a double or Doppelgänger with the same appearance, but usually with different character traits that is leading a life of its own.
Intermetamorphosis	The belief that people can swap identities with each other but appear the same.

Delusions of thought interference/control

One type of delusion that has importance is that in which the person believes that their thoughts are being interfered with by an external force. At the core of these experiences is the sense of a loss of integrity or control over one's thoughts (and therefore, private space and autonomy), which is referred to as 'passivity'.

Three main patterns occur: thought withdrawal, thought insertion and thought broadcast. In thought insertion, thoughts are ascribed to other people who intrude their thoughts. Patients often report that these thoughts have been 'put there by others' and do not recognize these thoughts as their own. In thought withdrawal, the person describes a sense (often as a sensation of feeling the thoughts being extracted) of their personal thoughts being removed by an external force and against their will 'my thoughts are being taken from me by others'. This is different from thought blocking where the person experiences a sense of being unable to generate thoughts and feeling mentally blank rather than that their thoughts being actively removed. Thought broadcast is the belief that one's private thoughts are accessible to others without having revealed them (i.e. that their internal thoughts are being broadcast to others who can therefore know what the patient is thinking). Patients will typically complain that 'others can read my mind'.

Eliciting these phenomena may seem daunting to the novice interviewer and patients who have not had these experiences may find the questioning strange or even upsetting. However, these phenomena can be gently probed for using the usual pattern of beginning with relatively open questions (e.g. 'do you ever feel that people are trying to influence your thoughts or feelings?' and 'have you ever experienced telepathy?'), subsequently proceeding to more specific questions, such as 'have you ever had the experience of feeling that the television or radio (or internet) is referring to you in particular or trying to influence your thoughts?'; 'have you ever felt that some of your thoughts are not your own or have been placed there by others?' or 'do you ever feel that people can read your mind?'

Delusions of thought interference are important phenomena as they are highly suggestive of schizophrenia and related conditions.

Thought-form

Disturbances to thought processes are often referred to as formal thought disorder. They involve a spectrum from excessively concrete thinking ('if it's raining cats and dogs, why cannot I see any animals' or 'I cannot explain what you mean by "a stitch in time saves nine" because I have no interest in embroidery') to thinking that is unusually loose with regard to the connection between thoughts, thus creating difficulties to converse coherently and understandably (so-called 'loosened associations').

A description of the more important abnormalities of thought-form is presented in Table III.2.

TABLE III.2 ■ **Examples of Types of Thought Disorder**

Flight of ideas/clanging	Abrupt changes from topic to topic but with discernible links between topics. This is frequently accompanied by 'clanging' whereby successive thoughts are linked by rhyming rather than meaning, e.g. 'Dr Marr, will go far, in his superfast car, ah ha ha' (classically associated with manic states).
Loosening of associations	The connection between thoughts is loosened and contains only remotely related ideas. The frame of reference of thoughts changing from sentence to sentence such that there is a rapid shifting from topic to topic without highly obvious connections. In a mild form, this can be considered as lateral thinking and underpins much good art (e.g. poetry). However, in psychosis, it can significantly impair the ability to conduct a coherent conversation in which case it is often referred to as 'tangentiality'. 'Knight's move' thinking refers to the nonlinear direction of thoughts that seem to move in two directions at once like the knight on a chessboard. 'Derailment' occurs where the person loses their train of thought and does not return to the original point.

(Continued)

TABLE III.2 ■ **Examples of Types of Thought Disorder—cont'd**

Poverty of thought/thought retardation	Thinking is slowed with fewer thoughts entering consciousness (classically associated with depression).
Thought block	Abrupt interruption to train of thought whereby the person feels that their thoughts suddenly stop and they 'draw a blank' (seen in psychotic conditions (especially schizophrenia) but also common in the general population at times of fatigue or stress (e.g. drawing a blank in an exam).
Perseveration	Persistent repetition of words or ideas beyond the point at which they are relevant (most frequently seen in organic illness and classically linked with frontal lobe pathology).
Circumstantiality	This is similar (but milder) to tangentiality whereby the pattern of thinking follows a nonlinear route with drifting focus but that eventually comes back to the point. Nonessential and irrelevant detail causing a delay in getting to the point (can occur in psychosis, temporal lobe epilepsy or as a manifestation of obsessional personality).
Incoherence	Thinking and its expression through speech becomes so lacking in structure as to be incomprehensible. The person voices actual words, but these do not allow for a coherent sentence and can result in what is essentially incoherent gibberish, referred to as 'word salad' or 'jargon aphasia' (seen in schizophrenia, severe mania and organic states, such as progressed dementia).

Abnormalities of perception

Abnormalities of perception can occur in any of the five senses—visual, auditory, gustatory, olfactory or tactile. The nature of any disturbances is defined by their relationship to external stimuli and the personal appreciation of their significance. In general, a perceptual experience may be a sensory distortion or deception. Sensory deceptions are further divided into illusions and hallucinations.

Sensory distortions

These occur when real objects are perceived as altered in some way—either in terms of their physical character (quantitative) or significance (qualitative). Qualitative distortions are frequently associated with drug toxicity and affect visual perception; for example, the colour of an object may seem altered. With quantitative alterations of perception, the size or shape may be altered. Micropsia occurs when an object is perceived as smaller than reality; macropsia occurs when an object is perceived as larger than reality; and dysmegalopsia occurs when the object appears altered in shape. These are associated with organic diseases, such as epilepsy, drug intoxication and withdrawal states. The main types of sensory distortion are listed in Table III.3.

TABLE III.3 ■ **Sensory Distortions**

Description	Diagnostic Significance
Changes in intensity (hyperaesthesia or hypoaesthesia)	
Increased sensitivity to sound (hyperacusis)	Anxiety, depression, migraine, alcohol withdrawal, autistic spectrum disorder, fatigue
Reduced sensitivity to sound (hyporacusis)	Delirium, depression, ADHD
Intensification of colour	Hypomania, LSD intoxication, intense normal emotion, e.g. romantic or religious experience
Reduced intensity of colour	Depression (everything is grey or black)
Reduced gustatory sensation	Depression (all food tastes the same)

(Continued)

TABLE III.3 ■ Sensory Distortions—cont'd

Description	Diagnostic Significance
Changes in quality	
Altered colour of the image (yellow, xanthopsia; green, chloropsia; red, erythropsia)	Intoxication with a variety of substances, especially hallucinogens, such as LSD or psilocybin, and also digoxin toxicity
Objects appear unreal and strange (derealization)	Mood and anxiety disorders, TLE, migraine, drug intoxication and withdrawal, states, fatigue
Change in form/shape (dysmegalopsia, metamorphopsia)	Visual problems, aura, epilepsy, schizophrenia

ADHD, attention deficit hyperactivity disorder; LSD, lysergic acid diethylamide; TLE, temporal lobe epilepsy.

Sensory deceptions

Sometimes called 'misperceptions' these involve a new perception that may (illusion) or may not (hallucination) be in response to external stimuli.

ILLUSIONS

Illusions are false perceptions of an external stimulus that are frequently associated with prevailing affect and occur when stimuli from a perceived object are combined with a mental image to produce a false perception. They are not necessarily indicative of psychiatric pathology. Three types are described: completion illusions, affect illusions and pareidolia. Completion illusions are when an incomplete or incorrect object, for example, an incomplete drawing or incorrect spelling, is perceived as complete or correct. We have an innate impulse to make sense of our experiences and as such, use experience and knowledge to fill in the gaps. Consequently, we perceive a different object to what has been presented. An example would be to see CCOK and perceive COOK as it makes more immediate sense. Affect illusions occur when the person's emotional state leads to misperceptions; for example, being frightened walking along a dark road may lead to the incorrect interpretation of a shadow from a tree as something more threatening, e.g. muggers. Pareidolia is when an individual perceives a meaningful image in a random or ambiguous visual pattern (such as flames of a fire, or in clouds). Examples would be the Rorschach test—seeing the man in the moon or the face of Jesus in a bowl of cornflakes.

HALLUCINATIONS

An hallucination refers to when perception occurs in the absence of a stimulus. Hallucinations are false perceptions. To the person, they seem to be occurring in external space ('without') even though they arise from 'within'. They are not under voluntary control and possess the substantiality of normal perception. They may be auditory, visual, olfactory, gustatory or somatic. Not all are of pathological significance. Auditory hallucinations are especially relevant to functional psychiatric conditions and have different characteristics according to the underlying diagnosis. Third-person hallucinations (e.g. where the person is referred to as he or she, discussed or commented on by voices) are suggestive of schizophrenia and related psychoses. Command hallucinations are important by their capacity to provoke behaviour, especially that which involves risk to self or others. The degree of compulsion to act upon command hallucinations must be clarified.

From a functional perspective, hallucinations may be classified as functional, reflex, extracampine or autoscopic. Different categories of hallucinations are described in Tables III.4 and III.5, below.

TABLE III.4 ■ Types of Hallucination

Hallucination Type	Description	Diagnostic Significance
Third-person auditory hallucinations	The patient hears voices referring to him/herself in the third-person, e.g. 'he/she is a bad person'	Highly suggestive of schizophrenia
Thought echo/echo de la pensée/Gedankenlautwerden	The patient hears his or her own thoughts aloud a short time after thinking them	
Running commentary	The voices consist of hearing a 'running commentary' on the patient behaviour, e.g. 'she is drinking tea'	
Second person auditory hallucinations	The voice addresses the patient in the second person, e.g. 'you are a bad person'	Occurs across a range of psychotic presentations, including affective schizophreniform and organic disorders
Visual hallucinations	Seeing an object that is not there, a false perception of vision	Suggestive of organic pathological conditions, such as delirium, dementia, tumour, hallucinogenic drugs
Olfactory hallucinations	False perception of smell	TLE, schizophrenia, depression
Gustatory hallucinations	False perception of taste	Schizophrenia, TLE
Somatic hallucinations	Sensations, e.g. heat, cold, electricity, visceral sensations affecting the skin, muscles, joint sense or internal organs; 'tactile' hallucinations describe sensation affecting the skin, and 'haptic' refers to hallucinations of touch; formication is a sensation of animals/insects crawling under the skin	Schizophrenia, organic psychoses, cocaine intoxication (formication)
Elementary hallucinations	Unstructured hallucinations, e.g. whirring noises (auditory), multicoloured spots (visual)	Not necessarily indicative of psychiatric illness
Negative hallucinations	The absence of perception despite the presence of a stimulus	Not necessarily indicative of psychiatric illness
Pseudo-hallucinations	Experienced in the inner subjective space. Lack of reality of true perception	Not necessarily pathological

TLE, temporal lobe epilepsy.

TABLE III.5 ■ Classification of Hallucinations

Hallucination	Explanation
Functional	Stimulus provokes the hallucination, and both are perceived in the same modality, e.g. hear the tap running and hear voices
Reflex	A stimulus in one modality provokes a hallucination in a different modality, e.g. seeing an angel when a bell rings; this may be a morbid form of synaesthesia, where one sees letters as colours

(Continued)

TABLE III.5 ■ Classification of Hallucinations—cont'd

Hallucination	Explanation
Extracampine	Hallucinations that are outside the normal field of the particular sense, e.g. seeing a person who is in a different country
Autoscopic	The experience of seeing oneself. The person 'remains' in their own body unlike with dissociative (or 'out of body') experiences where the person sees their own body from a vantage point outside their physical body; associated with migraine, epilepsy, organic psychoses and drug intoxication
Distinct formed	Elderly patients with normal consciousness and no brain pathology, but with reduced visual acuity due to ocular problems experience vivid, distinct formed hallucinations, often of men wearing hats. This is called Charles Bonnet syndrome
Lilliputian	Hallucinations involve seeing tiny people or animals. These can occur with alcohol withdrawal

FLASHBACKS

A flashback is a perceptual experience whereby the person has a sudden, usually powerful, re-experiencing of a past experience. They are sometimes referred to as 'daymares' or involuntary recurrent memories. Typically, flashbacks are triggered by psychologically symbolic experiences one encounters in the current time that stimulate intense recall of a previous event from memory. Flashbacks can involve a variety of emotions, including joy, sadness and fear and can occur as part of normal experience. However, in psychiatry, the term is predominantly used to describe perceptual disturbances of PTSD and related conditions where the person has re-experiencing phenomena relating to traumatic events. These can include intrusive recollections, nightmares and flashbacks that are associated with marked autonomic arousal. Flashbacks occur involuntarily. The person typically recognizes that the experience is not 'real' but it can be so intense that the person 'relives' the experience during which they may struggle to recognize it as memory and not something that is happening in real-time. As such, flashbacks can provoke marked distress and hyperarousal with actions to remove themselves from the triggering stimulus. Therefore, more severe flashbacks can appear very similar to hallucinations, although their situational character and close relationship to previous traumatic experience usually allow for them to be distinguished from hallucinations.

Derealization and depersonalization

Perceptual disturbances can also occur with qualitative alterations in consciousness. *Dissociation* is a mental process whereby the person becomes disconnected to their sense of self, including thoughts and feelings, and sometimes, can include a sense of being outside of oneself and watching themselves from above like an actor in a play. This can occur in states of extreme stress or trauma and with substance-induced states. Ketamine is an analgesic anaesthetic agent that can have marked dissociative effects with the so-called 'out of body experiences'. *Derealization* (a sense that the world around is not real) and *depersonalization* (a sense of detachment or being outside oneself as though watching a movie where one feels detached from other people). Both are frequently associated with a sense of the speed of time being altered and a general sense of fogginess or being in a dream. Deja and Jamais Vu can also occur. Derealization and depersonalization can be part of normal experience (e.g. when fatigued) and occur at elevated frequency across a range of mental disorders (e.g. mood and anxiety disorders) and in organic brain disorders where they are classically linked to temporal lobe activity and are a well-recognized feature of temporal lobe seizures.

Abnormalities of mood and affect (emotion)

Abnormalities of mood are the most common symptoms encountered in psychiatry. Mood is defined as a prolonged emotional state and can be characterized both subjectively by the patient and objectively by the clinician. Affect is the expression of emotional state at a point in time and is inferred objectively. These concepts are sometimes likened to the relationship between weather and climate—mood refers to a sustained emotional 'climate', while affect refers to more fluctuating changes in the emotional 'weather'.

Normal mood is referred to as euthymia or normothymia, while normal affect is often referred to as appropriate in expression and range (or resonance). A depressed mood is characterized by feelings of sadness often with a sense of hopelessness, despondency and/or apathy. An elated mood is character-ized by a sense of happiness or cheerfulness. These emotional states are part of the everyday experience but become pathological when they are excessive or not justified by circumstances. In mania, for exam-ple, the sense of happiness is frequently unshakeable even in the face of adversity (such as hospitalization or negative life events). Elated patients may, for example, describe hospital food as 'superb!'

Several other terms can be used to describe mood states, such as dysphoric, euphoric, dysthymic, hyperthymic and ecstatic. Dysphoria describes a negative mood state that reflects mental discomfort and unhappiness that is frequently used when a person is discontent for reasons that may not relate to a sustained lowering of mood as we would typically expect in depressive illness. Euphoria is a state of elated mood that implies an organic focus (e.g. frontal lobe lesions, end-stage dementia) where a sense of excessive well-being is expressed because of an apparent loss of emotional regulation. Ecstasy refers to a state of intense joy and contentment that relates to a religious experience or positive life events (victory in sports, success in examinations, childbirth). Furthermore, elation, euphoria and ecstasy all describe mood states that include happiness but differ in terms of their relationship to other factors, such as other aspects of psychopathology, the context in terms of life events and apparent cause. Dysthymia describes a state of persistent low mood that is less acute and less severe than depression that was previously considered as a 'depressive personality'. In recent times, dysthymic disorder has been viewed as closer to depressive illness than personality disorder in character. Similarly, hyperthy-mia relates to a sustained tendency towards exceptionally positive mood and disposition.

Mood can sometimes be described as anxious or irritable if they are the dominant emotional states of the person. Mixed affective states occur where there are contrasting elements that occur together simultaneously or over short periods. 'Dysphoric mania' is an example where there are fea-tures of mania and depression with restlessness, irritability, unhappiness and pessimism. Agitated depression is a similar concept where the person has depressed mood but with agitation rather than the classical psychomotor slowing that is associated with many depressive episodes.

Disturbances of affect can be in terms of its appropriateness of expression ('blunting'), stability ('lability') and resonance ('flattening'). Blunt (or incongruous) affect is one that lacks sensitivity to or consistency with circumstances, for example laughing in response to receiving news of a death or accident to a close one. It is seen in chronic schizophrenia, schizoid personality and autistic spec-trum disorder. Flat affect is where the range of affective expression has become reduced (or flat-tened) and is typical of depressive illness where the emotional state remains despondent even in the face of news that would usually be received positively and with joy (e.g. winning money or succeed-ing in an interview or examination). A labile mood is one that is prone to fluctuation. This is typical of manic states where an elated and jovial person can rapidly switch to marked irritability.

Abnormalities of consciousness

Consciousness can be thought of as awareness of experience and can be considered both quantitatively (arousal and alertness) and qualitatively (comprehension and awareness). Cognition refers to the men-tal processes involved in understanding and processing experience of the world around us. These include attention, orientation, memory, comprehension, visuospatial reasoning and problem-solving.

From a quantitative perspective, consciousness level falls along a continuum that ranges from being hyperalert to having full alertness and awareness to reduced arousal with stupor (where the person is minimally responsive) and ultimately coma (where the person is unresponsive to external stimuli). The impairment of consciousness is an important feature of organic illness. In delirium, for example, consciousness can be affected both qualitatively ('clouding') and quantitatively in terms of arousal, with both reduced arousal and hyperaroused states possible.

'Clouding of consciousness' is a descriptor that is used to describe qualitative changes to consciousness that impede the grasp of the environment. The person is in a cloud or fog that separates them from the clarity of usual awareness. The term is largely interchangeable with 'confusion'. These terms equate with a combination of impaired attention and diminished awareness. The fluctuation of consciousness refers to a pattern of consciousness that changes over time, for example, in delirium. The patient may become more disorientated in the evening when they are tired, and when the anchors of the day are less evident (diurnal fluctuation of consciousness sometimes called 'sundowning').

Consciousness and symptom generation: hysteria, factitious disorder and malingering

A further consideration is a relationship between conscious and unconscious factors in mental symptoms. Traditionally, the term 'hysteria' has been applied to symptoms where the person is not conscious of the origin of their symptoms which are deemed to occur unconsciously. Dissociative disorder, somatic symptom disorder and conversion disorder (CD) are examples of this phenomenon. CD relates to patients who present with neurological symptoms (e.g. blindness, seizures or fainting, weakness or paralysis, problems swallowing or dysphagia) which are not consistent with a well-established organic cause and relate to a psychological trigger, such as stress. CD has been relabelled as 'functional neurological symptom disorder' in the Diagnostic and Statistical Manual of Mental Disorders-5. The relationship between conscious and unconscious factors in such presentations is complex in that the level of visible distress of the person is frequently much less than one might expect given the symptoms, suggesting that the person has an awareness that their loss of function is not necessarily based upon serious physical pathology. This disconnect is sometimes referred to as 'La belle indifférence'. In simple terms, these presentations are thought to reflect the fact that the person is psychologically unable to deal with a stressor and thus expresses (or 'converts') their distress through often compelling physical symptoms. These presentations are less common in modern practice, perhaps reflecting a greater general psychological awareness in society and the destigmatization of mental illness. In-keeping with this possibility, they are more common in persons from lower socio economic groups, those who are less educated, from rural backgrounds and in developing countries. Of note, symptoms of hysteria should be distinguished from factitious disorder and malingering. While dissociation and conversion are unconscious and reflect an abnormal coping mechanism used, for example, to avoid a stressful or intolerable situation, factitious disorder and malingering are consciously mediated (i.e. the patient is purposely faking the symptoms). Factitious disorder and malingering differ in respect of motivations for the deception. In malingering, the reason for the deception is tangible and rationally understandable, such as evading criminal prosecution, obtaining financial compensation, avoiding work or military duty or as means of obtaining drugs. In factitious disorder, the motivation is a pathological need for the sick role. Moreover, factitious disorder is considered a mental illness, whereas malingering is not.

Abnormalities of speech and language

A patient's speech, language and ability to converse may give the examiner valuable clues as to their diagnosis. It is important to note that one's speech is the vehicle by which thoughts are communicated, and there is an overlap between abnormalities of speech and thinking. Formal thought disorder, for example, might be communicated through grossly disorganized speech that can at times be virtually incomprehensible and described as a 'word salad'. In addition, there are several abnormalities of speech production, organization and content that clinicians need to recognize.

Disturbed speech production includes dysphonia, dysarthria and dysphasia (with aphonia, and aphasia reflecting a total rather than partial loss of function). In dysphonia, there is difficulty in vocalization (e.g. speaking with a whisper) which can reflect lesions of the vocal cord or as a hysterical phenomenon. Dysarthria relates to motor difficulties in speech production that can occur after cerebrovascular accidents or can relate to muscular difficulties in the mouth and larynx, for example, extrapyramidal effects of medication. In dysphasia, the difficulty is with understanding or producing words and is thus primarily a language rather than speech disorder. Stuttering, also known as stammering, describes a disturbance in the flow of speech with repetitive jarring at certain words or syllables. It is frequently unrelated to mental disorder but also can occur as a manifestation of anxiety (especially in children) and in the aftermath of severe trauma later in life. The flow of speech is also frequently altered in mood disorders with fast and often loud 'pressure of speech' in hypomania and mania and slowing of speech, often with a soft-spoken voice in depressive states.

The organization of speech is closely related to thought processes. It can vary from characterologically determined overinclusive speech that may involve circumstantiality (a failure to get to the point with efficiency), logorrhoea (excessive wordiness, often with considerable repetition) and tangentiality (where the conversation repeatedly veers off the principal subject with oblique or irrelevant content). Perseveration is the persistent repetition of words or ideas beyond the point at which they are relevant. These disturbances are often an expression of obsessional or schizotypal personality traits but are also more common in people with schizophrenia and those with organic brain disease.

The content of speech is also impacted by mental disorders. In mania, there is often colourful or flamboyant content (sometimes with rhyming or musicality called 'clang associations') because of the expansive thinking that is typical of that state (e.g. 'Dr Marr, will go far, in his superfast car, ah ha ha'). In depressive illness and chronic schizophrenia, there can be a poverty of speech or even alogia or muteness. Psychotic disorders can also include unusual use of language with made-up words ('neologisms') or the use of recognized words but with a personalized meaning that is not usually attributed to them ('metonyms'). Neologisms (or 'new' 'words') can sometimes endure and then become part of the mainstream language (e.g. 'mansplaining' as a verb to describe a male talking down to a female in a patronizing way, or 'confubble', which means to confuse and befuddle). Neologisms are frequently cannibalized from two words which are spliced to create the new phrase. Metonyms are recognized words used in a way that communicates a new concept, e.g. 'Washington' when referring to the United States Government. Metonyms are frequently encountered in good poetry where they can bring lateral thinking to the content.

Cognition

Cognition is the process by which various cognitive functions allow a person to appreciate and respond to the world around them. These cognitive functions relate to different neuropsychological domains (attention, orientation, comprehension, memory and executive function) that can be tested during the psychiatric assessment. This should be distinguished from the concept of 'cognitive set' which relates to how a person perceives themselves in their interactions with the surrounding world and is typically altered in depressive states (so-called cognitive distortions that include an unduly negative self-perception). While the majority of mental disorders impact upon cognitive function in some way (e.g. attention and short-term recall, which are decreased in depressive states and the early phases of psychosis), in organic brain disorders cognitive disturbance is the primary or core feature (e.g. attention is particularly impaired in delirium, while impaired short-term memory is characteristic of dementia). In contrast, disturbances to mood, thinking and perception are considered as secondary aspects.

Attention is the focusing of consciousness on a stimulus. Therefore, consciousness is necessary for attention. Attention can be voluntary or involuntary, the former being associated with consciously focusing on an event and the latter when the event attracts the subject's attention (e.g., a car back-firing). Attention can be further subdivided into focused and sustained attention (sometimes called 'vigilance'), with the former relating to the ability to direct and focus attention over seconds, with the latter reflecting the ability to extend this attention to a task for sustained periods—typically more than 10 seconds and often extending to minutes and longer. This can be described as the 'attention span', which is typically between 10 and 20 minutes in teenagers and adults. The relevance of attention span to education was demonstrated in a classic experiment where it was found that the average duration that students could maintain attention from the start of a didactic lecture was 11 minutes! The ability to perform tasks that require sustained attention impacts various activities of daily life, such as watching a television programme to the conclusion, or reading an article in the newspaper in its entirety. Selective attention is a further aspect of attention that relates to the ability to direct our focus to relevant stimuli while ignoring irrelevant stimuli in the environment. This is a valuable ability as we have a limited capacity in terms of how much information can be processed at a given time, and selective attention allows us to focus on what is important while deprioritizing less significant elements.

Orientation is the ability to gauge time, place and person accurately. Orientation to time is generally disturbed first, followed by place and then the person. Disorientation to a person can relate to significant others (e.g. what does that person (key nurse) do for a living?) which is considerably more common than loss of orientation to self which usually relates to severe or highly progressed organic brain disease (the 'mirror sign') or hysterical 'fugue' states where the person loses conscious awareness of their previous identity. It is important to take a flexible stance in terms of the distinction between understandable inaccuracies in responses to questions regarding orientation, especially in elderly persons who have been in hospital for prolonged periods during which their normal daytime pattern and weekly routine do not occur. As a general rule, it is rare for a normal individual to misidentify the year or the month, but as many as 5% of older patients may misidentify the date (day of the month), especially when they have been in hospital for more than a week. Orientation to place reflects the ability to communicate one's location (including its significance), such as that they are in a hospital or an outpatient clinic or at home and can extend to naming the town or city where that location is. Impaired temporal and sometimes spatial orientation can occur in states of intoxication or fatigue.

Memory is a highly complex component of cognition that can be considered from a variety of perspectives, including temporal aspects and content. In crude terms, memory can be tested for registration, short-term recall and ability to remember events from the immediate past (intermediate memory) and distant past (long-term memory). Memory can also be autobiographical (relating to personal events and experiences) or procedural (relating to skills or knowledge of procedures sometimes called memory for 'how to'). Declarative memory can be divided into episodic and semantic memory. Episodic memory is for experiences and specific events in time in a serial form, including autobiographical events (times, places, associated emotions and other contextual knowledge) that can be explicitly stated or 'declared'. Of note, the context and associated emotions are included in this part of memory. Semantic memory is a more structured record of facts, meanings and knowledge about the external world that are acquired over time. It refers to general factual knowledge that is abstract, relational and independent of personal experience and of the context in which it was acquired. It includes things, such as vocabulary, capital cities, social customs, understanding of mathematics and functions of objects. Procedural memory relates to the store of knowledge that relates to being able to perform tasks. It is implicit and less readily stated or declared. Knowing how to drive a car, ride a bicycle or swim are examples of functions that exercise procedural memory. It typically operates at an unconscious and automatic level and without awareness of the previous experiences that shaped the memory.

The principal aspects of memory that are relevant to the practising clinician are impairments of short-term memory, which occur in patients with dementia, post-seizures (including after ECT) and in those with traumatic brain injuries, and a variety of presentations that include expression of memories that are not accurate. Disorders of memory can be divided into amnesia (where there is a loss of the content of memory) and paramnesia (where the content of memory is distorted or inaccurate). Some examples of clinical phenomena that reflect these types of memory disturbance are presented in Table III.6. Anterograde amnesia describes the failure to create new memory from a particular point (e.g. a head injury with loss of consciousness) and retrograde amnesia where memory for incidents prior to an event are lost. This is typically of the period immediately preceding the event but also sometimes of longer-term, stored autobiographical memory. Impaired registration with reduced short-term memory can occur in any mental disorder where registration is impeded by poor attention and distractibility (e.g. major depression, anxiety states, ADHD and delirium).

TABLE III.6 ■ **Disorders of Memory**

Memory Disturbance	Description
Amnesia	
Psychogenic/hysterical/ dissociative amnesia	Sudden retrograde episodic memory loss with amnesia for personal identity and personal events. Might be associated with a fugue state where the person travels away from their usual place in which they operate and may be found wandering and lost. Social skills and personality are maintained. It is said to occur in the context of extreme trauma and is usually short-lived (hours to days).
Blackouts	Discrete periods of anterograde amnesia particularly associated with alcohol intoxication.
Paramnesia	
Retrospective falsification	Deliberate or unconscious alteration of memory for past events or situations used as a mental mechanism for ego preservation and reflecting the current emotional, experiential and cognitive state. For example, in depression, a patient may describe all their past failures while ignoring their achievements.
False memory	A person will recall events that they strongly believe took place but did not take place.
Screen memory	A memory which is partially true and partially false. This is thought to occur when the entirety of the true memory is too painful.
Confabulation/falsification of memory	In confabulation, the patient may fabricate, distort or misinterpret memories without the conscious intention to deceive, rather, the patient is filling in gaps in memory with imagined or untrue experiences. It is associated with organic brain disease and classically with Korsakoff's syndrome.
Pseudologia fantastica/ pathological lying	This term describes confabulation in the absence of organic brain disease. The individual may describe major traumas or grandiose ideas. Munchausen's syndrome is a variant where the subject feigns illness or psychological trauma to gain sympathy or attention.

Visuospatial function refers to that aspect of brain function that identifies and integrates visual phenomena, such as shape, depth and spatial relations. It is the cognitive function that underpins understanding and navigating our environment and the structures contained therein. In clinical settings, it can be assessed through the ability of the patient to reproduce a visual image, including its component elements. Conventionally, this is assessed through drawing tests (e.g. the clock drawing test, the interlocking pentagons test), the ability to perform functional tasks, such as dressing, making a bed, assembling items and the patient finding their way around the environment. Disturbances to visuospatial abilities occur in the context of general cognitive impairment, but they are also disproportionately affected in delirium and in conditions that include lesions of the occipito-parietal cortex.

Executive functions are those aspects of brain function that underpin organization and planning, concept formation and word/idea generation. They involve several processes, such as working memory, cognitive flexibility, inhibitory control and other complex functions as planning, problem-solving and abstract reasoning. Deficits of the executive functions are observed in all populations to varying degrees, but more severe executive dysfunction occurs in organic brain syndromes, functional psychotic illnesses, ADHD and autism. These cognitive deficits affect routine functioning in personal, social and vocational activities, as well as worsen the clinical course of the disease by impacting upon treatment adherence. A scheme for assessing cognitive function while at the bedside is described in Box II.6, above.

Insight

Insight is a key concept in psychiatry that distinguishes many more serious mental illnesses from the rest of medicine, and that underpins the need to consider treatment that is without the person's consent. In this respect, psychiatry significantly differs from medico-surgical care, where most patients present actively seeking help. In contrast, approximately one in ten admissions for psychiatric care occur using procedures defined in law for involuntary treatment. In addition, insight is a key factor that impacts upon adherence to treatment plans. It is important to recognize that insight is not a static, fixed concept and can change as the patient's mental health improves or worsens. The following questions are useful in assessing insight:

- Does the patient recognize their current 'problems' as symptoms of being unwell or experiencing illness?
- Does the patient believe that the illness is a psychological/mental illness?
- Does the patient recognize the need for treatment?
- Is the patient willing to accept treatment?

Insight is thus a multidimensional construct that includes the ability to recognize that one has a mental illness, the capacity to label abnormal experiences as pathological, the specific attribution of one's symptoms to mental illness and willingness to accept help in the form of treatment.

Although classically associated with psychosis, insight can also be impaired in nonpsychotic illnesses, such as OCD, depressive disorders, eating disorders and even specific and social phobias. It impacts upon help-seeking and adherence in these conditions. The issue of insight is particularly challenging in anorexia nervosa where the body image distortions along with overvalued ideas about appearance and weight are held with a veracity that is akin to delusional ideation and has an impact upon well-being and behaviour that is similar to that with psychosis. While insight is primarily a medical term, 'capacity' is a related legal concept that reflects an inability to decide because of an impairment of the mind or brain. One's level of insight can thus impact upon one's legal capacity to decide about treatment or other personal matters.

Abnormalities of motor activity

Many psychiatric disorders and their treatments can result in disturbances to motor function that should be noted in the MSE, usually in the section that deals with appearance and behaviour. They may involve quantitative disturbances to the amount or speed of activity or can reflect qualitative deviations from normal motor activity. These alterations are important as in addition to providing clues to the diagnosis (e.g. psychomotor slowing in depression), on occasion they can reflect serious and potentially life-threatening pathology (e.g. muscular rigidity in neuroleptic malignant syndrome).

Decreased motor activity is most commonly seen in depression, chronic schizophrenia and various organic mental disorders (e.g. hypoactive delirium). In depression, it classically involves combined slowing of mental and physical activity sometimes referred to as 'psychomotor retardation'.

In chronic schizophrenia, the reduced activity can occur as part of the negative syndrome along with reduced motivation and social behaviour. It is important to consider the role of antipsychotic treatment through sedative effects and/or parkinsonism. In the latter, this may also be associated with cogwheel rigidity and mask-like faces.

Stupor is an extreme form of motor retardation characterized by akinesia (loss or impairment of the power of voluntary movement) and mutism (inability to speak), which together are termed 'akinetic mutism' with preserved consciousness. Stupor can occur in a variety of conditions that include affective disorders, psychosis and organic brain disorders. Unlike comatose states, the stuporose patient retains some degree of responsiveness to external stimuli.

Catatonia refers to an abnormality of movement and behaviour that relates to a disturbed mental state. It was commonly observed in psychiatry during the early and mid-20th century but is much less common nowadays, possibly because of the earlier treatment of mental disorders with effective antipsychotic interventions. It can involve a variety of unusual posturing and behaviours that may include repetitive or purposeless overactivity, or catalepsy (muscular rigidity and fixity of posture with reduced responsiveness to external stimuli, such as pain), resistance to passive movement and negativism (the tendency to either resist movement of a body part by another or to move in an opposite manner to a request, apparently without motive or purpose). In catatonia, the patient does not move normally despite the physical capability to do so. It is associated with schizophrenia, affective disorders, focal neurological lesions, intoxication and metabolic disturbances. The main features of catatonia are presented in Table III.7.

Increased motor activity can reflect anxiety, anger, agitation (e.g. agitated depression) or the hyperactivity of mania. Agitation or irritability may accompany many disorders (e.g. anxiety, depression, schizophrenia, organic disorders) and reflect distress. In such cases, movement may not be goal-directed. In the hyperactivity of mania, actions are usually goal-directed, albeit frequently in response to disinhibiting thoughts or impulses and are not necessarily rational. Catatonic excitement may be seen in schizophrenia wherein the individual engages in non-goal-directed overactivity.

TABLE III.7 ■ **Abnormalities of Motor Activity that can Occur in Catatonia**

Catatonic Feature	Description
Posturing/ catalepsy	The patient may maintain unusual and uncomfortable postures for extended periods; the psychological pillow is an example wherein the patient will hold their head above the pillow when lying down
Stereotypies	Nongoal-directed, repetitive movements
Mannerism	Seemingly goal-directed repetitive movements, but without any obvious purpose
Waxy flexibility	After being placed in an unusual position or pose, the patient will maintain this for an extended period
Automatic obedience	The patient will obey commands even when subsequently given instructions to the contrary
Echolalia	The patient repeats the speech of the examiner
Echopraxia	The patient repeats the actions of the examiner
Negativism	The patient will resist the examiners' attempts to make contact
Ambitendency	Alteration between resistance and cooperation

(IV) Martha: Enquiry-based Learning

LEARNING OBJECTIVES

- To appreciate how modern methods are increasingly being applied to medical education programmes, including their potential advantages.
- To be aware of the factors that promote student engagement with psychiatry teaching and the factors that are linked to students subsequently undertaking postgraduate careers in psychiatry.
- To understand the relative merits of large versus small-group teaching and how enquiry-based approaches to learning are applied.
- To recognize different types of inquiry-based teaching, including problem-based and case-based learning.
- To appreciate the importance of applying learning outcomes to ensure that the teaching programme is appropriately focused and comprehensive in content.
- To be aware of the different international bodies that provide learning outcomes that can be applied to teaching programmes.
- To recognize how the quality of a teaching programme can be assessed, both cross-sectionally and longitudinally.

1. Martha is a clinician educator who has just been appointed as the new Head of Teaching in Psychiatry at the University of Hope School of Medicine. She has been tasked with updating the teaching programme, which has been quite static in content and delivery style since the previous Head of Department retired three years previously. Upon reviewing the programme, she notes that it is mainly comprised of a series of lectures by invited expert clinicians from the local hospital. The department secretary tells her that the lecture schedule runs smoothly as it has remained unchanged for the past decade or so. She also confides that the teaching sessions are quite poorly attended by students and wonders if Martha might consider introducing a register of attendance to improve student engagement.
   1. What are your initial thoughts about the programme as described?
   2. What additional information might you seek about the teaching programme?

The existing programme as described seems very much like the 'traditional' model of medical education, whereby lectures are delivered by 'experts' to students, who attend as mostly passive participants (i.e. a 'teacher-centred' as opposed to a 'student-centred' approach). The lack of attendance is probably related to the predictable content of the lectures, and limited interaction with students such that students can simply circulate copies of the notes without having to attend the lectures. Given the increased focus upon performance in the assessment of medical student abilities, students are more likely to be excited by educational activities that involve active participation.

It would be useful to get information on the background expertise of lecturers, the constructive alignment (or lack of it) between the material covered in the lectures and assessment, the actual attendance rates, feedback on the lectures from students and teachers alike. It would also be informative to review the curriculum covered by the lectures and how the overall teaching programme aligns with the suggested learning outcomes stipulated by relevant international bodies involved in standard-setting for medical education. Some aspects of the programme may have become less relevant or even redundant and may need to be retired and replaced by other activities that are underemphasized in the existing programme. It may be necessary to engage faculty members in training around more student-focused teaching and learning practices (e.g. small-group teaching, flipped classrooms, online learning). These methods involve more active learning. It will also be important to gauge the level of support from students for changes to this type of learning, including gaining an understanding of how well they appreciate the value of actively engaging with more practical and PBL activities.

By ensuring a more interactive learning approach, and by increasing the relevance of the programme for students, i.e. outlining to students that the curriculum is covered by the programme and that the teaching programme will prepare them for examinations and the demands of real-world clinical practice, one can increase student interest in and ownership of the programme which in turn can result in a very valuable and engaging learning experience. Assessment can be a very powerful driver of learning. Cohen described how learners 'don't respect what you expect, they respect what you inspect'. Similarly, it has been observed that 'the assessment tail wags the curriculum dog, or more crudely, grab the students by the tests and their hearts and minds will follow'.

FURTHER READING

For a discussion of key issues in the reform of medical education, see: Cohen JJ. (2006) Professionalism in medical education, an American perspective: from evidence to accountability. Medical Education 40(7):607−617. doi:10.1111/j.1365-2929.2006.02512.x

Practically speaking, a move to a student-centred active learning approach will most likely result in a need for more teachers to meet the demand of small-group learning and more training. There will also be a requirement to introduce mechanisms for regular student and teacher feedback. This will allow the new Head of Department to optimize the programme as it evolves, while at the same time reassuring students that their input into the development of the programme is valued.

2. Martha contacts some recent graduates of the programme to gather feedback about their experience. They reveal that they frequently relied upon a student that was a good notetaker for lecture notes rather than attend in person, as they were busy with trying to keep up with other elements of the final medicine programme. They report that the main interactive opportunity was after the lecturer had finished and that often they ran over time with little opportunity to ask questions. They also reported that although the lecturers were 'very nice', often the content did not seem directly relevant to the students as the majority did not plan to undertake careers in psychiatry.
  3. What are the shortcomings of traditional didactic methods of teaching and what alternatives can Martha consider?
  4. How can Martha ensure that the content of teaching sessions is appropriate?

These observations from the former students capture some of the problems with traditional didactic methods of teaching. Although these methods can be an efficient means of communicating information to medium and large groups, their impact is often much less than with activities that require more active student participation and problem-solving to encourage the integration of information into their knowledge and skillset. It is well documented that maintaining learner attention over sustained periods is enhanced by having regular breaks in the flow of sessions that keep students focused. Activities, such as problem-based and case-based sessions, are ideally designed to address this issue and are often delivered in small-group settings. Modern medical education typically includes a combination of large and small-group activities which can optimize the need for the efficiency of volume while enhancing learning.

It is important in modern highly saturated medical programmes to monitor the content of teaching sessions to ensure adequate coverage of identified learning outcomes and to ensure that best use is made of the valuable face-to-face teaching time. Learning outcomes to guide the content of medical education (and psychiatry in particular) are available from a number of bodies that include the ADMSEP Association of Directors of Medical Student Education in Psychiatry (America), the AMC Australian Medical Council (Australia) and the RCP Royal College of Psychiatrists (UK), all of which are covered in this textbook.

FURTHER READING

For a review of evidence to support the positive impact of problem-based approaches upon the educational environment, see: Qin Y, Wang Y, Floden RE. (2016) The effect of problem-based learning on improvement of the medical educational environment: A systematic review and meta-analysis. Medical Principles and Practice 25(6):525–532. doi:10.1159/000449036

Faculty development can help to emphasize the importance of using stated learning objectives both at the commencement of each teaching session and to review the effectiveness of sessions prior to their conclusion. This requires careful attention to timekeeping during sessions so that there is adequate time to both complete and review the material covered. This process can be monitored through regular ongoing student feedback.

3. Martha decides to design a more student-focused programme and wants to replace the lecture programme with a series of highly interactive problem-based sessions. She uses the departmental grand rounds as a forum to introduce her plans and the rationale for reforming the teaching programme.
5. What is problem-based learning?
6. What key messages will Martha want to communicate to the faculty about her plans to reform the teaching programme?
7. How can Martha best engage faculty in the grand rounds session which is one hour in duration?

Problem-based learning (PBL) is an educational approach that uses real clinical problems as a context for students to acquire knowledge and develop skills. Developed in the late 1960s, it has been implemented in many medical school curricula and other professional training programmes around the world. The PBL approach is student-centred and emphasizes problem-solving in small groups that are facilitated by tutors. Effective implementation of PBL builds on students' prior knowledge and stimulates self-directed learning. It is believed to: (i) improve the retention of information by encouraging deep learning; and (ii) promote other skills and attributes, such as teamwork, professionalism and life-long learning, which are essential to future clinical practice. The early development of such skills is designed to enhance the confidence and performance of students and graduates. Some evidence suggests that PBL is also better at allowing students to develop problem-solving skills than traditional didactic curricula and that it allows for a better educational environment. However, there is also evidence indicating that the PBL learning model is not superior to the traditional approach with respect to the acquisition of factual knowledge, and it is often more time-consuming and resource-intensive than conventional approaches.

Case-based learning (CBL) is an enquiry-based pedagogy similar to PBL, with the main difference being that students are provided with learning objectives. It focuses on learning within a clinical setting, uses real-life problems and a guided enquiry method and provides structure during small-group sessions. It is more time-efficient with some evidence that students and faculty prefer it because of its heightened focus and greater opportunity for clinical skills application. It is particularly suited to students that have developed self-directed learning abilities and who are in time-pressurized programmes (e.g. later years of medical school).

FURTHER READING

For a review of modern approaches to medical education, see: O'Connell HP. (2009) Spicing up medical education. The British Medical Journal 339:b2779. doi:10.1136/bmj.b2779

Martha will need to convey the clear evidence base from general and medical education research of the power of student-centred approaches to learning, such as employed in PBL and CBL, with likely benefits for the university in terms of better student performance, enhanced student experiences, the better future success of graduates with an enhanced reputation for the university and enhanced retention of students on the programme because of improved quality of the teaching experience. There may be barriers to her ideas, as some more 'traditional' teachers may not see the merits of the new programme approach and there will be some higher costs involved, in terms of delivering the teaching in small-group settings, with the necessity for more teachers and the necessity for training them in the 'new' ways of teaching.

It might be useful for Martha to conduct a PBL/CBL session at grand rounds, to demonstrate the power of these methods, in terms of engagement, deep learning and integration of new learning. A structure similar to this section would be suitable on the benefits of PBL/CBL.

---

4. Just prior to the commencement of the academic year the student's final year class representative approaches Martha to inform her that many of the students are concerned about how the new teaching programme will work. They have asked that they receive some guidance on how to best use the teaching programme. Martha welcomes the request and delivers a guidance session to the incoming students detailing the changes to the programme and how she is hoping that they will allow for a more enjoyable and effective learning experience for students.
    8. What advice should Martha give to the students as to how they can make best use of the teaching session?

Martha can reassure the students by sharing with them findings from educational research. She can also highlight to them the more personalized approach involved in PBL/CBL, whereby students are 'brought along' regardless of background knowledge level and students are not 'lost' as sometimes happens in a traditional lecture-based didactic programme. She can also highlight to the students the fun and interactive nature of PBL/CBL, thus simulating real-world clinical team working scenarios and enhancing student relationships and overall morale. She can also reassure the students that the PBL sessions will have a clear examination focus and that they will cover all the required curriculum.

---

5. The following academic year is busy as the department delivers the new teaching programme. Attendance at protected teaching sessions improves considerably. Martha holds a party for the teaching staff to celebrate the end of the academic year which is attended enthusiastically by most colleagues who have contributed to the teaching programme during the year. One colleague who has had a little too much to drink is more sceptical about the curriculum redesign and challenges her as to what evidence there is that the programme has improved?
    9. What are the indicators that can be used to evaluate a teaching programme of this type?

There are multiple indicators to be considered, both cross-sectionally and longitudinally. These include satisfaction ratings by students and teachers (e.g. as measured on scales, such as the Dundee Ready Education Environment Measure [DREEM] or through bespoke surveys addressing key areas of feedback), student retention rates on the programme (i.e. fewer dropouts, hence financial savings for the programme), enhanced performance and pass rates at final examinations (teachers do not like failing students just as students do not like to fail). Longitudinal measures could be the success of the graduates in postgraduate training, examinations and career progression, students returning as teachers and the enhanced reputation of the University with improved research output and an increase in the number and quality of student applications.

Two other useful indicators are to get feedback on how much talking time is spent by students (overall and coverage across the group) than the facilitating tutor. Ideally, students should dominate talking time, with more than 50% attributed to them. A second useful marker is the percentage of students who undertake postgraduate training in psychiatry as a medical career because of the impact that the learning method had on their engagement with the discipline.

FURTHER READING

For a review of factors that influence recruitment of medical students into postgraduate careers in psychiatry, see: Farooq K, Lydall GJ, Malik A, et al. (2014) Why medical students choose psychiatry – a 20 country cross-sectional survey. BMC Medical Education 14(1):12. doi:10.1186/1472-6920-14-12

CHAPTER 1

Shane

Acute Mania

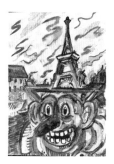

1. Describe the differential diagnosis of patients presenting with acute elation.
2. Outline the diagnostic features of a manic episode.
3. Understand the prevalence of bipolar illness.
4. Describe the evidence supporting bipolar illness as a predominantly genetic condition.
5. Understand the legal principles that underpin the involuntary treatment of mental illness.
6. Outline the criteria for treatment (including hospitalization) for those unable to commit to treatment voluntarily, i.e. involuntary treatment under mental health legislation.
7. Outline in detail the principles for the management of acute mania.
8. Understand the uses of lithium in the management of bipolar illness.
9. Describe the role of other mood stabilizers in the management of bipolar illness.
10. Be aware of the magnitude of risk for suicide in patients with bipolar affective disorder.

1. Shane, a 19-year-old trainee garage mechanic, is brought to the emergency department one Monday morning by his work colleagues. They report that he is usually a quiet and reserved person but has been acting strangely all morning: looking 'spaced out', pacing around the repair area of the garage reciting a pop song, and insisting that all the cars are being *'fixed by the power of the tune'*. When asked to commence his usual duties, his workmates report that he became angry and argumentative, shouting that he had *'more important things to do'*. After some persuasion, he had agreed to accompany them to the hospital in the belief that he could 'heal' some of the patients.
   1. What are your initial thoughts regarding this presentation? Is Shane 'psychotic'? What are the potential challenges of this assessment process?

BOX 1.1 ■ Suitable questions to explore for the presence of elated mood

- How has your mood been lately? How good has it been?
- Has your mood been changeable?
- Does anything upset you?
- How have your energy levels been?
- Have you felt low in between times of feeling great?
- How have your confidence levels been?
- Have you been feeling special/talented/empowered?
- Have you been talking about/demonstrating this to people?
- Have you put yourself in harm's way?
- Have you been sleeping enough? Have you been needing less sleep? Do you feel tired or reenergized in the morning?

This presentation includes behaviour that is grossly bizarre and appears to be occurring in the context of unusual beliefs that are being acted upon and, thus, likely to be delusional in nature. These ideas are grandiose in quality, with Shane believing that he has special healing capabilities. His behaviour is of concern because it is socially inappropriate and out of character, both of which suggest a morbid process. This may reflect a primary psychiatric disorder or could be secondary to an underlying physical condition. It is important to think about the kind of risks involved with such a behaviour. Efforts at engagement will need to be sensitive to his apparent affective lability and recent verbal aggression. It will be important to try and avoid direct confrontation to explore his recent experiences and beliefs. The interview should occur in a setting that allows for a safe exit if he becomes excessively agitated or challenging. Suitable questions to explore for the presence of an elated mood are shown in Box 1.1.

---

2. At the time of the interview, Shane insists that you converse in the waiting area and repeatedly breaks into the Irish language. He appears agitated and excited. After initially challenging you to provide evidence of your medical qualifications, he becomes more chatty and agreeable and explains that he has found his vocation in life and believes that he can '*fix things by using virtual powers of healing bestowed by the great one*'. This realization occurred over the previous weekend during a visit to a local music festival. When you enquire about other relevant details (such as how this all started), he suddenly becomes confrontational and demands to see the hospital manager. At this point, the nursing staff inform you that his mother has phoned and wishes to speak with you.

   2. List some suitable questions that would help you to establish Shane's current mood state.

   3. What key information would you seek from his mother?

   4. What is the differential diagnosis for this presentation and what investigations would you order? Does Shane need an urgent brain scan?

Shane's mother is likely to be able to shed light on many important aspects of his presentation, including when his behaviour first appeared to be unusual and whether the onset was sudden or gradual. Any recent events that may be relevant should be explored together with any history of mental or physical illness. This is an ideal opportunity to clarify his usual pattern of behaviour and premorbid personality, any known history of substance use, and any family history of psychiatric illness (Box 1.2). It will also be important to ascertain her perception of how this situation should be handled and to inform her of the mechanisms by which he can receive appropriate assessment and treatment, including whether this behaviour requires involuntary procedures.

This presentation includes grossly disturbed and socially inappropriate behaviour with labile affect, elated mood, irritability, agitation, and delusional ideas. Together, these features indicate a psychotic process with associated disturbance of mood. Therefore, the differential diagnoses include mania (rather than hypomania, which is less severe, does not include psychosis, and results in less functional

---

BOX 1.2 ■ Key elements of collateral history

- First appearance of symptoms
- Acuity of onset
- Recent stressors (physical, psychological)
- Previous history of mental or physical illness
- Possible indicators of substance misuse, including alcohol
- Premorbid personality
- Family history of psychiatric illness

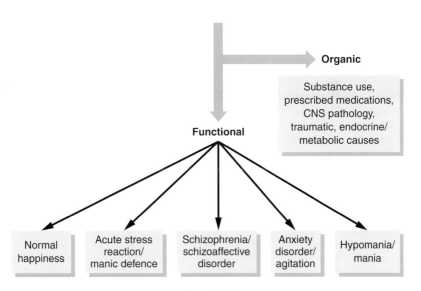

Fig. 1.1 Differential diagnosis of a patient presenting with elation.

impairment), manic phase of schizoaffective disorder or acute schizophrenia (although schizophreniform features have not been elicited), any of which may have an organic basis (see Fig. 1.1).

Shane's presentation is more severe than that which could be considered within the spectrum of normal happiness. Anxiety disorders do not involve psychotic features. An acute reaction to a stressful event is a possible cause (so-called psychogenic psychosis), and the term 'manic defence' is sometimes used to describe a state of apparent elation occurring in response to a severe adverse circumstance or life event. However, in current thinking, adverse events are usually conceptualized as precipitating factors for patients with a biological vulnerability towards serious mental illnesses, such as bipolar affective disorder.

The criteria for the diagnosis of a manic episode are outlined below. Essentially, a sustained period of abnormal, elated, or irritable mood is accompanied by disturbances of thinking, behaviour, and biological function that substantially impact adaptive functioning and are not better explained by a physical or substance-related cause (Box 1.3).

Careful observation can help to assess Shane's ongoing mood state and presence of specific symptoms (delusions, hallucinations, and schizophreniform symptoms). The physical examination will need to be thorough as the physical differential diagnosis is quite broad.

Box 1.4 shows an approach to investigations that are applicable to most patients who present with acute major psychiatric problems. The range and timing of investigations depends on the

---

BOX 1.3 ▪ The diagnosis of an episode of mania is based on the following:

1. An abnormal mood that is elated, expansive or irritable in nature
2. An elevated sense of confidence, ability, self-importance or grandiosity, increased activity, accelerated or pressurized speech and thinking, diminished judgement, disinhibition with heightened engagement and risk-taking, spending, substance use or sexual activity that are noticeably out of character, excessive or irrational
3. An episode that is associated with significant functional consequences (e.g. requires intervention by others and/or hospitalization) or includes overt psychotic features (e.g. grandiose delusions or hallucinations)
4. An episode that is evident over a sustained period (e.g. not better explained as primarily relating to the acute effects of substance use), and that is not secondary to physical illness (e.g. an endocrine disorder or an organic brain lesion)

BOX 1.4 ▪ Investigations applicable to most patients who present with acute major psychiatric problems

1. First-line investigations
   Complete blood count
   Urea and electrolytes
   Liver function tests
   Thyroid function tests
   Fasting lipids
   Erythrocyte sedimentation rate
   C-Reactive protein
   Blood glucose
   Drug screen
   Urinalysis
   Electrocardiogram
2. Second-line investigations (as indicated)
   Auto-antibody screen
   Anti-N-methyl-D-aspartate antibodies
   Cerebrospinal fluid examination
   Structural neuroimaging (computed tomography/magnetic resonance imaging)
   Functional neuroimaging (single-photon emission computerized tomography)
   Electroencephalography
   Anti-human immunodeficiency virus antibodies
   Syphilis serology
   Urinary porphyrins

---

severity of symptoms, background history, the ability of the patient to cooperate with investigations, and in some cases, availability, e.g. single-photon emission computerized tomography. All patients who present with major psychiatric symptoms warrant brain imaging to rule out possible organic central nervous system causes. The presence of any neurological signs adds to the urgency of testing.

---

3. Shane's mother reports that he has been acting strangely since returning from the festival the previous evening. He seemed unusually cheerful and had woken the family in the middle of the night by playing music in the sitting room. The following morning, his mother noted that he had already left the

house and had not slept on his bed. Shane had some difficulties two years previously, while still at school, when he seemed to lose interest in his studies and sporting activities, stopped attending school for a month, and started to inflict superficial lacerations on his forearms. His general practitioner arranged for an assessment by a private psychiatrist who suggested that he commence antidepressants, but he refused and seemed to gradually return to his normal self. He successfully completed his exams before leaving school to commence an apprenticeship to become a mechanic. She confirms earlier impressions that he is normally shy and introverted with few friends and has not had a serious girlfriend.

5. What is the likely explanation for the episode two years prior to the current episode, and what diagnostic significance does it have?

The diagnosis of bipolar affective disorder (BPAD; previously referred to as manic depression) is frequently delayed, and in many cases, a definitive diagnosis is not established until five years or more after the initial presentation. This is often because the principal pattern of illness suggests a unipolar depressive illness and the bipolar nature of symptoms is not apparent until mania or hypomania occurs. However, it is also evident that in many cases, there are previous 'silent' episodes of elation that are not recognized because they are relatively mild and/or brief and resolve spontaneously.

Careful consideration of the nature of previous episodes is important in all patients presenting with mood disturbance, as it can provide important insights into likely diagnosis and treatment response. Such episodes may present as feelings of excessive well-being, increased energy, unusual confidence or creativity, overspending and disinhibition, behaviour that is out of character, and impulsive or flamboyant behaviour. Collateral sources of information are vital in this regard. In addition, a possible bipolar nature to illness is suggested where there is a family history of bipolar illness, the presentation of depressive illness is atypical or involves mixed affective features, a younger age of onset, and relative treatment resistance.

From a diagnostic perspective, the International Classification of Diseases (ICD)-10 and Diagnostic and Statistical Manual of Mental Disorders (DSM)-5 somewhat differ in their criteria for diagnosis of BPAD. In ICD-10, a diagnosis of BPAD is based on at least two episodes of illness, one of which has involved hypomania, mania, or mixed affective symptoms. In DSM-5, a single manic episode suffices. Furthermore, in DSM-5, BPAD is subclassified into type I (where there has been at least one manic episode) and type II (where there have been hypomanic rather than manic symptoms).

4. When you return, Shane has wandered into the treatment area and has placed his hands on the forehead of an elderly man to whom he is singing that he will soon be *'forever healed, signed and sealed'*. You suggest that he should be admitted to the hospital, but he becomes annoyed and refuses, shouting *'get lost you jerk, let me do my work, or I will go berserk'*.
6. What can you do now?
7. How is treatment provided to persons who refuse to accept help voluntarily? What principles underpin involuntary treatment?

At this stage, it is important to consider issues of safety for Shane and those around him as his behaviour is grossly bizarre and potentially interfering with the care of other patients, many of whom are likely to be seriously ill and vulnerable. Shane's mental state is such that he appears to have little capacity to appreciate reality at present. The severity of his symptoms suggests that he will need to be managed in a safe place for ongoing assessment, investigation, and stabilization of his mental state.

Involuntary treatment procedures are particular mechanisms that permit the administration of necessary treatment for mental disorders in situations when the patient is unwilling or unable to consent to treatment voluntarily. Major mental illnesses differ from mainstream medical conditions in their capacity to impact insight levels and seeking care. Involuntary treatment is indicated when the patient has a mental illness that requires treatment, which is likely to be of benefit, and that cannot be provided by less restrictive means than through hospital admission. Involuntary procedures allow for detention in a recognized treatment centre and short-term administration of treatment against the person's will. An important element of mental health legislation is that it includes procedures to ensure that any detention is reviewed by an independent body in-keeping with international human rights conventions.

Shane's current mental state indicates that he lacks insight. Furthermore, he is behaving in a bizarre and grossly inappropriate way. While elated patients can sometimes be managed voluntarily, in many cases, the volatile nature of mental illness and/or inability to give informed consent makes voluntary treatment unrealistic. In addition, the risk of non-adherence to prescribed treatment is high.

---

5. An emergency department doctor initiates the process for involuntary admission to the psychiatric unit, which is located at the rear of the hospital. With much persuasion and with the assistance of security staff, Shane agrees to go to the acute admission unit.
   8. What should happen now?
   9. What treatment would you suggest, and what are the options if Shane refuses oral medication?

Modern mental health legislation seeks to uphold the rights of patients to receive treatment in the least restrictive environment possible and to be informed of the therapeutic plan and their rights throughout. Unfortunately, the nature of acute mania is such that a significant percentage of patients have seriously impaired judgement with diminished insight and are unpredictable and labile in their affective expression and attitude towards treatment. For many patients, the optimal course of action is to ensure a safe environment in which their mental state can be stabilized so that they can participate more meaningfully in the therapeutic process and treatment decisions. As much as possible, a more complete history should be determined and a physical examination with appropriate investigations should be conducted. This may need to be postponed until Shane is more cooperative.

With more minor disturbances of mental state, it is sometimes prudent to observe progress without pharmacological intervention. However, in reality, it is common to prescribe antipsychotic medications at this stage, which will help to stabilize his mental state and behaviour. In Shane's case, the severity of his symptoms would suggest that a 'wait and watch' approach may not be in his best interests. If Shane refuses oral treatment, it may be necessary to administer his treatment intramuscularly, always bearing in mind the increased bioavailability (typically doubled) of psychotropics when administered through this route. In addition, when possible, agents with potentially stimulant actions should be discontinued (e.g. antidepressants, steroids).

---

6. Shane is informed of his admission status and proposed treatment. He refuses oral medication and is given 5 mg of haloperidol and 2 mg of lorazepam intramuscularly with a prescription for these drugs to be repeated twice per day if needed.
   10. What is the rationale for this treatment combination?
   11. What are the pharmacological alternatives to this approach?

The treatment of acute mania is guided by extensive experience from everyday clinical practice, but there is a relative lack of high-quality evidence to compare different approaches, and treatment can vary considerably across different centres.

FURTHER READING

For a review of the evidence underpinning the pharmacological management of acute mania, see: Goigolea J, Vieta E. (2010) Treatment guidelines for acute mania. Annals of General Psychiatry 9(Suppl 1):S62. doi:10.1186/1744-859X-9-S1-S62

In general, treatment involves either an antipsychotic agent (classically, haloperidol, but more recent evidence supports the use of atypical antipsychotic agents) or sometimes a mood stabilizer. In both cases, a benzodiazepine agent may also be used for acute alleviation of agitation. Lorazepam is the preferred agent because of its predictable bioavailability and rapid onset of action relative to other benzodiazepines. Mood-stabilizing agents are not available in an intramuscular form for patients who refuse oral medication.

Some evidence suggests that acute treatment with an atypical antipsychotic is less likely to be followed by a depressive phase than treatment with typical antipsychotic agents. In addition, many of these agents are available as rapidly dissolving formulations (oro-dispersible) that can allow for better monitoring of compliance and reduced risk of so-called 'cheeking', whereby patients hold a tablet in their cheek so that they can remove it later.

When a mood stabilizer is used, it is important to recognize that lithium has a relatively delayed onset of action (that is not suited for the acute management of more severe illness), and that both lithium and valproate have teratogenic potential. It is recommended that the combination treatment of an antipsychotic with a mood stabilizer be considered where there is a poor response with either drug administered alone. Valproate is more inherently sedative than lithium and, therefore, is frequently preferred when a mood-stabilizing agent is used for acute treatment.

---

7. Shane gradually settles, switching to oral risperidone after four days. His investigations are essentially normal, except a positive urinary screen for cannabinoids. After a fortnight, Shane's symptoms have improved greatly and he describes feeling embarrassed about his behaviour around the time of admission. He is keen to clarify what caused this to happen and how he can avoid experiencing similar episodes in the future. He wants to know if his use of cannabis caused the episode. He also informs you that a paternal aunt was 'manic depressive' and, ultimately, died because of suicide.

   12. How will you explain his diagnosis, including the relevance of cannabis use?

   13. What do we know about the genetic aspects of bipolar affective disorder?

   14. What are your thoughts regarding the ongoing treatment?

   15. What is the prognosis of bipolar affective disorder, and what is the risk of Shane ending his life by suicide?

Shane experienced an episode of depression two years ago, followed by the current manic episode. Therefore, his preferred diagnosis is BPAD (Type I). It is likely that his exposure to cannabis was a precipitating factor for this episode, and that this helped to aggravate an underlying vulnerability towards mood disturbance. There could be some debate as to whether this episode might be primarily attributed to cannabis use, but the severity of symptoms, the mood-congruent nature of the psychotic features, the previous documented affective episode, and the family history all indicate a likely diagnosis of BPAD.

Both acute and chronic use of cannabis are associated with psychological and behavioural problems. In particular, cannabis use is linked to schizophrenia, anxiety and mood disorders. The principal mechanism of these interactions is through the effects of tetrahydrocannabinol (THC) on the endogenous cannabinoid system, which has important and extensive modulatory interactions with most neurochemical systems implicated in major mental disorders. Interestingly, THC is a psychotomimetic and is considered to be the primary compound of *Cannabis sativa* and is responsible for most of the effects of the plant. Another major constituent is cannabidiol (CBD), formerly regarded to be devoid of pharmacological activity, but recently licensed for sale in many parts of the world. Emerging evidence suggests that CBD may have antipsychotic effects and appears to have a pharmacological profile similar to that of atypical antipsychotic drugs.

FURTHER READING

For an overview of the relationship between cannabis use and mental disturbance, see:
Available at: https://www.rcpsych.ac.uk/expertadvice/problemsdisorders/cannabis.aspx

The direction of causality in these relationships has been the source of much historical debate—cannabis use is common in individuals with psychiatric illness (e.g. any use is twice as common in patients with BPAD than in the general population) and may reflect a form of self-medication for psychological distress—'*it helps me chill*'. In addition, studies over the past decade have highlighted that the use of cannabis may be associated with an increased incidence of major psychiatric disorders, especially in patients who are genetically vulnerable to psychiatric disorders.

The relationship between cannabis and schizophrenia has been studied in reports linking an increased risk of schizophrenia in patients with particular polymorphisms of the catechol-O-methyltransferase (*COMT*) polymorphism Val158Met (*COMTVal158Met*) gene (an enzyme involved in dopamine catabolism), and specifically, in those with the *COMT* valine allele who are exposed to early and intense cannabis use. However, its role in mood disorders is less clear, but at the very least, cannabis use can aggravate the course of both bipolar and unipolar illnesses.

FURTHER READING

For a review of the genetics of bipolar disorder, see: Kerner B. (2014) Genetics of bipolar disorder. The Application of Clinical Genetics 7:33–42. doi:10.2147/TACG.S39297

Bipolar affective disorder is considered to be a condition with strong genetic predisposition. Numerous studies have indicated that it aggregates in families with the lifetime risk in first-degree relatives, which is increased by almost 10-fold when compared with the general population (1%). Some evidence suggests that bipolar types I and II disorders 'breed true', with relatives of those with bipolar I disorder more likely to experience bipolar I rather than a bipolar II illness pattern. Relatives of patients with BPAD also have an elevated risk of unipolar depressive illness (but not vice versa). Concordance rates for BPAD I are 2–3 times greater in monozygotic than in dizygotic twins (30%–90% versus 23%, although the rates vary).

Overall, the heritability of BPAD (i.e. the proportion of risk that is attributed to genetic factors) is estimated to be between 80% and 90%, emphasizing that it is strongly a genetic condition. Therefore, careful assessment of family history is important for the accurate and early recognition of bipolar illness.

A manic episode comprises one phase of BPAD, which is typically a recurrent condition in which further episodes of hypomania, mania, or depression are likely to occur. Therefore, prophylactic maintenance treatment is strongly recommended. The relationship between acute and maintenance treatment warrants careful consideration. In some cases, the agents used for acute management are selected according to their potential role in longer-term prophylaxis (e.g. mood stabilizers). However, other studies have suggested that the high discontinuation rates with lithium may be reduced by initiating such treatments when patients have recovered and are better able to participate in treatment decisions. The commitment to long-term lithium therapy, for example, includes regular monitoring of serum levels and potential adverse effects. Many patients are more likely to adhere to such treatments if they are better aware of this requirement when treatment is initiated.

The majority of the people who experience a manic episode will experience further episodes in the future. The term 'bipolar' reflects the fact that the vast majority of persons who experience manic episodes also experience depressive phases. In reality, most bipolar patients experience greater morbidity from depression than from mania. Indicators of a poor longer-term prognosis include early-onset, severe episodes with psychosis, concomitant substance abuse, comorbid personality disorders, or intellectual disability.

Bipolar affective disorder is an often severe and recurring illness with elevated lethality largely because of suicide. The suicide rates average 1% annually and are 30–60 times higher than that of the international population rate in developed countries, which is 15/100,000 persons annually. It is estimated that 15% of patients with BPAD ultimately end their lives by suicide. Suicidal acts typically occur early in the course of illness and are associated with severe depressive or mixed states. The high lethality of suicidal acts in bipolar disorder is suggested by a much lower ratio of suicide attempts (3:1) than the general population (30:1). Effective acute treatment is essential to managing short-term risk, but there is a lack of evidence to support the impact of longer-term interventions. A notable exception is lithium prophylaxis, which has been consistently found to substantially (80%) reduce the relative risk of suicide and attempted suicide.

Aaron

Acute Psychosis

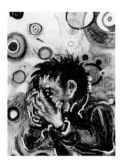

1. Perform an initial evaluation, history and mental state examination of a patient with psychotic symptoms.
2. Provide medical and psychiatric differential diagnoses for psychotic presentations.
3. Appreciate the epidemiology, diagnostic criteria, clinical features and course of psychotic disorders.
4. Perform an assessment of risk to others in the context of psychotic illness.
5. Recognise the initial management of acute psychotic illness.
6. Describe the construct of insight and how this relates to prognosis in psychotic illness.
7. Recognise prognostic indicators at first episode psychosis.
8. Understand the rationale for early intervention services.

1. A local general practitioner faxes you a letter on a Monday afternoon requesting that you see a patient urgently who has a relatively sudden onset of 'acute paranoia'. Unfortunately, the general practitioner is unavailable when you request additional information. Aaron, a 22-year-old single apprentice electrician, presents. The letter from his general practitioner states that Aaron has been acting 'bizarrely' and has 'questioned his identity' in recent weeks, causing concern to his family. On assessment, Aaron is a little vague and detached but generally cooperative. He says he has no real understanding of why he has been referred to the clinic but has no problem 'having a chat'. He is mildly agitated, but there is no evidence of major affective disturbance, hallucinations or thought disorder. When directly questioned about the content of the referral letter, Aaron shows you what appears to be a photograph of himself as a child, alongside his sister and parents. He seems to be slightly perplexed about the identity of another child who appears to have accidentally strayed into the line of the photographer's lens. Nonetheless, he tells you that he is no longer concerned about this occurrence and laughs it off and says that the child must have 'photobombed' the family. You contact Aaron's father, Joseph. He mentions that Aaron has

Continued on following page

(Continued)

recently been spending a considerable amount of time in his bedroom, has missed work on occasion and socializes less than usual. He suspects that Aaron has been smoking cannabis. At times, Joseph has thought that he heard Aaron talking to himself in his room. However, on entering, it appears that Aaron is talking on his mobile phone. He is happy for Aaron to return home and agrees to keep a close eye on him until the morning when you will review the situation again in the outpatient clinic.

    1. What are your initial thoughts about this presentation?

Although the correspondence lacks detail, this is an urgent referral raising concern about Aaron's recent behaviour. Despite his general practitioner's concerns about acute paranoia, it is not clearly apparent that Aaron is experiencing hallucinations, thought disorder or bizarre delusions. Although he exhibits some agitation, you do not note any objective evidence of mood disturbance and Aaron reports that his mood is 'fine'. He does seem to be preoccupied about the photograph to the extent that he is carrying it around on his person but he is not forthcoming about his concerns. It should be considered unusual that Aaron presented willingly to the mental health services in the absence of any subjective symptoms or distress.

Assessment of first-episode psychosis (FEP) requires a thorough history and longitudinal evaluation alongside collateral information. At this stage, there is a long list of differential diagnoses, including the first presentation of a psychotic illness (either nonaffective or affective) and no psychiatric illness (see Fig. 2.1).

2. The following morning you meet Aaron and his father—who is visibly distressed—in your clinic. Aaron was brought to the emergency department overnight by the police but was discharged so that he could attend this morning's appointment. Joseph had entered Aaron's room the previous evening after he had heard Aaron talking animatedly. He had been shocked to find that Aaron had wired together a number of electronic devices in a very haphazard and disorganized manner. He had placed a number of basins of water in the room and had shouted to his father that he 'just wanted everything in this family to stop'. The walls of the bedroom were covered with photographs of Aaron as a child. When Joseph confronted him about this, Aaron had stated that 'none of those pictures are of me'.

On assessment, Aaron is initially agitated, although not overtly aggressive. His mood is labile, but he is cooperative. He denies having any desire to harm himself or others but seems unwilling to provide any explanation for his behaviour. Nonetheless at one stage he states 'you will see in time' when asked about his actions. Despite insisting that 'doctor, there is nothing wrong with me', he agrees to a brief admission to the psychiatric unit for assessment.

    2. What is the association between psychosis and risk of harm to others?

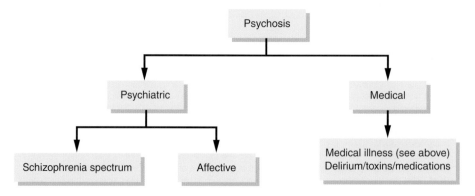

Fig. 2.1 Differential diagnoses in first-episode psychosis (FEP).

FURTHER READING

For a review of violence and psychosis, see: Douglas KS, Guy LS, Hart SD. (2009) Psychosis as a risk factor for violence to others: A meta-analysis. Psychological Bulletin 135 (5):679–706. doi: 10.1037/a0016311

Despite his reassurances, it should be assumed that Aaron may present risk to himself and others. The association between psychosis and risk to others is complicated. However when delusional themes include ideas of violent action, the risk must be considered to be significant. Of note, Aaron is acting upon his escalating delusional beliefs in a way that is extremely dangerous and potentially lethal.

Risk assessment

Methods of risk assessment include unaided clinical judgement, actuarial methods and structured clinical risk assessments. Unaided clinical judgement has been demonstrated to be no better than chance in terms of assessing risk. Actuarial assessments focus on relatively small numbers of risk factors that are known or thought to predict violence. These tend to be static/historical factors, such as offending history, juvenile delinquency, previous treatment failure and noncompliance. Actuarial assessments are used extensively in the criminal justice system to make parole decisions.

Structured clinical risk assessment examines risk in three different areas: historical, clinical and future/speculative. The historical clinical risk management-20 (HCR-20) is a commonly used tool that provides a structure for assessing the combined role of current clinical, historical and contextual factors that are known to be associated with a risk of violence (Table 2.1).

The relationship between psychosis and violence is complex and controversial. In general, patients with a psychotic illness are no more likely than the general public to engage in violent behaviour. Nonetheless, random acts of disorganized violence are more common in the context of psychosis. Despite a lack of consistency across individual studies, a large meta-analysis concluded that psychoses are associated with violence and violent offending. However, it is noteworthy that much of the excess risk appears to be mediated by comorbid substance abuse. Other studies have demonstrated that in psychotic individuals the increased violence rates can be linked to factors such as previous criminality, impulsivity, poor insight and non-adherence to treatment.

3. Aaron is admitted to the ward. He settles in well and establishes a superficial rapport with a number of other patients. He appears to enjoy the company of his roommate, John, who is soon to be

Continued on following page

TABLE 2.1 ■ **HCR-20**

Historical	Clinical	Risk Management
• Previous violence	• Insight	• Plans lack feasibility
• Young age at first offence	• Negative attitude	• Exposure to destabilizers
• Relationship instability	• Active mental illness	• Lack of personal support
• Unemployment	• Impulsivity	• Noncompliance with remediation attempts
• Substance abuse	• Unresponsive to treatment	• Stress
• Mental illness		
• Psychopathy		
• Early maladjustment		
• Personality disorder		
• Supervision failure		

(Continued)

discharged after a drug-induced psychotic episode. Despite this, nursing staff note that Aaron is reluctant to engage in any structured activities and can be quite animated on occasion. When questioned about the events prior to admission, he says, 'I am all over that now. It was a mix-up'. Initial routine blood investigations, screening for illicit drugs, brain magnetic resonance imaging (MRI) and electroencephalogram (EEG) are all normal. He agrees to a trial of antipsychotic medication (olanzapine), although he does not feel that he is unwell.

   3. What is the rationale for these investigations?

   4. What are your initial thoughts about Aaron's level of insight?

Evaluating a patient with FEP requires consideration of a broad range of differential diagnoses. The absence of a family history of major mental illness, an acute illness onset and age at onset beyond the middle 30s will heighten concern that psychotic symptoms are secondary to an organic disorder. Even when suspicion is low, careful consideration should be given to the possibility that an index presentation may be the result of a neurological or medical condition.

Differential diagnoses include the following: head trauma, infections, brain tumours, seizures, multiple sclerosis, metachromatic leukodystrophy, Huntington's disease, Wilson's disease, endocrinopathies (thyroid, adrenal, pancreatic), autoimmune disorders (e.g. anti-N-methyl-D-aspartate (NMDA) receptor body encephalitis and systemic lupus erythematosus), vitamin deficiencies and disorders of metabolism, such as acute intermittent porphyria. A relatively common precipitant of psychotic symptoms is an adverse reaction to prescribed medication, including steroids, L-dopa, anticholinergics and H_2 blockers. Therefore, all FEP individuals should undergo a thorough medical and neurological evaluation. Initial investigations include a full blood count, urea and electrolytes, thyroid function tests, an autoantibody screen (including anti-NMDA receptor antibodies), urinalysis and a toxicology screen. In most cases, a brain MRI scan should be obtained along with an EEG.

Although Aaron appears to have limited insight, does not feel that he is unwell and does not wish to be in the hospital, he is accepting medication. Many individuals concord with treatment despite a denial of their illness. Conversely, others are not concordant despite a good awareness of their illness. Several factors, including one's personality, social milieu and perceived coercion, may affect either one of the constructs and not the other. A more detailed consideration of insight is provided later in this chapter.

4. At your multidisciplinary team meeting on Thursday morning, the inpatient staff raise concerns about Aaron. The previous night he had been observed outside the treatment store attempting to gain access. When prevented from doing so, he requested a tourniquet and some phlebotomy needles. At the subsequent assessment, he told staff that his roommate John had absconded and been 'replaced by a similar-looking patient'. Aaron demanded that the nurses take blood from his roommate for 'DNA analysis'.

  When this suggestion was refused, Aaron asked if he could gain access to the 'shock therapy' room, as he was concerned—'as an electrician'—about the 'interference' it was causing to his radio and laptop. He told the staff that he had needed to wear earphones to 'drown out the political messages' coming through his devices because of this interference. He stated that if his requests were not granted, he would discharge himself as a voluntary patient the following morning.

   5. How would you proceed?

As Aaron appears to represent a risk to John, and has impaired judgement, underpinned by delusional beliefs, it would be unsafe for him to be discharged from hospital. In these circumstances, when the criteria for 'mental disorder' are met, a voluntary patient may be detained under Section 23 of the Mental Health Act.

5. During your ward round, you find Aaron to be markedly dishevelled. He tells you that he believes that 'the real Aaron disappeared as a child' and that he was, in fact, Aaron's twin brother and was unsure of his own name.

When you ask him when he became aware of this, he reports 'I noticed some peculiarities in the family photographs displayed in our house' and that 'they were acting strangely for a few months' until 'the final proof' had come with finding the photo he had shown you at your initial meeting. Although he had initially felt relief, he had become increasingly distressed by 'static' that had started emanating from his mobile phone, which subsequently 'spread' to all of his devices, becoming more formed until he started hearing 'political messages' from a number of voices.

These voices had talked to each other about a number of disappearances of individuals who had been replaced by 'doubles', but recently they had become 'more like instructions'. He believes that his thoughts and actions are being both controlled and monitored: 'they comment on everything I do'. He had attempted to 'block' these messages by interfering with the electronics in his bedroom and assures you that he did not mean to cause himself or his family any harm.

Throughout this description, Aaron is smiling, and he laughs on occasion. He does not want to be in hospital, but after some reassurance, he is willing to stay and to continue taking olanzapine as he admits to being under severe stress and feels the medication has a relaxant effect.

6. How would you describe Aaron's presentation in terms of its psychopathological features?
7. What are the so-called first-rank symptoms of schizophrenia?
8. Broadly outline the main diagnostic categories included in the differential diagnosis of Aaron's presentation.
9. What are the pharmacological considerations for first-episode psychosis?

Aaron describes a delusional mood or atmosphere, where he appears perplexed that 'something weird' was happening before his uncertainty is resolved by a delusional perception when he observed the photographs. Within this primary delusion, a false meaning is attributed to the normal percept of the photo. His beliefs are false, appear to be held with strong conviction and cannot be easily explained by cultural factors so are correctly defined as delusional. Definitions of the term 'paranoid' are inconsistent across phenomenologists (ranging from self-referential to persecutory beliefs). However, Aaron's thought content is clearly bizarre, self-referential and persecutory. Specifically, he has delusions of misidentification, whereby he believes that the identity of people around him have been interfered with.

He demonstrates passivity phenomena where he believes that external agents are controlling his actions (passivity of volition) and thoughts (thought insertion). He also has a possible passivity of emotion, which is demonstrated by his grossly incongruous affect.

After initial elementary hallucinations ('static'), as the psychosis becomes more overt, Aaron is experiencing more complex, third person auditory hallucinations in the form of running commentary. Although they are not referenced in the Diagnostic and Statistical Manual of Mental Disorders (DSM)-5, the so-called first-rank symptoms of schizophrenia (as first defined by Schneider in 1959), continue to be viewed as useful markers for the presence of schizophrenia in the International Classification of Diseases-10 classification system (Box 2.1).

BOX 2.1 ■ First-rank symptoms of schizophrenia

1. Audible thoughts (thought echo)
2. Third person auditory hallucinations
3. Voices heard commenting on one's actions (running commentary)
4. Somatic/thought passivity experiences (passivity of impulses, actions, feelings, somatic sensations)
5. Thought withdrawal
6. Thought insertion
7. Thought broadcasting
8. Delusional perception

PSYCHIATRIC DISORDERS

Aaron has had a comprehensive battery of medical investigations, and no acute medical cause for his symptoms has been identified. His presentation at this stage can be viewed as 'functional'.

Emil Kraepelin's historical classification of functional psychoses into nonaffective (dementia praecox, later termed 'schizophrenia') and affective (manic-depressive psychosis, later termed 'bipolar affective disorder') continues to dominate psychiatric practice. However, patients with FEP frequently also demonstrate significant manic or depressive symptoms. As such it can be challenging to differentiate a primary psychotic disorder from a mood disorder with psychotic symptoms in the early stages of the illness, especially if the picture is complicated by issues such as alcohol or substance use. A careful history and collateral information should be obtained because differentiating between these syndromes has significant treatment and prognostic implications.

SCHIZOPHRENIA AND NONAFFECTIVE PSYCHOSES

Regarding schizophrenia, three diagnostic criteria must be met according to the DSM-5 (Box 2.2).

If signs of disturbance are present for more than a month but less than six months, the patient is considered to have a schizophreniform disorder. Psychotic symptoms lasting less than a month may be diagnosed as brief psychotic disorder. Extremely transient psychotic episodes, lasting minutes to hours, can sometimes occur in individuals with borderline or schizotypal personality disorder.

AFFECTIVE DISORDER

Psychotic symptoms are common in both the manic and depressed phase of bipolar disorder (BD) type I, with greater than half of all individuals diagnosed with BD experiencing psychotic mood symptoms in their lifetime. The DSM supports the clinical assumption that BD with psychosis represents a more severe form of illness than BD without psychosis. Individuals with BD commonly endorse grandiose delusions and relatively few of them experience the Schneiderian first-rank symptoms traditionally evident in schizophrenia. Furthermore, psychosis in BD tends to be mood-congruent and of briefer duration than in schizophrenia.

Epidemiological research suggests that 15%–19% of patients with major depression exhibit psychotic symptoms, such as delusions or hallucinations, with even higher rates observed in hospitalized samples. The similarities between schizophrenia and BD in terms of their clinical and neurobiological features is further complicated by the diagnosis of schizoaffective disorder. This is defined by mood disorder and schizophreniform symptoms that are both prominent throughout an episode of illness. In such cases, patients may be described as 'schizo-manic' or 'schizo-depressed' depending on the pattern of affective disturbances.

BOX 2.2 ■ The diagnosis of schizophrenia is based upon the following:

1. The presence of characteristic symptoms, such as psychotic symptoms that have a schizophreniform character (e.g. Schneiderian first-rank symptoms), formal thought disorder, grossly disorganized or catatonic behaviour or negative symptoms.
2. Symptoms that have significant functional impact in terms of reduced self-care, interpersonal interactions and the ability to engage with occupational activities.
3. Symptoms that occur over a sustained period and are not better explained by substance misuse, schizoaffective or affective disorder.

SUBSTANCE ABUSE

A significant proportion of patients presenting with FEP report current or past substance abuse. Illicit substance abuse often presents a diagnostic challenge. Strict adherence to DSM requires that the psychotic symptoms persist for at least 1 month to exclude a diagnosis of substance-induced psychotic disorder. The effects of substance abuse on the onset, treatment response, course and outcome of psychotic illnesses remain poorly understood. There has been a particular focus on the role of cannabis in recent years. In short, early, frequent use of high potency cannabis appears to have a role in precipitating psychosis in genetically vulnerable individuals. Consideration of the impact of illicit drugs on precipitating and perpetuating psychosis is covered in detail in Chapter 12. Drug testing is discussed in Chapter 25.

Pharmacological interventions in first-episode psychosis

A detailed discussion with the patient and their family should be held, around the nature, process, benefits and potential adverse effects of any proposed treatment. In the acute presentation, this may be impractical, and if there is significant behavioural disturbance that does not respond to psychological or behavioural strategies, rapid tranquillization (RT) may be necessary. RT is discussed in Chapter 1 and typically involves the combination of an antipsychotic agent with benzodiazepine. A treatment algorithm for FEP is outlined in Fig. 2.2).

For a review of interventions in first episode psychosis, see: Liu P, Parker AG, Hetrick SE, et al. (2010) An evidence map of interventions across premorbid, ultra-high risk and first episode phases of psychosis. Schizophrenia Research 123(1):37–44. doi:10.1016/j.schres.2010.05.004

6. Aaron remains as a voluntary patient, and his phone is taken away for safe-keeping. He is compliant with his medication regime, and over the following 10 days, his condition appears to settle. He continues to talk about 'doubles' for a number of days. However, he becomes considerably more subdued and at times is reported by the nursing staff as appearing depressed.

At this point, Aaron admits to habitual cannabis use, but claims that he had stopped smoking the drug a fortnight prior to admission as it had been making him feel 'uneasy'. He recalls having a profound feeling that 'something very weird was going on' and 'realizing' that he had a different identity. On further questioning, he consistently says that 'it must have been the drugs'. He does mention that an uncle of his was treated in a large psychiatric institution on a number of occasions for 'breakdowns'. He becomes upset when recalling his own initial presentation and appears to have an understanding of the social fall-out and that a number of his friends have failed to visit him, saying that 'they must think I'm a psycho'. He is dysphoric but does not display the biological features of a depressive syndrome.

10. What do you feel about Aarons's insight, and how would you formally assess it?
11. What are the main diagnostic considerations at this point?
12. What is known about the cause of schizophrenia?

Aaron appears to have gained genuine insight as his interpretation seems considered and has resulted in (realistic) pessimism. There are a variety of proposed mechanisms which may contribute to diminished insight in psychosis, with most research focusing on psychological theories, other psychopathology and neuropsychological deficits.

Historically, poor insight has been thought to relate to psychological defence mechanisms. There is an evidence base for this interpretation, as high levels of insight are repeatedly associated with increased levels of depression. This suggests that 'denial' of illness may be self-protective. Insight impairment has been associated with higher levels of general psychopathology, however this, relationship is not particularly strong and insight may remain chronically impaired despite successful

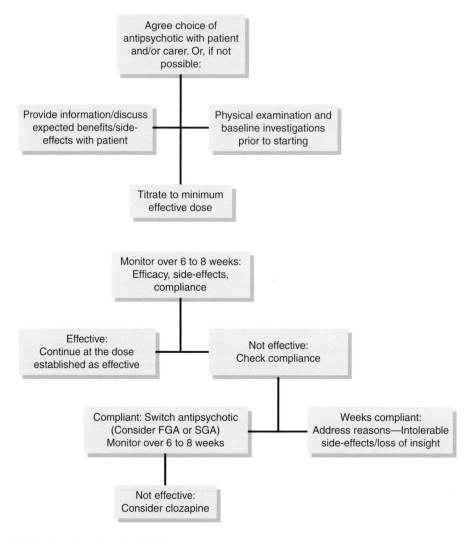

Fig. 2.2 A treatment algorithm for FEP.

treatment of psychotic symptoms. This has led some researchers to believe that insight impairment is a primary symptom caused by a neuropsychological deficit, analogous with anosognosia, which is sometimes observed in stroke victims (see Box 2.3 for model questions for assessing insight).

In terms of Aaron's risk, the relationship between suicide, deliberate self-harm and insight is complicated. Diminished insight in schizophrenia has been associated with a poor prognosis and reduced compliance with treatment, both of which are risk factors for suicide. However, some studies have suggested that the presence of insight is, in itself, a risk factor for increased suicidal ideation in psychosis.

The additional information provided by Aaron raises the possibility of drug-induced psychosis. The symptoms presented relatively quickly, with a clear temporal relationship with cannabis use (and abrupt cessation) and appeared to have settled very quickly with antipsychotic medication. However,

---

BOX 2.3 ■ Model questions for assessing insight in psychosis (adapted from the Schedule for the Assessment of Insight)

1. Do you think you have been experiencing any emotional or psychological changes or difficulties?
2. If the doctor(s) and/or others think you have been experiencing emotional or psychological changes or difficulties, do you think there must be something wrong with you even though you do not feel it yourself?
3. How do you explain your condition/disorder/illness?
4. Has your condition led to adverse consequences or problems in your life?
5. Do you think that the belief is not really happening (could you be imagining things)?
6. Do you think the 'voices' you hear are actually real people talking, or is it something arising from your own mind?
7. Have you been able to think clearly, or do your thoughts seem mixed up/confused?

---

the family history of psychosis may be significant. Furthermore, Aaron's symptoms were relatively systematized and included a number of classical components of a schizophrenia-spectrum illness.

Importantly, longitudinal studies of FEP have observed changes in diagnosis over time. In particular, persons with a label of drug-induced psychosis frequently receive more long-term diagnostic labels, such as schizophrenia, as their situation evolves over time.

The cause of psychosis, like many other mental health-related disorders, is not fully understood. The current explanatory models cite a combination of genetic and environmental factors. For example, an individual with a first-degree relative suffering from schizophrenia has a 10% chance of developing the disorder. By comparison, the risk of schizophrenia in the general population is about 1%. Furthermore, this risk rises to 50% for monozygotic twins, providing clear evidence of a genetic basis. Indeed, multiple susceptibility genes have been identified. Some of the environmental factors known to be associated with schizophrenia are early, frequent use of high potency cannabis, prenatal infection or malnutrition, birth trauma, and history of spring or winter births. However, it is unclear how these factors interact with genetic factors to cause schizophrenia.

---

7. After a six-week admission, Aaron is discharged from the hospital on olanzapine, with a comprehensive discharge plan, including cognitive behavioural therapy with his clinical nurse specialist, family therapy with his social worker, and input from an occupational therapist.

Initially, he dismisses any of his symptoms as being a result of his drug use. At subsequent visits, Aaron becomes more distressed when discussing his initial presentation, and voices concerns about returning to work and socializing again. However, he does not appear overtly depressed. He presents regularly for his medication despite some weight gain and mild sedation. He is worried about the possibility of a relapse.

13. What do we know about the outcome predictors in first-episode psychosis?

Psychotic illness has a varied prognosis. For example, the majority of patients with schizophrenia experience a course of multiple episodes and increasing impairment and a smaller proportion (20%–50%) experience recovery or significant improvement. More than 50% of sufferers can hold down meaningful day-to-day vocational activity. Factors predicting poor outcome in psychosis include male gender, single marital status, insidious onset, predominant negative symptoms, poor insight and poor premorbid adjustment. There is now a growing body of evidence supporting the association between a long duration of untreated psychosis (DUP) and poor outcomes.

Good prognostic indicators in FEP

- The onset of prominent symptoms within 4 weeks of the first noticeable change in usual behaviour or functioning

- Confusion or perplexity at the height of the episode
- Good premorbid social and occupational functioning
- Absence of negative symptoms
- Female gender
- Later age of onset
- Short DUP
- Compliance with antipsychotic treatment
- High premorbid functioning
- Absence of 'soft' neurological signs
- Originating from a country in the developing world (because of postulated lower levels of stigma and better social support).

Historically, studies of outcomes in psychosis have been over-represented by patients with chronic, treatment-refractory schizophrenia and poorly represented by recovered patients at follow up. These factors have contributed towards a biased perception of poor prognosis and outcomes and may have influenced current clinical and public perspectives on the prognosis of schizophrenia.

Furthermore, 'recovery-focused' research suggests that remission of illness based on symptom criteria alone is a weak predictor of outcome function. 'Outcome' is a multifaceted area and should include consideration of a range of different measures, including social relations, employment, symptoms and duration of hospitalization.

Early intervention in psychosis

There has been increased interest in the concept of the prodromal phase prior to presentation with FEP. The prodromal phase may be represented by a variety of symptoms, including vague perceptual disturbances, anger or irritability, derealization, ideas of reference, anxiety and social withdrawal.

Patterns of the prodrome or at-risk mental state generally fall into those with the following:

1. Attenuated psychosis—characterized by odd beliefs, ideas of reference and vague perceptual disturbance
2. Brief symptoms lasting less than one week
3. Social decline with a family history of psychosis.

Early intervention services aim to intervene at an earlier stage to reduce the number of patients developing chronic disabilities. It is consistent with the 'toxic psychosis' theory, which proposes that psychosis is neurotoxic and that an increased DUP is associated with poorer outcomes. Evidence-based strategies in early intervention include anxiety management, cognitive behavioural therapy, family interventions and occupational therapy. There is some evidence that low dosage second-generation antipsychotics and fish oils may prevent the development of a full psychotic syndrome, but further research is necessary to substantiate these findings.

FURTHER READING

For a review of the relationship between the duration of untreated psychosis and outcomes, see: Pentilla M, Jaaskelainen E, Hirvonen N, et al. (2014) Duration of untreated psychosis as predictor of long-term outcome in schizophrenia: systematic review and meta-analysis. British Journal of Psychiatry 205(2):88–94. doi: 10.1192/bjp.bp.113.127753

CHAPTER 3

Anna

Recurrent Depressive Disorder

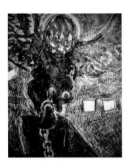

1. Define the key clinical diagnostic features of depression.
2. Understand relevant differential diagnoses and comorbid disorders, including illicit drug use.
3. Outline the main treatment strategies for depression considering biological, social and psychological approaches.
4. Understand the mode of action of the main classes of antidepressants.
5. Understand how one selects an appropriate antidepressant agent.
6. Understand when referral to specialist mental health services is appropriate.
7. Describe the natural history of recurrent depression and the role of maintenance treatment.

---

1. Anna is a 22-year-old single mother of two children who presents to her general practitioner with abdominal discomfort. At consultation, the general practitioner notes that this is the third occasion that she has attended the surgery in as many weeks, having complained previously of back pain. Upon discussion, he notes that her complaints are quite vague and that she is 'quiet' throughout. When he asks how her mood has been, she begins to weep. She then explains that she has been upset since her recent split with her boyfriend.
    1. What are your initial thoughts about this presentation?
    2. What are the symptoms of 'clinical depression' and how is the severity of illness ascertained?

This presentation involves a combination of somatic symptoms and psychological distress. There are many possible interactions between physical and psychological complaints, and it is important to remain open-minded to the significance of either as a primary complaint. Pre-existing physical problems are often aggravated by psychological factors, while major psychological distress is often communicated through physical complaints (so-called 'somatization'). This can lead to a delayed or misdiagnosis.

FURTHER READING

For a key study that addresses the detection of depressive illness in primary care, see:
Arroll B, Khin N, Kerse N. (2003) Screening for depression in primary care with two verbally asked questions: cross sectional study. The British Medical Journal 327(7424):1144–1146. doi: 10.1136/bmj.327.7424.1144

Screening for possible depression is an important element of assessing patients with physical complaints, and this can be effectively managed by probing their recent mood and interest/enjoyment levels. These two symptoms (low mood and anhedonia) are especially useful for identifying depressive illness in patients presenting to primary care.

'Clinical' depression is a term used to distinguish an abnormal state of sustained low mood as part of a wider syndrome of psychological and physiological disturbance that warrants specific therapeutic (or 'clinical') intervention rather than an expectation that time will allow for normal readjustment.

In considering whether a patient has a clinical depressive illness, it is important to consider a range of symptom clusters that include: (1) low mood with loss of enjoyment and interest; (2) disturbed cognitive 'set' (negative self-regard, feelings of guilt or hopelessness); (3) somatic or biological features that reflect disturbance of biological rhythms (sleep/appetite/energy/libido); and (4) risk of self-harm. This constellation makes up the syndrome of clinical depression.

The terminology used to describe depressive disorders in the International Classification of Diseases (ICD)-10 and Diagnostic and Statistical Manual of Mental Disorders (DSM)-5 is somewhat different. ICD-10 categorizes depression as a depressive episode for single events and recurrent depressive disorder where two or more episodes occur. DSM-5 describes a spectrum of depressive disorders that includes major depressive disorder (including a major depressive episode), persistent depressive disorder (dysthymia), disruptive mood dysregulation disorder, premenstrual dysphoric disorder, substance/medication-induced depressive disorder, depressive disorder because of another medical condition, other specified depressive disorder, and unspecified depressive disorder. The common feature of all these disorders is the presence of a sad, empty, or irritable mood, accompanied by somatic and cognitive changes that significantly affect the individual's capacity to function. However, they differ in terms of duration, timing, or presumed cause.

ICD-10 includes three key symptoms and seven associated symptoms of depression. The key symptoms are: (1) persistent sadness or low mood; (2) loss of interest or pleasure; and (3) fatigue or low energy. The associated symptoms are disturbed sleep, poor concentration or indecisiveness, low self-confidence, poor or increased appetite, suicidal thoughts or acts, agitation or slowing of movements and guilt or self-blame. In ICD-10, the severity of depression is defined as not depressed (fewer than four symptoms), mild depression (four symptoms), moderate depression (five to six symptoms) and severe depression (seven or more symptoms, with or without psychotic symptoms) (Box 3.1).

---

2. Anna reports that she has had a low mood for most of the day, every day of the previous month. She describes feeling guilty because she has been struggling to care for her children and at times has been 'snappy' and irritable with them. She reports problems getting to sleep, poor appetite and concentration, loss of interest in her usual activities and that she has stopped going out except for essential trips (e.g. shopping for groceries). She denies any feelings of hopelessness or thoughts of self-harm.

> ## BOX 3.1 ■ Diagnosis of major depressive disorder
>
> 1. Depressed mood and/or anhedonia (loss of interest or pleasure) that is present for most of the time and is pervasive in terms of personal, occupational and social functioning domains.
> 2. Associated symptoms that include:
>   - An altered sense of self with negative self-regard, feelings of worthlessness or guilt that can progress to include psychotic symptoms.
>   - Impaired thinking with reduced concentration and indecisiveness that can progress to the poverty of thought.
>   - Disturbed sleeping patterns (either insomnia or hypersomnia).
>   - Reduced energy with fatigue and/or reduced motivation.
>   - Reduced activity levels and/or agitation.
>   - Significant weight loss because of reduced interest in food or weight gain because of comfort eating.
>   - A sense of pessimism and hopelessness that can progress to a passive death wish, thoughts of self-harm, suicidal ideation or intent.
> 3. That causes significant distress and/or impairment in functioning in social, interpersonal and occupational activities.
> 4. Symptoms are not better explained by substance use, medical illness or another functional psychiatric disorder (e.g. schizophrenia, schizoaffective disorder).
>
> The severity of an episode is graded as mild, moderate and severe according to the number of the above features that are evident, with the presence of psychosis implying severe illness.

Her general practitioner suggests that she might benefit from antidepressant therapy, but she indicates that she would prefer to avoid 'going down the medication route'. She agrees to contact the practice counsellor and return for another assessment in three weeks.

3. What are some suitable questions to explore for features of a major depressive illness?
4. What are the possible explanations for patients presenting with sadness, and how are they distinguished?
5. What is 'counselling', and what is the evidence to support its effectiveness in depressive illness?

Suitable questions to explore for features of a major depressive illness include:

- How have you been feeling in your mood?
- Does your mood change over the day?
- Have you been able to enjoy things?
- How have you been feeling about yourself?
- How do you see the future?
- Describe your sleep pattern?
- What is your appetite like? Have you lost weight recently?
- How are your energy levels? Can you perform your usual activities?
- How has your concentration been? Can you follow a television programme or a newspaper article?
- Has there been any change in your libido?

It is a normal part of human experience to feel sadness in a variety of circumstances, but it is important to distinguish adjustment symptoms from more severe pathological states that warrant specific therapeutic interventions. While it is normal to experience sadness in response to adverse experiences and loss events, where such responses are more prolonged or symptomatically severe, this is likely to indicate psychological illness. A key consideration is to recognize that pathological states are usually precipitated by life events but also reflect a biological vulnerability towards illness. The 'understandability' of low mood needs to be carefully considered in the context of the

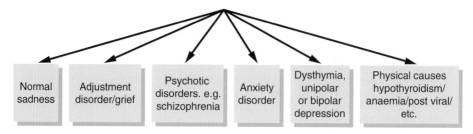

Fig. 3.1 Differential diagnosis of sadness.

possibility that such states may have progressed to become so severe as to now be beyond that which can be viewed as a normal reaction to adversity. In particular, the social divide between clinicians and patients from lower socioeconomic groups has been highlighted as a major obstacle to accurate detection of pathological states such as depression in such populations ('I would feel depressed if I had to deal with their day-to-day problems').

In the differential diagnosis, it is important to establish whether there are features of depressive illness, as this will take diagnostic precedence over adjustment reactions and requires therapeutic consideration (Fig. 3.1).

Depressive illness commonly occurs in the context of physical illness (especially conditions that are chronic and/or impact upon neural function), and a comorbid physical cause is particularly important to consider where depressive illness first occurs in patients over 40 years of age.

Anxiety symptoms commonly complicate depressive illness and the appearance or a worsening of anxiety symptoms should always raise the possibility of an underlying depressive condition.

Bipolar depression is suggested by a personal history of elation (this should be carefully explored for in the previous history as undiagnosed milder episodes are not uncommon), a family history of bipolar illness, atypical clinical features (e.g. mixed mood states), severe illness and/or relative treatment resistance.

Dysthymia is a condition that presents with a persistent low mood of milder severity. Dysthymic individuals are often described by friends as 'grumpy', 'negative' or 'pessimistic'. 'Double-depression' relates to the occurrence of major depression in the context of long-standing dysthymia.

FURTHER READING

For a review of the effectiveness of psychological interventions (including counselling) in depression, see: Cape J, Whittington C, Buszewicz M, et al. (2010) Brief psychological therapies for anxiety and depression in primary care: meta-analysis and meta-regression. BMC Medicine 8:38. doi:10.1186/1741-7015-8-38

Counselling is the term used to describe talk therapy that can include a variety of elements (supportive, educational, coping skills enhancement) that assist and guide individuals in resolving personal, social, or psychological problems and difficulties. Therefore, counselling covers a wide range of possible supportive interventions, and the experience and training of the counsellor can vary widely. Evidence supports the effectiveness of counselling for mild and moderate depressive illness and subthreshold depression. Pharmacological interventions (often combined with psychological interventions) are recommended for more severe illness. The effectiveness of antidepressant agents in milder forms of depression is increasingly questioned as to whether they are superior to a placebo in clinical trials.

3. Anna attends the counsellor on a single occasion but fails to keep subsequent appointments. She returns for review three weeks later and describes some worsening of symptoms. At this point, she agrees to commence escitalopram 10 mg per day. Four weeks later, her condition has worsened, and she now confides that she has been feeling that she cannot shake the depression and having intermittent thoughts of harming herself because she feels *'useless'* and *'a burden'*. Upon questioning, she reassures the general practitioner that she could not harm herself because 'I love the children too much'. The general practitioner increases the dose of escitalopram to 15 mg per day, but after a further four weeks, she remains depressed and despondent about the future.

    6. How does one select an appropriate antidepressant agent, and what is the recommended first-line pharmacological treatment for depressive illness?

    7. What are the key messages to give to a patient commencing antidepressant therapy?

    8. What are the indications for referral of depressed patients to specialist mental health services?

The choice of antidepressant agent is determined according to the severity of illness, previous history of antidepressant therapy and the potential for adverse effects and interactions with other medications. For the first episode of depression, a medication from the serotonin specific reuptake inhibitors (SSRI) family is generally considered appropriate because of their tolerability profile. If this strategy is not successful (with an adequate dosage for an adequate trial period), an agent from a different class, for example, a serotonin and noradrenaline reuptake inhibitor (SNRI), such as venlafaxine, should be considered. The National Institute for Clinical Excellence offers guidelines on the selection of antidepressants (see Box 3.2).

FURTHER READING

A good source of information for patients commencing antidepressant therapy can be accessed at: http://www.rcpsych.ac.uk/mentalhealthinfoforall/problems/depression/antidepressants.aspx

Nonadherence to antidepressant therapy is a common problem in everyday practice and is in part related to misinformation about the treatment process, including the timing of response and possible adverse effects. Patients commencing antidepressants should be encouraged to discuss their treatment expectations.

In particular, it is important to emphasize that antidepressants are not addictive, not known to have major long-term adverse effects, have a delayed onset of action of 10–14 days, should be continued for at least six months after symptom resolution (longer in patients with severe or recurring episodes) and should not be abruptly discontinued since they can have discontinuation effects. This latter problem is especially common with agents with short half-lives, such as paroxetine and venlafaxine.

Although most patients with a depressive illness can be managed in primary care, referral to specialist mental health services is appropriate for patients with a depressive illness where:

- there are urgent concerns regarding safety for the patient or others.
- the severity of illness is such that specialist opinion regarding management is required.
- the patient has a history of treatment resistance.
- there are diagnostic uncertainties or significant complicating factors, such as comorbidities or situational factors.

FURTHER READING

For an overview of the management of depression, see: Timonen M, Liukkonen T. (2008) Management of depression in adults. BMJ 336:435–439. doi: 10.1136/bmj.39478.609097.BE

BOX 3.2 ■ Selecting antidepressants

Assess likely tolerability, including the following:

Anticipated adverse events, for example, side-effects and discontinuation symptoms.
Potential interactions with concomitant medication.
Comorbid physical illness.
The person's perception of the efficacy and tolerability of any antidepressants they have previously taken.

Usually choose a serotonin specific reuptake inhibitor in the first instance

Take the following into account:

Serotonin specific reuptake inhibitors are associated with an increased risk of bleeding. Consider prescribing a gastroprotective drug in older people who are taking nonsteroidal antiinflammatory drugs or aspirin.
For people who have a chronic physical health problem, consider using citalopram or sertraline as these have a lower propensity for drug interactions.
Paroxetine is associated with a higher incidence of discontinuation symptoms.

Consider toxicity in overdose for people at significant risk of suicide

Be aware that venlafaxine and especially tricyclic antidepressants are associated with a greater risk of death from overdose.

When prescribing drugs other than serotonin specific reuptake inhibitors, consider the following

The increased likelihood of the person stopping treatment because of side-effects, and the consequent need to increase the dosage gradually with venlafaxine, duloxetine and tricyclic antidepressants.
Specific warnings, contraindications and monitoring requirements for some drugs.

Some treatments should generally be prescribed by specialist mental health professionals

Monoamine oxidase inhibitors (such as phenelzine).
Combination therapy with antidepressants.
Lithium augmentation of antidepressants.

When prescribing antidepressants for older adults

Adjust dosage, considering their physical health and concomitant medication.
Monitor carefully for side-effects.

---

4. Anna's general practitioner makes a referral to the local mental health services where she is assessed and noted to have moderate-to-severe depression because of the presence of marked lowering of mood and widespread disturbance of biological function. She agrees to try a different antidepressant treatment.
    9. What is an adequate trial of antidepressant treatment?
   10. What are the main classes of antidepressants, and how do they compare with regard to their mechanisms of action?

An adequate trial of antidepressant treatment involves administering a therapeutic dosage for six weeks as long as the patient remains fully compliant with the treatment. An advantage of the SSRI family of agents is that the starting dosages are typically at the lower end of the therapeutic dosage range. In contrast, the older tricyclic agents require a number of dose escalations to reach the therapeutic range and are often prescribed at subtherapeutic dosages. Venlafaxine shares this

TABLE 3.1 ■ Antidepressant Medications and Mechanism of Action

Name	Mechanism of Action	Example
SSRI	Selective serotonin reuptake inhibitors	Fluoxetine, Paroxetine, Sertraline, Citalopram Escitalopram
SNRI	Serotonin and noradrenaline reuptake inhibitors	Venlafaxine, Duloxetine
NaSSA	Noradrenergic and specific serotonergic antidepressants	Mirtazapine
NaRI	Selective noradrenaline reuptake inhibitor	Reboxetine
SARI	Serotonin antagonist and reuptake inhibitor	Trazodone
NDRI	Noradrenaline and dopamine reuptake inhibitors	Bupropion
Melatonergic agents	Enhances noradrenaline and dopamine release	Agomelatine
TCA	Serotonin and noradrenaline reuptake inhibitors	Clomipramine, Nortriptyline, Amitriptyline
MAO-I	Monoamine oxidase inhibitors	Moclobemide, Phenelzine, Tranylcypromine

SSRI, serotonin specific reuptake inhibitor; SNRI, serotonin noradrenaline reuptake; NaSSA, Noradrenergic and specific serotonergic antidepressants; NaRI, noradrenaline reuptake inhibitor; SARI, Serotonin antagonist and reuptake inhibitor; NDRI, Noradrenaline and dopamine reuptake inhibitor; MAO-I, Monoamine oxidase inhibitors; TCA, tricyclic antidepressants

potential for failure of response because of the use of low/subtherapeutic doses, with 150 mg per day considered the lowest therapeutic dose in healthy adults.

The main classes of antidepressant agents are shown in Table 3.1.

The monoamine hypothesis of depression postulates that a deficiency or imbalance in monoamines is a primary factor in the pathophysiology of depressive illness. Antidepressant agents increase synaptic monoamine availability by three principal mechanisms: (1) blockade of reuptake molecules; (2) inhibition of monoamine catabolism by monoamine oxidase; and (3) enhancement of monoamine release by reducing feedback inhibition to presynaptic auto-receptors.

SSRIs inhibit 5HT reuptake and block 5HT-1a auto-receptors, and thus, increase serotonin availability and release. They have minimal effects upon H1, alpha-adrenergic and muscarinic receptors with negligible effects on sodium channels and are thus relatively safe in case of an overdose. The major side-effects of SSRIs are nausea and gastrointestinal upset, early agitation, sexual dysfunction and an increased propensity for bleeding.

SNRIs inhibit the reuptake of both serotonin and noradrenaline (and dopamine at higher doses). They have minimal effects on H1, alpha-adrenergic and muscarinic receptors.

Noradrenergic and specific serotonergic antidepressants block alpha-2 adrenergic receptors, and thus, increase the release of both noradrenaline and serotonin. They also block alpha-1 adrenergic receptors, leading to orthostatic hypotension, and H1 receptors, leading to sedation and weight gain.

Noradrenaline reuptake inhibitors specifically block noradrenaline reuptake.

Serotonin antagonist and reuptake inhibitors increase serotonin and are often used for their sedative properties.

Noradrenaline and dopamine reuptake inhibitors block noradrenaline and dopamine reuptake, e.g. bupropion, which is also used to reduce cravings in smoking cessation.

Agomelatine is an antidepressant agent that antagonizes 5HT-2 receptors (enhances the release of noradrenaline and dopamine) and is an agonist at melatonergic receptors (M1 and M2).

Tricyclic antidepressants act principally by blocking the reuptake of both noradrenaline and serotonin (and dopamine). The relative balance of noradrenaline versus serotonin effect varies (e.g. clomipramine is principally serotonergic while nortriptyline is mainly noradrenergic). They have many other neurochemical effects that cause unwanted effects, for example:

Blockade of muscarinic cholinergic receptors potentially causing dry mouth, blurred vision, urinary retention, constipation and impaired attention.

Alpha-1 adrenergic antagonism potentially causing orthostatic hypotension and dizziness.

Histaminic-1 receptor blockade potentially causing sedation and weight gain.

Sodium channel blockade potentially causing cardiac arrhythmia and seizures.

Currently, they are not commonly used because of their side-effect profile.

Monoamine oxidase inhibitors are irreversible blockers of MAO-A, and thus, can cause the accumulation of amines (e.g. tyramine) with hypertensive effects. This requires careful dietary management to avoid certain foodstuffs (so-called 'wine and cheese' interaction) and has implications for drug interactions. They are reserved for atypical depressive illness. Examples include phenelzine and tranylcypromine. Moclobemide is a reversible monoamine oxidase inhibitor carrying a reduced risk of major food and drug interactions. However, patients should still be advised to avoid large quantities of tyramine rich foods and sympathomimetic drugs.

FURTHER READING

For a meta-analysis comparing antidepressant agents, see: Cipriani A, Furukawa TA, Salanti G, et al. (2019) Comparative efficacy and acceptability of 21 antidepressant drugs for the acute treatment of adults with major depressive disorder: a systematic review and network meta-analysis. The Lancet 391(10128):1357–1366. doi:10.1016/S0140-6736(17)32802-7

The use of agents as first- or second-line treatments is generally dictated by the severity of illness and propensity for side-effects. Although in clinical practice it is noted that agents with dual monoamine action (e.g. SNRIs) are more effective for more severe illness, the evidence from large studies (e.g. the STAR–D trial) and meta-analyses do not indicate major differences in their efficacy.

---

5. Anna commences venlafaxine 75 mg per day with a plan to escalate the dose over a week to 225 mg. After a month, she has improved somewhat, but still complains of low mood, anergia and low confidence. In particular, she continues to experience initial insomnia and believes that this is the cause of her low energy levels. She asks if she could be prescribed a 'sleeper' to overcome this problem.
  11. What is the impact of increasing doses of venlafaxine?
  12. How can depression-related insomnia be managed?

The dosage at which antidepressants have a therapeutic effect is a key consideration in treatment. The SSRIs can generally be commenced at dosages that have a therapeutic effect. However, for other agents, such as venlafaxine, duloxetine and the older antidepressants (e.g. tricyclic agents), there is a need to escalate dosages to minimize the propensity for adverse effects. Venlafaxine is an example where increasing effectiveness is linked to dose escalation. This has been explained in terms of neurochemical activity: at doses of 75 mg and 150 mg per day, the principal neurochemical effect is serotonergic, while at doses of 200 mg and over, the dual action is more evident with enhanced noradrenergic and serotonergic activity. With even higher doses, such as 300 mg and above, dopaminergic effects also occur.

Insomnia is a frequent problem in patients with depression and may involve any of a number of patterns, most commonly initial insomnia and early morning wakening, but also middle insomnia and, in some cases, hypersomnia. It is important to note that both the amount and quality of sleep are affected. Sleep problems improve as depression resolves, but short-term symptomatic management of insomnia is frequently required. It is worth noting that depression has been described as a sleep disorder such that restoring a healthy sleep pattern can be a key step in resolving overall symptoms of depression. Careful attention to sleep hygiene, emphasizing daytime exercise and avoiding stimulants (e.g. caffeine) can be helpful. In addition, many antidepressants are inherently sedative (e.g. mirtazapine, TCAs, agomelatine). However, where these are not preferred (e.g. risk of overdose with TCAs), it may be prudent to use a short-term course of a hypnotic agent (preferably one with less propensity for dependency and/or a 'hangover' effect) or an antipsychotic sedative agent (e.g. low dose quetiapine) if there are concerns about dependency potential.

---

6. Anna's psychiatrist increases the dose of venlafaxine to 300 mg per day and prescribes a short (two week) course of a hypnotic (zolpidem). Over the following month, her depressive symptoms settle, and she discontinues the hypnotic. At follow-up review, Anna is keen to discuss how long she will need to continue treatment, and whether she can decrease the dosage now that she is feeling better and how she can prevent a recurrence.
   13. How would you address her questions regarding how long she should continue treatment, and at what dosage?
   14. How does the risk of recurrence relate to the number of previous episodes?

Continuation pharmacotherapy for 6—12 months after the symptoms resolve is recommended for all patients with depression who respond to acute treatment with antidepressants. In addition, maintenance phase pharmacotherapy has demonstrated efficacy in preventing depressive recurrence for up to five years. The risk of further episodes with treatment discontinuation is predicted by the previous episode frequency with a relapse rate of 50% after one episode, 70% after two episodes, and 90% or more after three previous episodes. In general, studies suggest that maintenance treatment doses are similar to those that establish initial response ('the dose that gets you well keeps you well').

However, recurrent depressive disorder should be considered a dynamic state where the risk of further episodes is a function of the interaction of predisposing risk factors and exposure to precipitating environmental factors (e.g. major life events, loss experiences) (Fig. 3.2). Consequently, careful attention to baseline risk relating to lifestyle (exercise, diet, substance use), social and

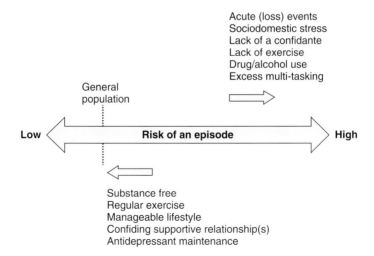

Fig. 3.2 A model of recurrent depressive illness showing the relationship between risk of recurrence and patient lifestyle.

relationship issues and other ongoing stresses allows for a greater sense of empowerment and ownership of illness. Depression can thus be conceptualized as a vulnerability towards depressive symptoms when exposed to stressful precipitants.

---

7. Anna discontinues medications after six months but re-presents a year later with symptoms of a severe depressive illness associated with marked biological disturbance, but without thoughts of self-harm or psychosis. She is commenced on venlafaxine, and the dose is increased up to 300 mg over the following 4–6 weeks. Unfortunately, however, this has a minimal effect on her symptoms.
    15.   What are the treatment options at this point?
    16.   What is the implication of this episode for maintenance treatment in the future?

Treatment-resistant depressive illness is defined as the failure to respond to two adequate trials of antidepressant therapy (or one antidepressant trial and electroconvulsive therapy). In such cases, it is important to review the diagnosis carefully to establish if depression is the primary issue. It is important to review the aetiological model for depression, focusing on possible perpetuating factors (e.g. substance use, physical illness, unresolved psychological or social factors). In addition, one should explore the patient's perspective of the treatment and likely adherence. Psychological interventions can be useful.

If a treatment-resistant depressive illness is the preferred diagnosis, then a range of possible therapeutic options are available. The sequence by which these options are used is generally determined by patient factors and the preferences and previous experiences of the treating team. There is little robust scientific evidence to favour one intervention over another, and a process of trial and error often follows. Options include the following:

1. Increasing to high dosage therapy
2. Changing antidepressant agent/class
3. Augmentation with a mood stabilizer, such as lithium
4. Electroconvulsive therapy
5. Combination antidepressant therapy (e.g. venlafaxine–mirtazapine combination)
6. Augmentation with an antipsychotic, T3 or psychological therapies
7. Use of an MAOI (especially if atypical features, such as hypersomnia, hyperphagia or reversed diurnal mood variation, are present)
8. Light therapy (especially if the illness follows a seasonal pattern)

FURTHER READING

For a systematic review of the impact of antidepressant maintenance therapy, see:
Machmutow K, Meister R, Jansen A, et al. (2019) Comparative effectiveness of continuation and maintenance treatments for persistent depressive disorder in adults. Cochrane Database of Systematic Reviews 5:CD012855. doi:10.1002/14651858.CD012855.pub2

This second episode, with severe illness and treatment resistance, emphasizes the need for sustained treatment when her symptoms ultimately resolve. It is estimated that continued antidepressant therapy reduces the odds of relapse by 70%, but the optimal duration of such treatment remains unclear.

Laura

Posttraumatic Stress Disorder

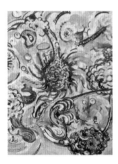

1. Describe the key clinical diagnostic features of posttraumatic stress disorder (PTSD), including differential diagnoses, common comorbid mental and physical disorders.
2. Briefly describe the epidemiology of PTSD, including its incidence, prevalence and gender differences.
3. Describe the key potential aetiological factors in PTSD and classify these in terms of medical/biological, social and psychological factors.
4. Describe the assessment of a suspected case of PTSD, beginning with a detailed history, mental state examination and collateral history, and appropriate biological investigations.
5. Describe the main treatments for PTSD and consider these in terms of medical/biological, social and psychological approaches.
6. Briefly describe the key prognostic factors for PTSD and compare its prognosis with other major mental health disorders.

1. Laura, a 22-year-old physical education student with no prior psychiatric history, is referred by a doctor at the university student health centre. She presented in a distressed state having failed her second-year summer examinations, and notably, did not turn up for two oral examinations. Previously, she has been a very focused student who achieved honours marks in her first-year examinations, but of late, admits to poor attendance at classes, social withdrawal and increased alcohol intake. She complains of a low mood, aggravated by persistent tension and anxiety punctuated by episodes of panic and upsetting nightmares.
   1. How would you summarize the main elements of this presentation?
   2. What additional information will you seek during the consultation?

The key elements to consider in this history are that there has been a recent change in Laura's behaviour in the context of her reporting significant and disabling psychological distress that includes a disturbed mood and associated anxiety symptoms. The presence of nightmares is a significant clue as to a possible cause of her symptoms as it is a more specific symptom. The role of substance use needs to be explored as this may be a primary contributing factor, a secondary maladaptive response, or both.

Key immediate information that should be explored includes clarifying when these problems first started and any possible precipitating factors at that time. This may need to be probed for gently, initially allowing Laura to volunteer information, but with more specific prompts, if needed.

The specific reasons underlying the change in her usual behavioural pattern need to be explored, as these may represent a general disinterest and withdrawal or a specific avoidance strategy.

A key element of the assessment will be to explore the character of psychological disturbances with a focus on assessing the extent (range and severity) of anxiety and depressive symptoms.

The assessment of anxiety symptoms includes the following:
- Characterizing the range of psychological and somatic symptoms evident.
- Clarifying the pattern of symptoms (generalized and persistent versus more discrete severe episodic).
- Exploring the relationship between anxiety and specific stressors.
- Exploring for specific symptoms, e.g. depersonalization/derealization, nightmares, intrusive thoughts and recollections, flashbacks, obsessional ruminations, compulsive behaviours, dissociative episodes.
- Determining the extent of avoidance and maladaptive behaviours, e.g. self-medication.

---

2. Laura confides that she was 'raped' while returning from an evening swimming session four months previously. She felt too humiliated and ashamed to tell anybody as she hoped that 'it would all just go away, and I could forget about it'. However, since then, she has been having recurring thoughts about the rape, including experiences where she has felt like she is reliving the experience all over again. She also reports nightmares ('a few times most nights'). She has been avoiding situations that involve mixing with others, especially men, and she has lost interest in and been unable to maintain her studies. She feels unable to cope and is constantly afraid of being overpowered or made to feel helpless again. She is irritable in social interactions and reports 'exploding' at the college administrator who asked her to provide a time to meet with her supervisor to discuss her performance in the examinations.

3. What are these symptoms, and what do they suggest?
4. What distinguishes posttraumatic stress disorder from other mental health disorders?
5. How should you probe for posttraumatic stress disorder symptoms during a patient consultation?
6. What is the broader differential diagnosis?

Laura has described significant psychological symptoms occurring after a serious traumatic event. These are referred to as 're-experiencing phenomena'. The recurring thoughts are termed 'intrusive recollections', while the reliving experiences during wakefulness are often called flashbacks or 'daymares'. She also reports avoidance behaviours and loss of normal interests with diminished stress tolerance, irritability and anger outbursts. This constellation of symptoms is indicative of posttraumatic stress disorder (PTSD) both in its context (acute trauma) and character of symptoms (Box 4.1).

> **BOX 4.1 ■ Diagnosis of PTSD**
>
> 1. Exposure to a stressor that is perceived as threatening to the integrity of the person (e.g. life-threatening or associated with a serious injury or sexual/physical violence). The experience typically involves a sense of helplessness or loss of control for the person.
> 2. Re-experiencing phenomena that are linked to the traumatic experience, including the following: intrusive recollections, marked anxiety when exposed to psychologically significant triggers, nightmares, flashbacks or other dissociative episodes.
> 3. Avoidance behaviours that relate to people, places, conversations, activities, objects, situations that may provoke thoughts, memories or feelings of the incident.
> 4. Negative symptoms that may include: memory loss of the incident, reduced interest in everyday life, feelings of estrangement, persistent negative emotional state (that can include fear, guilt, anger or shame), exaggerated negative beliefs or expectations (e.g. 'I can never be safe' or 'bad things are inevitable') and reduced capacity to emotionally engage with positive experiences.
> 5. Marked alterations in arousal and reactivity associated with the traumatic experience that can include hypervigilance with exaggerated startle reflexes, hyperreactivity to negative experiences, outbursts that can include verbal or physical aggression and reckless or self-destructive behaviour.
> 6. These difficulties are persistent and temporally related to the traumatic incident, causing significant distress and/or impairment in social, interpersonal and occupational activities.
> 7. Symptoms are not better explained by substance use, medical illness or another functional psychiatric disorder (e.g. panic disorder or psychosis).

PTSD occurs in response to a traumatic event that is exceptionally threatening or catastrophic, and that would cause severe distress to almost anyone. Typical events include combat-related trauma, sexual or physical assault, accidents and disasters. Less restrictive descriptions focus upon the response of the sufferer whereby the event is particularly stressful for that person at that time. The person may be a victim or a witness to the event. A recurring theme among sufferers of PTSD is that the incident involved a sense of helplessness with a loss of control over events.

In the assessment of this presentation, it is important to not only clarify the presence of PTSD but also explore other conditions as possible differential or comorbid diagnoses. The traumatic nature of the event is consistent with PTSD, while phobic disorders tend to be associated with stressors that are perceived as threatening by the sufferer but would not be considered so by most people. Panic episodes share the physiological arousal that can occur with re-experiencing phenomena of PTSD but tend to lack a specific previous traumatic experience. Sometimes, the re-experiencing phenomena of PTSD can be difficult to distinguish from psychotic features (e.g. distinguishing between flashbacks and visual hallucinations). However, in general, people with PTSD retain insight into the nature of flashbacks and intrusive recollections and recognize that they are abnormal events that are not based upon current reality. In addition, the clinical features of PTSD typically relate quite specifically back to the traumatic incident. Moreover, the presence of depressive features, such as a sustained lowering of mood with distorted cognition, disturbed biological function and possible thoughts of self-harm, need to be carefully assessed for as depressive illness is a key differential diagnosis of PTSD (Fig. 4.1).

Diagnostic and Statistical Manual of Mental Disorders (DSM)-5 requires that symptoms be present for at least one month for a diagnosis of full PTSD to be made. The International Classification of Diseases (ICD)-10 mandates that symptoms should usually appear within six months of the event. However, the onset of symptoms is delayed in approximately 10% of cases, sometimes for many years, only to be awakened by a symbolic event often at a time of psychological vulnerability.

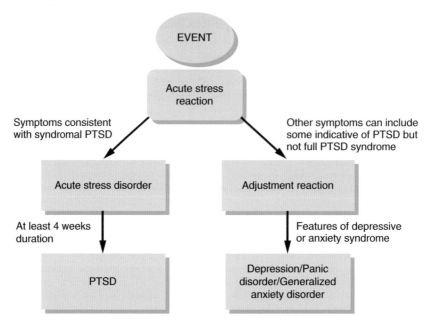

Fig. 4.1 Differential diagnosis of psychological disturbances occurring after an acute stressful event

---

3. Laura finds the consultation stressful, especially when recounting the actual rape experience, but feels relieved that she is addressing her problems. You explain to her that she is in control of the consultation and that she can stop or take a break at any point if she feels that she is becoming upset or overwhelmed. She feels less helpless and is keen to learn about the range of available treatment options. She agrees to stop drinking as this makes her feel more anxious the following day. She prefers to explore nondrug related options in the first instance because her mother was a 'Valium addict' and she is afraid that she might get 'hooked on pills'.

  7. How common is posttraumatic stress disorder?
  8. Why do certain people develop posttraumatic stress disorder in response to stressors while others do not?
  9. What investigations are indicated?
  10. What are the treatment options for posttraumatic stress disorder, and how should treatment be sequenced?

Most humans experience at least one stressor serious enough to precipitate PTSD during their lifetime, but only a minority develop full syndromal PTSD. The frequency of PTSD is closely related to the frequency of exposure to precipitating traumatic events, but lifetime prevalence is estimated at approximately 8% of the general population, with a 1%–3% 12-month prevalence.

PTSD occurs twice as frequently in females due to the combined effect of a higher frequency of exposure to traumatic events and greater susceptibility to develop PTSD in response to such exposures. Other factors associated with an elevated risk of developing PTSD include the severity of the trauma (duration, perceived threat, loss of integrity or helplessness), dissociative experiences around the event, poor social support, lower socioeconomic status, lower educational attainment, being from an ethnic minority, prolonged litigation and premorbid vulnerability because of previous psychological difficulties and a history of mental illness. Comorbid affective, anxiety and substance misuse problems are extremely common, and are prevalent in more than half of cases. They appear to be secondary in most cases, for example, as maladaptive coping or reactive features.

FURTHER READING

For a clinical review of posttraumatic stress disorder, see: Bisson JI, Cosgrove S, Catrin L, Roberts NP. (2015) Posttraumatic stress disorder. British Medical Journal 351:h6161. doi:10.1136/bmj.h6161

Although Laura's presentation indicates a psychological disturbance in response to an identifiable and discrete stressful event, all patients with anxiety symptoms should be investigated for other possible contributing factors, including physical or 'organic' factors.

More common factors include evidence of medication or substance use (steroids, stimulants such as caffeine and diet pills, thyroid dysfunction and disturbed glucose metabolism), and substances of abuse (both through acute intoxication and withdrawal effects). Less common possibilities include hormonal causes, such as stress axis disturbance (e.g. Cushing's disease) and pheochromocytoma. A typical workup includes a detailed history of medication and substance use along with a full blood count, urea and electrolytes, liver function tests, thyroid function and fasting blood glucose.

The treatment of PTSD involves a combination of: (1) supportive measures aimed at managing symptoms, for example, anxiety management strategies, and advice regarding any practical problems that have emerged (e.g. reporting the incident to police, dealing with college procedures), any substance use issues; (2) specific psychological interventions (e.g. trauma-focused psychotherapy) to address the symptoms of PTSD; and (3) pharmacological interventions (which are often considered as second-line interventions).

Psychological therapies that have a trauma focus, such as eye movement desensitization and reprocessing or trauma-focused cognitive behavioural therapy, are especially effective and associated with symptom resolution in two-thirds of recipients. These therapies involve addressing the psychological impact of the experience, including challenging aberrant beliefs regarding the ongoing threat and feelings of guilt or shame. Controlled re-exposure to trauma-related experiences can assist in alleviating feelings of helplessness or loss of integrity without being overwhelmed. In some cases, the patient's recollection of events is impaired such that re-experiencing the event can facilitate the processing of the experience.

Pharmacological therapies can also assist in recovery. The use of antidepressant agents, especially serotonin specific reuptake inhibitors, is supported by meta-analyses. Variable evidence exists for other agents such as clonidine and various antipsychotic agents. Benzodiazepines are best avoided as they can aggravate problems with impulse control or dissociation and have the potential for dependency.

FURTHER READING

For more information on treatment strategies for posttraumatic stress disorder, see: Lee DJ, Schnitzlein CW, Wolf JP, et al. (2016) Psychotherapy versus pharmacotherapy for posttraumatic stress disorder: systemic review and meta-analyses to determine first-line treatments. Depress Anxiety 33(9):792–806. doi:10.1002/da.22511

In establishing a coherent treatment plan, it is important to recognize that the timing of different interventions is important (e.g. initial interactions are often predominantly supportive to allow for symptom control and establishment of a sound base for a functional therapeutic relationship) and that treatments can act synergistically (e.g. pharmacological control of symptoms can facilitate psychological interventions). Patients must have a sense of control over treatment choices as the helplessness and loss of control around the traumatic incident is often a prominent theme, and many patients have a sense of resentment at having to seek treatment for something that they did not cause.

---

4. Over the next two months, Laura attends anxiety management sessions and engages with the clinical psychologist for trauma-focused cognitive behavioural therapy. During this time, she reveals that she was sexually abused as a child (over two years, aged 9–11) by an elderly neighbour. She indicates that she has been having recollections and nightmares of this incident along with the more recent rape. The alleged abuser has now died, and she does not want to progress the matter from a legal perspective. She continues to experience intrusive recollections, flashbacks and nightmares, albeit less frequently and at a severity that is less distressing. She remains hypervigilant in social settings and avoidant of social interactions. She reports being especially upset when watching a television soap that featured a sexual assault. She wants to continue to attend the psychological therapy sessions, but now also wishes to consider pharmacological treatments as she has deferred her repeat examinations but has returned to college and is finding it hard to keep up with the demands of her course.

11. What is the postulated mechanism of posttraumatic stress disorder?
12. What advice would you give her regarding combination treatment?

PTSD occupies a particularly interesting position at the psychological–biological interface, whereby environmental stressors are thought to induce acute and chronic changes in brain function and behaviour. The symptoms of PTSD are thought to reflect disturbance of interactions between the thalamus (a sensory gateway), hippocampus (short-term memory processing), amygdala (fear responses) and the medial prefrontal cortex (modulates subcortical responses).

Cognitive theories of PTSD postulate that symptoms occur because of classical conditioning whereby psychologically symbolic events trigger a fear response similar to the original stimulus. Avoidance and emotional numbing are responses produced by operant conditioning that reduce likely exposure to future stress. Other theories suggest that people with PTSD have excessively negative appraisals of the event and its implications for future threat and personal integrity as evidenced by beliefs that there is an ongoing threat or that they were in some way responsible for the events that occurred.

Studies of people with chronic PTSD indicate smaller hippocampal volume, reduced hippocampal N-acetylaspartate activity (a marker of neuronal integrity) and decreased hippocampal activation in response to memory tasks. Studies in children and adults with new-onset PTSD have not shown decreased hippocampal volume, suggesting that these changes occur in response to chronic PTSD rather than reflect a biological vulnerability to developing the condition.

FURTHER READING

For a more detailed discussion of the neurobiology of posttraumatic stress disorder, see:
Sherin JE, Nemeroff CB. (2011) Post-traumatic stress disorder: the neurobiological impact of psychological trauma. Dialogues in Clinical Neuroscience 13(3):263–278.

Noradrenergic systems are dysregulated with elevated levels of catecholamines in patients with PTSD. Other work has focused on the stress axis. This has indicated enhanced negative feedback on the HPA-axis with decreased cortisol levels in chronic cases and an opposite dexamethasone suppression test response than major depression, with hypersuppression of cortisol in response to dexamethasone administration. These disturbances have been postulated to occur because of overactivation of the stress axis during traumatic events, with reduced hippocampal volumes linked to exposure to high levels of glucocorticoids.

Paroxetine can reverse many of these pathophysiological changes with some evidence that successful treatment is associated with increased hippocampal volume. Other mechanisms for the therapeutic effect of antidepressant agents are mediated by anxiolytic or antidepressant effects which provide symptom control that allows for adaptation to the experience and/or engagement with psychological treatments.

The relative effectiveness of combined psychological and pharmacological therapy versus either treatment alone is poorly studied. However, good clinical sense dictates that the targeted use of pharmacological interventions can assist the overall therapeutic process and may facilitate engagement with psychological therapies.

---

5. Laura commences on paroxetine and continues the sessions with the psychologist (now extended to monthly appointments). Her original symptoms gradually diminish, and she does well in her end of term tests at Christmas. However, she is contacted by the local police who have detained a suspect for the alleged rape incident and have asked if she is willing to give evidence.

    13.   What advice would you give regarding her participation in the legal proceedings?

Involvement in legal proceedings relating to PTSD (either criminal or compensation-based) can sometimes result in symptoms being prolonged, while for others it can assist in their recovery by allowing closure. The stress of impending court appearances and other court-related activities can be unhelpful, while the process can also be re-traumatizing and trigger re-experiencing phenomena. Therefore, decisions regarding participation in such activities need to be highly individualized. However, clinicians have a reporting obligation if the alleged perpetrators of sexual assaults may still pose a risk to others. Prolonged litigation is a recognized, poor prognostic factor. These issues need to be explored with Laura to assist her in deciding what is best for her recovery.

---

6. Six months later, you meet Laura for a routine outpatient review. She decided to decline participation in the legal case as she felt that it would adversely affect her progress, and she felt that it was better to put the incident behind her and focus on her studies. She now has a boyfriend and is worried as to how her experiences might impact upon the physical aspect of the relationship. She only occasionally experiences nightmares and recollections, and the flashbacks have now ceased. However, she reports a sense of emotional detachment from some aspects of life. She lacks motivation and feels that she has not recovered her previous levels of interest in life.

    14.   What are the possible causes for her continued difficulties?

    15.   How would you assess her prognosis?

Laura's ongoing difficulties include a constellation of symptoms that may reflect persisting PTSD with prominent features from the C and D cluster as described in DSM-5 (see above). These are sometimes referred to as the 'negative symptoms' of PTSD and include a sense of emotional numbing with feelings of estrangement and disconnectedness from everyday life, often with reduced enjoyment.

Depressive illness is a possible differential diagnosis, and distinction of these states requires careful assessment for other features of major depressive illness. If the latter is the favoured diagnosis, then an altered dosage or switching antidepressant agent (e.g. to a dual-acting compound) is recommended. The optimal management of chronic PTSD is unclear, but it is important to note that therapeutic gains can occur with psychological and pharmacological interventions long after the initial traumatic event. Moreover, a review of treatment history can reveal new approaches.

Many people who develop symptoms of PTSD will recover spontaneously over time. Rates of probable PTSD in Manhattan, New York, after the 9/11 bombings reduced from 7.5% after one month to 1.6% after four months and 0.6% after six months. Other studies suggests that 30%−50% of those who experience trauma will experience more persistent illness. In Laura's case, the prognosis can be assessed after the consideration of factors associated with more prolonged difficulties, engagement with treatment, ongoing support mechanisms and socio-adaptive functioning.

The prognosis of PTSD is related to a range of factors that reflect the personal characteristics of the victim (prior traumatic experiences, inherent resilience, robustness of the premorbid personality, social capital and exposure to further stresses) and the severity of the incident. Notably, child abuse and neglect are recognized risk factors for the development of adult personality disorders, affective disorders, substance abuse and medical problems.

Jane

Alcohol Use Disorders

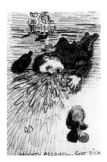

1. Discuss typical presentations of substance use disorders in general medical and psychiatric clinical settings.
2. Obtain a thorough substance use history using empathic, non-judgemental interviewing techniques.
3. Determine past and recent abuse (amount and frequency), features indicating dependence, withdrawal symptoms, complications, past treatment history, readiness to change, support network and socio-forensic issues.
4. Understand the role of screening questionnaires (e.g. CAGE) and physical and laboratory investigations (e.g. toxicology, liver function test).
5. Recognize the clinical features of alcohol intoxication.
6. Determine the need for emergency care because of substance intoxication or withdrawal.
7. Recognize the clinical signs and recommend management strategies for substance withdrawal from sedative-hypnotics, including alcohol and benzodiazepines.
8. Understand the epidemiology, course of illness, and the medical and psychosocial complications of common substance use disorders.
9. Discuss management strategies for substance abuse and dependence, including detoxification, 12-step programmes, support groups, pharmacotherapy, rehabilitation programmes, psychotherapies and family support.

1. Dr Crowley is the new general practitioner (GP) in Ballybeg. Martin Doherty, a local businessman, invites Dr Crowley to a dinner party at his house. The party is well attended by local business people and professionals, and everyone has an enjoyable evening. Dr Crowley notices that Martin's wife, Jane, drinks heavily throughout the party and ends up singing loudly and embarrassing her husband towards

Continued on following page

(Continued)

the end of the evening. Some of the locals brush this off by saying that she is 'great craic'. A week later, Jane visits Dr Crowley to renew her oral contraceptive pill prescription. She is 38-years-old and has three children, aged twelve, eight and six. Dr Crowley checks her blood pressure and finds it to be mildly elevated. He also notices that she has a faint smell of alcohol from her breath. 'We were partying again last night Doc, so the blood pressure could be up a bit today'.

1. Define the criteria for alcohol use disorders.
2. Outline the assessment approach in an individual with suspected alcohol use disorders.
3. What are the main screening tools for alcohol use disorders used in everyday clinical practice?
4. What is the prevalence of alcohol use disorders?

Criteria for diagnosis of alcohol use disorders (AUDs)

FURTHER READING

For a useful overview, see: Carvalho AF, Heilig M, Perez A, et al. (2019) Alcohol use disorders. Lancet 394(10200):781−792. doi:10.1016/S01406736(19)31775-1.

Harmful use of psychoactive substances involves a pattern that is causing damage to physical or mental health or social function (e.g. hepatitis or episodes of depressive illness secondary to heavy consumption or marital breakdown). Dependence syndrome describes a combination of physiological, behavioural and cognitive strata, which dominate other behaviours that hitherto had greater priority. In the Diagnostic and Statistical Manual of Mental Disorders (DSM)-5, there is a single category called AUDs, which is further divided into mild, moderate and severe. This reflects the perception of AUDs as a single continuum that typically escalate over time (Box 5.1).

Screening tools

The use of screening tools can improve the identification of AUDs. The CAGE, Michigan Alcohol Screening Test (MAST) and Alcohol Use Disorders Identification Test (AUDIT) are commonly used screening tools that can be readily completed in most clinical settings.

BOX 5.1 ■ Alcohol use disorders are diagnosed according to the following:

1. Excessive intake of alcohol
2. A strong desire to consume alcohol (craving)
3. Inability to control alcohol intake, even with the efforts to do so
4. Excessive time spent around alcohol use, both in terms of consumption and recovery from its effects
5. Interference with social or occupational functioning, with evidence of increasing primacy of alcohol over other activities
6. Continued use despite adverse effects that may be social, psychological or physical
7. Evidence of physical addiction with increasing tolerance to acute effects
8. Evidence of physical addiction with symptoms of withdrawal upon cessation of use

The severity of alcohol use disorder is graded as mild, moderate or severe according to the number of the above features that are evident.

CAGE: More than two positive responses suggest possible at-risk drinking and indicates the need for further assessment:

1. Have you ever felt the need to **C**ut down on your alcohol consumption?
2. Have you felt **A**nnoyed when criticized about your alcohol use?
3. Have you felt **G**uilty about your drinking?
4. Have you ever had a drink first thing in the day, to steady your nerves or get rid of a hangover? (**E**ye-opener)

MAST

In this 25-item screening test, five to six positive answers indicate a possible AUD with seven or more positive answers indicating a probable AUD.

AUDIT (World Health Organization, 2nd edition)

The AUDIT is a ten-question self-report survey developed by the World Health Organization to screen patients for possible AUDs. A score of eight or more identifies both heavy drinkers and those with AUDs. A score of 20 or more warrants further diagnostic evaluation for alcohol dependence syndrome (ICD-10).

Assessment approach

A detailed psychiatric history should focus on areas where alcohol is adversely affecting daily life in terms of social, occupational or recreational activities and functioning. 'Primacy' is a concept that is central to AUDs, whereby consumption of alcohol takes precedence over all other priorities and activities. A collateral history may be particularly revealing (see Box 5.2). In addition, emphasis should be given to assessing evidence of mood disorders, and where present, establish the relationship to alcohol use to assess whether it is primary or secondary. Alcohol is a well-recognized depressant that is also commonly associated with post-alcohol dysphoria after significant consumption. Most mood disturbances that occur in the context of excessive alcohol consumption resolve with successful discontinuation of alcohol use. However, it should also be noted that alcohol misuse is common as a significant comorbid issue in all major psychiatric disorders.

BOX 5.2 ■ Questions relating to features of alcohol use disorder

1. Have you had recurrent problems or failed to fulfil your role in your work or personal life because of your drinking?
2. Have you ever been in trouble with the law because of your drinking?
3. Have you repeatedly driven a car or a machine under the influence of alcohol?
4. Have you found that you need to drink more (or less) to get the same effect as before (indicating changes in tolerance)?
5. Have you ever had a drink to help deal with a hangover or withdrawal symptoms (e.g. 'the shakes?')
6. Have you ever experienced severe alcohol withdrawals, seizures or the delirium tremens (DTs)?
7. Do you ever have difficulty stopping drinking once started?
8. Do you have episodes of absent memory related to drinking ('blackouts')?
9. Have you experienced physical health problems because of your drinking, such as stomach or liver problems or accidents, falls or fractures?
10. Do you want to stop drinking (establishing readiness for change)?
11. Have you had previous treatment or rehabilitation?
12. Are you taking other prescribed or illicit drugs?

TABLE 5.1 ■ Clinical Features Associated with Alcohol Use Disorders

System	Examine for:
General appearance	Tremor, alcohol foetor, facial capillarization, obesity or malnutrition
Cardiac	Hypertension, cardiac arrhythmias, cardiomyopathy
Endocrine	Pseudo Cushing's syndrome
Respiratory	Chest infection
Hepatic	Hepatomegaly (or small cirrhotic liver in chronic/severe AUDs, jaundice, spider naevi, ascites)
Gastrointestinal	Abdominal tenderness, melaena
Central nervous system	Ataxia, delirium, coma
Peripheral nervous system	Neuropathy
Musculoskeletal	Myopathy

AUDs, alcohol use disorders

A mental state examination should be performed, exploring for evidence of acute intoxication, withdrawal features, affective disorder, anxiety issues, psychotic symptoms and cognitive impairment.

A focused physical examination should be performed, looking for signs of acute intoxication, withdrawal and features suggestive of longer-term alcohol misuse, including neurological problems, hepatic impairment/failure and physical stigmata (see Table 5.1).

The following blood investigations are helpful:
- Full blood count (looking for macrocytic anaemia)
- Liver function test (looking for raised gamma-glutamyl transferase (GGT) and other liver enzyme abnormalities, such as raised aspartate transaminase and alanine aminotransferase)
1. Urea and electrolytes
   - Blood glucose
   - Carbohydrate Deficient Transferrin (CDT).

CDT is also a useful test to identify heavy alcohol use. Healthy individuals with low reported alcohol consumption and a negative AUDIT will typically have a CDT% <1.7% (95th percentile for the social drinking population). Elevated levels of CDT suggest recent alcohol abuse, especially if other liver-associated enzymes (such as GGT) are elevated. Certain rare liver disorders can also increase CDT levels. Elevated GGT is a good indicator of recent alcohol misuse, while other liver enzyme abnormalities and raised mean corpuscular volume may be indicative of a longer-term pattern of misuse.

Prevalence

The prevalence of AUDs varies depending on the strictness of the diagnostic criteria used and the population being studied. Higher levels are seen in certain cultures, such as northern and Western Europe, where alcohol use is ubiquitous, whereas AUDs are uncommon in many Islamic countries where alcohol use is largely prohibited on religious and cultural grounds. High national per capita alcohol consumption is linked with adverse health outcomes, such as a high number of hepatic cirrhosis cases per year. Drinking styles may also be relevant, for example, in Ireland and the United Kingdom, there is a more harmful binge drinking culture that contrasts with the more moderate 'café style' consumption in Mediterranean countries.

In Ireland, it is estimated that more than 150,000 people are dependent drinkers, more than 1.35 million are harmful drinkers and 30% of people interviewed say that they have experienced some form of harm because of their drinking. The report also revealed that 75% of alcohol consumed in Ireland is done so as part of binge drinking and that people underestimate their own intake by about 60%.

Furthermore, 58% of the population in the United Kingdom reported drinking alcohol in the previous week. Almost 1 in 5 (18%) of higher earners drink alcohol at least five days a week. In detail, 77% of those earning over £40,000 drank alcohol in the last week compared with 46% of those earning up to £9999. In 2015, 1.4% of all deaths in the United Kingdom were alcohol-related, representing a 13% increase from 2004. Alcoholic liver disease accounted for nearly two-thirds of all alcohol-related deaths.

Prevalence of lifetime and 12-month alcohol abuse in the United States have been reported as 18% and 5%, respectively.

---

2. Dr Crowley takes a detailed history of Jane's alcohol use. She is initially reluctant to give details but volunteers that she drinks 2–3 bottles of red wine during a 'normal' week and that she can have an additional 5–6 glasses of wine along with 'a few' vodkas when they are 'entertaining'. *'But sure, I wouldn't worry about that. The last GP here before you used to drink us all under the table. Did you ever meet Dr Kelly? God, he was great fun. But he did go a bit overboard. I think there was trouble with the Medical Council. His files were a bit of a mess. He really was a great GP though. He never worried about my drinking'.* Dr Crowley then performs a physical examination after obtaining her consent and with his practice nurse present. He finishes by taking some blood tests.

  5. How would you go about taking a comprehensive history of alcohol use?
  6. How is a unit of alcohol defined, and what are the recommended 'safe limits' of alcohol consumption?
  7. Describe an approach to dealing with alcohol use disorders in the workplace and a medical colleague.
  8. How does alcohol exert its effects at a neurotransmitter level?

The history should focus on onset, quantity and pattern of alcohol intake. If problems are evident, then the history should proceed to include questions about AUDs. It is vital to also ask about other substance use, such as prescribed and illicit drugs, and the level of engagement with and response to previous treatments, if relevant.

Suggested questions are as follows, and an empathic and non-judgemental approach should always be used.

Questions relating to lifelong alcohol use

  1. When did you first start drinking regularly?
  2. When, if ever, did you think you had an alcohol problem?
  3. What has been your pattern of drinking throughout your life until the present?
  4. What are the most common alcoholic beverages you consume and how much (of each)?
  5. Describe your current daily and weekly drinking (establish the number of units per week).
  6. Has someone close to you (e.g. spouse, family or friends) ever expressed concern at your drinking?

Safe limits and alcohol units

Alcohol is the most used mood-altering substance in Western society, used by 90% of the population. It is rapidly absorbed with peak levels being reached 30–60 minutes after ingestion. It is estimated that one-third of the population in the United Kingdom consume more alcohol than the recommended safe limits. Alcohol intake can be conveniently measured by units, with one unit (8 g) of alcohol being metabolized by the body per hour. A binge is defined as consuming over six units in one sitting. At time of writing, the Health Service Executive (HSE, Ireland) recommends safe levels of alcohol intake are no more that 17 standard drinks or units per week for men and no more than 11 for women.

Clinical findings

Regular use of alcohol above the recommended safe limits can have a detrimental effect on every physiological system. These effects are more pronounced in females and with advancing age.

Gastrointestinal: Gastritis/gastric erosions, haematemesis, oesophagitis, Barrett's oesophagus (metaplasia of the lower third of the oesophagus), Mallory—Weiss oesophageal tears because of vomiting, peptic ulceration, chronic diarrhoea, chronic pancreatitis with chronic fluctuating abdominal pain and steatorrhoea, portal hypertension.

Cardiovascular: Hypertension, cardiac arrhythmias (atrial fibrillation and ventricular extra-systoles), dilated cardiomyopathy, cerebrovascular accident.

Metabolic: Hypoglycaemia, ketoacidosis, hyperuricaemia, hypertriglyceridemia, hypomagnesaemia.

Haematological: Anaemia (B12, folate deficiency), thrombocytopenia, disordered clotting.

Endocrine: Hypercortisolaemia, hypogonadism, infertility, impotence.

Alcohol-related liver disease: fatty change, alcoholic hepatitis and cirrhosis, hepatic encephalopathy, haemochromatosis (in the genetically vulnerable). Fatty change can occur after a single episode of heavy drinking and can be asymptomatic. Such change can be reversed with abstinence. It may present with lethargy and a painful swollen liver. Alcoholic hepatitis and cirrhosis occur in over 30% of heavy drinkers after 10—30 years.

Respiratory: Bronchiectasis, atypical pneumonia (*Klebsiella, Streptococcal*), tuberculosis. Up to 80% of alcohol-dependent people are regular smokers.

Neurological: Mild anterograde amnesia (blackouts) are common, Wernicke—Korsakoff syndrome (severe anterograde amnesia in fewer than 1% of those with alcohol dependence syndrome), peripheral neuropathy, central pontine myelinolysis, cerebellar degeneration, optic atrophy, alcoholic myopathy/polyneuropathy.

Bone and musculoskeletal: Decrease in bone density, increase in falls, vulnerability to bone fractures, gout, osteoporosis, avascular necrosis, proximal myopathy, Dupuytren contracture.

Dermatological: Spider naevi, palmer erythema, acne rosacea, discoid eczema.

AUDs are associated with a four-fold increase in premature mortality. The most common causes are heart disease, stroke and cancers (hepatocellular, oesophagus, stomach, mouth, tongue and pharynx, rectum and breast). The risk of suicide, accidents and liver cirrhosis also increase the risk of premature death.

Dealing with AUDs in the workplace

Several behaviours regarding job performance indicate a high likelihood that an employee has problematic alcohol or drug use, such as a pattern of poor-quality work, workplace accidents, attendance problems (classically Monday morning absenteeism) and problems related to interaction with clients, customers and colleagues. Employees, even doctors, may need education on recognizing the signs and symptoms of AUDs. Education campaigns should include information on alcohol and substance misuse and specific information on obtaining confidential counselling. Additionally, support can be provided through programmes such as Alcoholics Anonymous or Al-Anon and the availability of counselling, diagnosis and treatment services. Worksite health promotion programmes (often called 'employee assistance programmes' that include access to free counselling), such as physical activity or nutrition programmes, can reduce alcohol and drug misuse as encouraging healthy behaviours is an appropriate adjunct to standard therapies for alcohol and substance use disorders.

Dealing with a medical colleague who may have an AUD requires sensitive handling. Guidelines are available from the Irish Medical Council's website.

Doctors are subject to the same illnesses as their patients. Most doctors who suffer from an illness will recognize that they have an illness, seek treatment and comply with the appropriate treatments and recommendations. This may include taking time off work or indeed changing the nature of their work, either temporarily or permanently. Doctors with health problems may recover with the appropriate treatment and where necessary, with the involvement of the relevant regulatory authority. Therefore, most doctors with health problems will not need to have any involvement with the Medical Council or its Health Subcommittee. Unfortunately, some ill doctors will lack such insights, because of denial, or delay seeking treatment for some other reason. In such cases, their illness may impair their practice and pose a potential risk to patients. It is this latter group of doctors who should be reported or referred to the Medical Council on the grounds of patient safety (Irish Medical Council).

Effects of alcohol at the neurotransmitter level

Alcohol has euphoriant, anxiolytic, sedative and disinhibiting effects and impairs judgement and cognition. It releases dopamine from the nucleus accumbens within the limbic ventral tegmental area dopamine (VTA—DA) system. It also works on serotonin pathways involved in priming and reinforcing effects. Besides, alcohol also promotes the release of endogenous opioids, contributing to its euphoriant effects.

The effects of alcohol are primarily mediated through glutamate and γ-aminobutyric acid (GABA) receptor-gated channels to which alcohol binds directly. Alcohol acts as an agonist at neuroinhibitory GABA receptors and an antagonist at glutamate receptors. Over time, this leads to downregulation of GABA receptors and upregulation in N-methyl-D-aspartate (NMDA)/glutamate receptors. The acute potentiation of the inhibitory neurotransmitter GABA at GABA-A and taurine account for the anxiolytic effects of alcohol. Alcohol inhibits the excitatory neurotransmitters glutamate and aspartate. The action of alcohol on the NMDA glutamate receptor is thought to contribute to intoxication and impaired cognition. Upregulation of NMDA receptors is seen with chronic alcohol use. Increased glutamate release accounts for the excitotoxic effects on acute withdrawal from alcohol. Alcohol, via L-type $Ca2+$ and G-coupled $K+$ channels, activate 5HT3 receptors resulting in an increased release of dopamine and glutamate. Alcohol cessation leads to unopposed glutamate neuroexcitation. Benzodiazepines ameliorate the effect of withdrawal because of cross-tolerance with alcohol at the GABA-A receptors.

Approximately 2%—10% of consumed alcohol is excreted through the lungs, urine and sweat, and the remaining alcohol is broken down by alcohol dehydrogenase to acetaldehyde, with most metabolism occurring in the liver.

In 50% of Asian people, an inactive genetic variant of *ALDH2* is expressed, and these individuals exhibit a 'flushing' reaction with alcohol consumption, because of an impaired ability to metabolize acetaldehyde (see Fig. 5.1).

3. A week later, Dr Crowley asked Jane to come back to his clinic. 'Your blood tests suggest that alcohol is taking its toll on your body. You need to see a counsellor. I know a local lady who is very good. Here is her card'. Jane reluctantly attends the counsellor on a few occasions only. She is suspicious of the whole process and has no intention of cutting down her alcohol intake. At the third session, she breaks down in tears. *'How can I possibly hold dinner-parties and meet my husband's business associates and our neighbours when I'm sober? He's been having affairs up and down the country for years and I'm so ashamed that I have to be fortified with drink. It's all I've got to keep sane'*. The counsellor subsequently meets with Jane and Martin together. Martin admits to having affairs some years back but nothing recently. *'That's a bloody excuse for your drinking, Jane'*.
　9. Describe the aetiological factors in the development of alcohol use disorder.
　10. Describe the main treatments available for alcohol use disorder, using a bio-psycho-social approach.

Aetiology

It is estimated that 40%—60% of the risk of AUDs is explained by genetics (more than 50 genes have been implicated) and the rest through gene—environment associations such as the availability of alcohol, alcohol pricing, peer pressure and attitudes towards drinking and drunkenness.

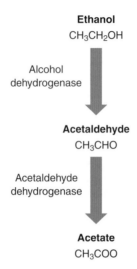

Ethanol
CH$_3$CH$_2$OH

Alcohol
dehydrogenase

Acetaldehyde
CH$_3$CHO

Acetaldehyde
dehydrogenase

Acetate
CH$_3$COO

Fig. 5.1 How ethanol is metabolized.

Children of alcoholic parents have an increased rate of AUDs. Concordance rates in twin studies for males and females are MZ:DZ 70%:43% and 47%:32%, respectively. Adoption studies show a four-fold increase in AUDs in male adoptees who were adopted away from alcoholic parents with AUDs.

Genetic effects may also determine the susceptibility to alcohol-related physical damage (e.g. psychosis, cirrhosis, brain damage) and the age of onset of dependence. To differentiate familial versus nonfamilial alcoholism, the former has a younger age of onset, more severe dependence and antisocial personality traits. Childhood aggression, inattention, hyperactivity and conduct disorders are also implicated.

FURTHER READING

For a detailed review of the genetics of alcohol use, see: Edenberg HJ, Gelernter J, Agrawal A. (2019) Genetics of alcoholism. Current Psychiatry Reports 21(4):26. doi:10.1007/s11920-019-1008-1

As with other drug dependence, the ventral tegmental dopaminergic reward pathway is likely to account for the development of dependence.

Variants of three genes (*ALDH2, ADH1B, ADH1C*) have been associated with reduced rates of AUDs.

The psychoanalytical theory accounts for dependence in terms of traumatic early-life experience, the need for oral gratification and the death-wish (self-destruction) theory. Classical and operant conditioning theories with relief drinking and cued response relapse are central in directing some therapeutic interventions, for example, relapse prevention.

Treatment

Generally, once significant dependence becomes evident, the preferred approach to alcohol use is to aim for total abstinence rather than controlled reduction of intake. Where the patients underestimate the extent of the problem, it can be useful to suggest a trial period of one month of abstinence.

If the patient is unable to stop for a month, it can be a powerful indicator to them that their alcohol intake is problematic and not under their control.

Individual counselling can promote problem-solving skills, cognitive restructuring, relapse prevention and social skills training. Voluntary agencies, including Alcoholics Anonymous (the 12-step programme), encourage group self-help and provide a voluntary sponsor to call at times of need when the patient is having difficulty controlling their drinking. Al-anon and Alateen provide support to family members and teenage children of problem drinkers, respectively. Residential units provide an opportunity to have a period of abstinence. Some provide detoxification, while others require detoxification to occur prior to admission. There are several overlapping approaches to successful management of problematic alcohol use that include harm reduction, motivational interviewing and methods to promote abstinence.

Several Pharmacological Interventions May Help Facilitate Abstinence

Several pharmacological interventions may help facilitate abstinence.

Disulfiram inhibits the action of acetaldehyde dehydrogenase so that alcohol consumption is followed by an unpleasant reaction comprising flushing, tachycardia, hyperventilation and considerable distress because of excessive acetaldehyde accumulation in the bloodstream. The therapy is used as a behavioural adjunct. However, it is not generally harmful. It can cause a variety of unpleasant side-effects, including a bad taste, sedation, rash and temporary impotence. Rarer, yet serious effects, include neuropathies, depression with psychotic features and an increase in liver enzymes and hepatitis. Because of concerns regarding this side-effect profile, along with effects that occur with long-term use (such as peripheral neuropathy) the use of disulfiram has declined considerably in recent years.

Naltrexone is an opioid antagonist that is used mainly in the United States for the treatment of AUDs. It reduces alcohol-induced reward. Acetaldehyde may combine with neurotransmitters to form tetrahydroisoquinolines, with opiate-like qualities, and naltrexone may blunt or block this effect, thus explaining its antieuphoriant effects.

FURTHER READING

For a review of pharmacological approaches to managing alcohol use disorders, see:
Kranzler HR, Soyka M. (2018) Diagnosis and pharmacotherapy of alcohol use disorder. JAMA 320(8):815–824. doi:10.1001/jama.2018.11406

Acamprosate is an NMDA receptor antagonist that is structurally similar to GABA, used to treat alcoholism. It is thought to act by balancing the glutamate–GABAergic activity in the brain, and works by decreasing cravings and urges to use alcohol. If necessary, it can be commenced while still using alcohol to help to maintain abstinence and is maintained if relapse occurs. Side-effects include gastrointestinal upset and diarrhoea, which rarely cause discontinuation.

---

4. Jane returns to her GP several weeks later. She is accompanied by her youngest child, 6-year-old Adam. She apologizes for bringing him but did not have anyone to mind him. Dr Crowley is aware from Dr Kelly's partially and alcohol-fuelled clinical notes that Jane was consuming alcohol during her pregnancy. Hence, Dr Crowley carefully examined Adam for outward signs of Fetal Alcohol Syndrome. Dr Crowley also asked Adam and his mother about how he is doing at school, and there appear to be no issues. Jane has presented as she is experiencing fatigue, abdominal discomfort and nausea, which has been worsening over the past week. The examination is normal, a pregnancy test is negative and Dr Crowley arranges some basic blood investigations and also commences Jane on daily oral thiamine as her symptoms, although nonspecific, could be because of thiamine deficiency related to her drinking. Dr Crowley is conscious of discussing alcohol-related issues with a child in the room, so he gives

Continued on following page

(Continued)

Jane some written information and asks her to commit to reading it before her next visit. Jane is agree-able to this plan and makes an appointment in three weeks.

11. What are the potential problems associated with consuming alcohol during pregnancy?
12. What is the role of thiamine in the body, and what are the symptoms of thiamine deficiency?
13. What is Wernicke's encephalopathy, and how does it relate to Korsakoff's syndrome?

Pregnancy

The use of alcohol during pregnancy is associated with increased rates of spontaneous abortion, pre-mature birth, low birth weight, growth deficits and mild learning disability. Babies born to mothers who consume alcohol can present with signs of withdrawal in the neonatal period, and these include irritability, hypotonia, tremors and seizures.

Fetal alcohol syndrome (FAS) is a potentially serious and lifelong problem in babies born to mothers who misuse alcohol during pregnancy. FAS varies in severity and features may include microcephaly, poor coordination, poor growth, reduced intelligence and behavioural problems. Abnormal facial features can be present with a smooth philtrum, thin vermilion, short palpeb-ral fissure, small maxillae and mandibles, cleft palate, small eye fissures and ear abnormalities.

Thiamine

Thiamine (vitamin B1) facilitates several key functions, including axonal conduction, muscle functioning, carbohydrate metabolism, enzymatic processes and the production of hydrochloric acid needed for digestion. Symptoms of thiamine deficiency include headache, nausea, fatigue, irritability, depression and abdominal discomfort. Thiamine deficiency can occur in AUDs because of reduced dietary intake, impaired absorption, impaired hepatic storage and impaired utilization.

Wernicke's encephalopathy

Wernicke's encephalopathy (WE) occurs as a result of thiamine deficiency and is characterized by a classic triad of confusion, ataxia and nystagmus, even though it is rare to see all three co-occurring (only 20% of cases). The condition generally develops over a period of days. Untreated WE is asso-ciated with high mortality and a high risk of progression to Korsakoff's syndrome. In those who recover, one-third have ongoing nystagmus, 50% have ataxia and 75% have some memory deficit (as part of Korsakoff's syndrome).

Nystagmus (horizontal more commonly and because of impaired lateral rectus muscle activity associated with a sixth cranial nerve palsy) and sluggish reaction times can be noted. These tend to resolve quickly with appropriate treatment, often within hours. Patients will often present as disorientated to time and place. Seizures, stupor and coma can all occur. Treatment is with parenteral thiamine until there is a significant improvement, at which time oral thiamine should be continued. Importantly, thiamine is important in the metabolism of glucose. Administration of glucose prior to the correction of thiamine deficiency can further deplete thiamine and aggravate WE. As a result, fluid replacement is sequenced to avoid a sudden depletion in thiamine.

Korsakoff's syndrome

Korsakoff's syndrome presents with a striking inability to form new memories, although the patient is alert and attentive with gaps typically filled with confabulation. While digit span is unimpaired, recall even after a few minutes is grossly affected. Long-term memory is relatively spared. Furthermore, 75% of patients do not significantly improve and may require residential care. In practice, most individuals with cognitive impairment in the context of AUDs have dementia of mixed causation.

Alcohol can induce a dementia-like picture without Korsakoff's syndrome because of its direct neurotoxicity.

---

5. Jane continues to drink heavily. She refuses to stop drinking completely, despite the strong advice of her GP and counsellor. Early one Sunday morning she is driving to the village and is stopped by Gardaí. They breathalyse her and find her alcohol levels to be four times above the legal limits for driving. She is arrested, and her husband is called to the Garda station. Sergeant Murphy is a family friend and a frequent attendee at the Doherty's parties. 'She'll have to do something, Martin, go in for treatment or something'. Dr Crowley interviews and examines Jane at the Garda station, taking a blood sample to test her alcohol levels. Jane is released and does not drink alcohol at all the next day. Her husband notices her pacing agitatedly around the house. He calls the surgery, and Dr Crowley agrees to see Jane. She is found to be orientated but hyperalert and distractible. Her BP, pulse and respiratory rate are increased, her reflexes are exaggerated, and she is displaying clear withdrawal symptoms. Dr Crowley prescribes her chlordiazepoxide 20 mg four times a day, reducing to zero over the next five days.

14. What are the features of alcohol withdrawal, and how does it compare to DTs?

Alcohol withdrawal is common in those with AUDs. Symptoms typically emerge 4—12 hours after the last drink and may include anxiety, palpitations, irritability, coarse tremor, sweating, headache, dry mouth, nausea and vomiting. Most will experience poor memory and concentration. Alcohol withdrawal can be accompanied by seizures, generally of the tonic-clonic type, and are more common in those with repeated episodes of withdrawal. The risk of seizures tends to peak one to two days after the last intake of alcohol.

DTs is a severe form of alcohol withdrawal that manifests as delirium. It is characterized by severe tremor and autonomic signs, confusion, disorientation and hallucinations. Symptoms generally peak at 2—3 days after the last alcohol intake. Visual hallucinations and frightening images are very common and can include seeing things, for example, insects, snakes and rats. Tactile hallucinations may also be present, for example, insects crawling on the skin or electric shock-like sensations. Auditory hallucinations are sometimes a feature and may include either simple sounds or voices, often accusatory or persecutory. Persecutory delusions may also be experienced. Disorientation to time and/or place is always a feature, as is memory disturbance. The level of confusion varies throughout the day and is often worse at night. The prevailing mood states of DTs include dysphoria, fear and even terror.

DTs is a medical emergency and is fatal in 5%—20% of cases, mainly because of cardiac, respiratory or hepatic complications. As such, treatment should involve specialist inpatient medical care. While most recover over 2—3 days, the condition can persist for weeks. Long-acting benzodiazepines (e.g. chlordiazepoxide or diazepam) are the mainstay of treatment, with gradually tapering dosages. High potency IV B-vitamins should be given for three days, followed by oral thiamine. Maintaining adequate fluid and electrolyte balance is important, and the general principles of management are the same as for a patient suffering from other causes of delirium.

---

6. Jane subsequently agrees to a referral to a residential alcohol treatment programme at St. George's Hospital, a private hospital that specializes in the inpatient treatment of addictions. She does well after her discharge from St. George's. She remains abstinent from alcohol for six months. However, she starts to drink heavily again after her first son leaves home for college in Dublin. Again, she attends her

Continued on following page

GP and counsellor. She quickly stops drinking this time. She receives a two-year ban from driving for her drink-driving offence. With the impact of the economic recession, her husband has less business and travels less than before. This turns out to be a positive development for everyone involved. The Doherty's grow closer, and Martin helps to support Jane through different stressful episodes in their lives.

15. Describe the role and interplay of primary, secondary and tertiary levels of care in the treatment of alcohol use disorders.

Primary, secondary and tertiary levels of care

Only about a quarter of people with AUDs ever seek help, with women having higher levels of treatment engagement. Most receive care from their GP, that is, in the primary care setting. Failure to identify an AUD can complicate the management of other medical and psychiatric disorders. GPs treat most cases of AUDs, with the referral of a small number of patients on to psychiatry or alcohol treatment services, along with input from voluntary and private agencies.

Typically, multidisciplinary psychiatric teams, that is secondary care level, have addiction counselling input through specially trained counsellors who can provide ongoing assessment and support for individuals with AUDs.

Tertiary care in a specialized alcohol treatment facility may be required when the individual develops medical complications secondary to their drinking, when a safe environment for detoxification is required and when the normal primary and secondary care levels of input have failed.

CHAPTER 6

Marguerite

Delirium

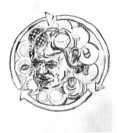

1. Give a clear clinical definition of delirium.
2. Understand how to approach cognitive assessment at the bedside.
3. Describe the epidemiology of delirium in different clinical settings.
4. List the predisposing and precipitating factors for delirium.
5. Describe the underlying pathophysiology involved in delirium.
6. Describe the key clinical features of delirium, distinguishing delirium from other disorders such as dementia and depression.
7. Describe the investigations required in the comprehensive assessment of an individual with delirium.
8. Describe the main approaches to managing and preventing delirium using a biopsychosocial approach.
9. Understand the factors that impact the decision to use pharmacological interventions in delirium.
10. Describe the prognosis of delirium.
11. Understand the relationship between delirium and dementia.

1. You are mid-way through a busy night on call when you are summoned to the geriatric medicine ward to review Marguerite, a 79-year-old woman, who is restless and wandering into adjoining beds. When 'confronted' by nurses, she seems disconnected and 'confused'. The nurses say that she was admitted from home yesterday for investigation as 'she has not been herself' and appears 'confused'.

    1. What are your initial thoughts regarding possible explanations for this presentation?
    2. What additional information might you seek?
    3. How would you approach a bedside assessment of her cognitive functioning?

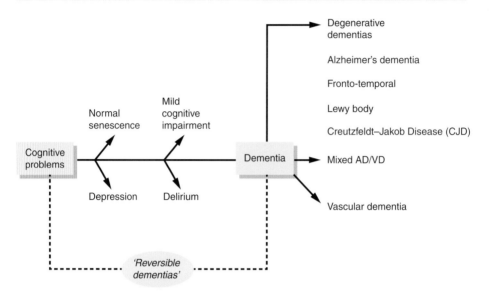

Fig. 6.1 The differential diagnosis of an elderly person presenting with cognitive impairment.

Confused older adults are a common problem in hospitalized populations. The confusion can range all the way from a situationally determined misunderstanding of circumstances in an older person with reduced cognitive flexibility because of normal senescence to frank delirium. In general, the principal differential diagnosis is between the so-called 3 Ds of delirium, depression and dementia, although these states are by no means mutually exclusive and frequently occur comorbidly.

The context of difficulties is key for establishing an accurate diagnosis (Fig. 6.1). The acuity of symptoms can be determined through a careful review of case notes and obtaining a collateral history from a reliable informant, such as a family member. In many cases, routine screening for cognitive function is performed at admission using instruments such as the Mini-Mental State Examination or the Montreal Cognitive Assessment tool. In addition, it is essential that the patient's baseline cognitive functioning is clarified (from a reliable informant). In the present case, this can be explored by probing about Marguerite's usual day-to-day pattern in terms of functional independence; for example, does she live alone, manage her own affairs, cook, drive, exercise or read the paper? Any changes to this usual pattern are important to document, including their timing and relationship to physical illness or life events. There are three general patterns: acute (suggesting delirium); acute on chronic (suggesting delirium in dementia); and insidious (depression typically evolves over weeks or months, dementia over months or years). The most typical causes of acute neuropsychiatric problems in the elderly are active infection; exposure to anticholinergics, opioids or benzodiazepines; and a previous medical or surgical procedure. Importantly, delirium is a more urgent diagnosis and is frequently considered to be an acute medical emergency as it can be a sign of a serious central nervous system or other pathological condition (e.g. stroke). Therefore, delirium takes diagnostic precedence such that Marguerite should be presumed to have delirium until otherwise established.

Being 'confused' suggests that she may be disoriented and may have a reduced awareness of her environment. This can be readily examined at the bedside by enquiring about the patient's understanding of where they are, the reason for being in a hospital and the identity of their care providers. It is essential to assess attention because this is fundamentally impaired in patients with delirium. This will be evident through engaging in a simple conversation with the patient about their circumstances and background, while paying attention to their ability to engage coherently and without distraction. Formal testing of attention can be achieved by asking the patient to recite the months of the year in reverse order (intact attention requires that the patient can successfully get back at least to July) (Box 6.1).

---

2. Upon examination, it emerges that there is limited information about Marguerite's background because her daughter with whom she has regular contact is away on holiday at present. No formal testing of cognitive status was performed at admission. At the bedside, Marguerite appears perplexed and distracted, says that she is not sure where she is and wants to go home to feed her cats. She is unable to identify the day or date but correctly identifies that it is winter in 2020. She is confused as to why you, a policeman, would want to question her. For the months backwards test, she replies 'December. . .September...January....'.

    4. What are the criteria for delirium and how can we clarify whether she meets these criteria?

    5. How common is delirium and why is it important?

    6. What are the possible aetiological factors for delirium and what investigations would you perform?

Delirium is a complex neuropsychiatric syndrome that can include a wide range of cognitive and psychiatric features. These include disturbances to consciousness, awareness of the immediate environment, thinking, language, perception, affective regulation, sleep–wake cycle and motor behaviour.

In terms of cognitive features, delirium involves generalized impairment of cognitive abilities but with particular disturbance to consciousness and attention. Consciousness can be affected both qualitatively ('clouding') and quantitatively in terms of arousal, and both reduced arousal and hyperarousal states are possible. Where the level of arousal renders formal testing of cognition impossible, this is considered evidence of severe inattention, and thus, consistent with a diagnosis of delirium. The exception is coma, whereby the patient is unrousable, which is considered to be a separate phenomenon to delirium. The primary cognitive disturbance is in *the ability to focus, sustain and shift*

BOX 6.1 ■ How we can assess cognition at the bedside:

- Approach the patient and introduce yourself (noting their level of arousal and ability to engage in conversation).
- Ask them their name and why they are in a hospital, followed by general questions regarding how long they have been in the hospital, what care they have received to date and who is that person (nurse) (noting their orientation and awareness of their environment and their focus and organization of thoughts).
- Ask them if you can do some short tests to assess their concentration and recall. Proceed by asking them to remember three objects (ideally that are in the vicinity and that can be cued for recall).
- Then ask that they recite the months of the year forwards, and then backwards—beginning with December (elderly patients should be able to recite back to July without omissions).
- Test their executive function by asking them to say as many words as they can beginning with the letter 'F' (at least 10 words within 60 seconds is normal).
- After approximately a three-minute delay, ask that they recall the three words. If necessary, you can cue them with prompts, for example 'I am wearing it' for a watch. A normal performance includes recalling all three words (if necessary, with cueing).
- If needed, long-term memory can be tested by inquiring about verifiable facts from the past, such as date and place of marriage, significant events documented in their case notes (operations, the birth of children, etc.).
- Visuospatial abilities can be assessed by clock drawing or copying overlapping pentagons, or more practically by asking directions to the bathroom or exit and specific queries regarding the proximity or shape of objects in their vicinity ('which is closer—the door or the window?').

The interpretation of performance in these tests is discussed in more detail in the chapter on the Mini-Mental State Examination.

attention, and is evident in terms of difficulty in orienting to salient stimuli, poor concentration, reduced vigilance, distractibility and impaired awareness of the immediate environment. Attentional abilities are disproportionately affected, but there are typical disturbances to other cognitive abilities, including orientation, visuospatial ability, executive function and short-term memory, which can usually be demonstrated with simple bedside tests.

A variety of neuropsychiatric symptoms can also occur, including disrupted circadian integrity (sleep and motor function) and disturbances to thinking, perception, affect and behaviour. Around 50% of patients have psychotic features. Delusions are typically simple persecutory ideas and relate to the immediate surroundings (e.g. that the hospital is a prison or that their medications are a poison). Perceptual disturbances include illusions and hallucinations and are most commonly visual or tactile. Affective lability, with unpredictable shifts in mood, anger and/or increased irritability, is common, but some patients present with a more sustained lowering of mood and reduced activity that is easily mistaken for depressive illness.

Establishing a diagnosis requires that the patient has evidence of:
1. inattention (e.g. failed the months backwards test), along with
2. disturbance to other cognitive domains (e.g. disorientation)
3. that disturbances are of relatively recent onset—either acute (hours/days), subacute (days/weeks) or that there has been a recent worsening of longstanding difficulties (acute or chronic) or that the patient has evidence of highly fluctuating consciousness/mental state.
4. The disturbances should not be attributable to established dementia or depressive illness, and
5. typically occur in the context of physical illness.

In reality, it can be useful to consider, apart from delirium, what else can cause a previously intact person to develop acute neuropsychiatric and cognitive difficulties suddenly. The concept of delirium can be used to capture this clinical presentation (Box 6.2).

The importance of delirium is emphasized by its frequency and impact upon outcomes. Delirium is common in most clinical settings, occurring in approximately one in five general hospital patients, and with rates of up to 90% reported among patients in palliative and intensive care settings. Delirium has a considerable impact on patient outcomes and healthcare costs. Patients with delirium are associated with prolonged hospitalizations, more complications, greater costs of care, reduced subsequent functional independence and increased in-hospital and subsequent mortality. Importantly, these adverse health and social outcomes are predicted by the presence of delirium and are relatively independent of confounding factors such as morbidity level, baseline cognition, age and frailty. In addition, delirium may be accelerating and possibly a causal factor in the development of dementia. No other psychiatric disorder has such penetration across healthcare settings. The frequency, along with the complexity of clinical presentation where typically 50% of the cases are not detected, makes delirium a key target for improved management within our healthcare services.

BOX 6.2 ■ The diagnosis of an episode of delirium is based upon:

1. Disturbance in attention (i.e. reduced ability to direct, focus and sustain attention) and awareness (reduced orientation to the environment).
2. Evidence of generalized disturbance in cognition (e.g. disorientation, executive or visuospatial ability).
3. The disturbance develops over a short period of time (usually hours to a few days), represents an acute change from baseline attention and awareness and often fluctuates in severity during the day.
4. The disturbances are not better attributed to another disorder (e.g. dementia).
5. The disturbance is associated with an underlying physical cause(s) (i.e. a medical condition and physical or pharmacological insult).

Delirium Aetiologies

- Drug-related
- Endocrine-metabolic
- Traumatic
- Epilepsy
- Cerebrovascular
- Tumour
- Infection
- Organ failure
- Not otherwise specified (heavy metal/insecticide poisoning)

Identifying and treating the underlying causes of delirium is at the core of delirium care. Delirium is usually multifactorial with typically three to four significant causative factors relevant during any single episode, which interact and overlap sequentially to produce or sustain delirium symptoms. The assessment of a delirious patient thus requires comprehensive assessment for multiple causes, beginning with a thorough history and examination, obtaining a collateral history to clarify baseline status and course of symptoms and review of recent medication exposure. The most typical causes are infection, polypharmacy and metabolic abnormalities. No identifiable cause is identified in 10% of cases. Box 6.3 shows a scheme of investigations that should be considered in

---

BOX 6.3 ■ Investigation of suspected delirium

1. Careful history and physical examination
2. Collateral history
   Baseline cognition
   Presence of sensory impairments
   Exposure to risk factors
   Review of medications, procedures, tests, intraoperative data
3. First-line investigations
   Complete blood count
   Electrolytes, Mg, Ca, PO_4
   Liver function test
   Urinalysis
   Electrocardiogram
   Erythrocyte sedimentation rate
   Blood glucose
   Chest radiograph
   Urinalysis
4. Second-line investigations (as indicated)
   Drug screen
   Blood cultures
   Cardiac enzymes
   Blood gases
   Serum folate/B12
   Electroencephalography
   Cerebrospinal fluid examination
   Computed tomography of the brain
   Magnetic resonance imaging of the brain
   Prolactin level
   Human immunodeficiency virus antibodies
   Syphilis serology
   Urinary porphyrins

all delirious patients along with other second-line investigations that are appropriate where clinical assessment and findings from preliminary tests suggest.

---

3. The following day, Marguerite undergoes a variety of tests and is noted to have a respiratory infection. Her mental state fluctuates from being lucid and aware of her surroundings to periods of acute agitation during which she appears disoriented as to where she is and has to be prevented from leaving the ward, which she describes as 'a prison'.
   7. What advice would you give nursing staff about ongoing care to the patient?
   8. Do other aggravating/risk factors need to be considered in managing her difficulties?
   9. What is the significance of clinical subtyping of delirium and how is it defined?

> **BOX 6.4 ■ The key principles of ward management of patients with delirium:**
>
> 1. Ensuring the safety of the patient and those in their immediate surroundings.
> 2. Minimizing the potential for complications such as falls, self-injury and hypostasis.
> 3. Simplifying the care environment to avoid excessive sensory stimulation.
> 4. Addressing any sensory impediments, while promoting patient efficacy in terms of orientation and functional abilities.
> 5. Promoting healthy sleep—wake patterns.
> 6. Minimizing pain.

The key principles of ward management of patients with delirium are shown in Box 6.4. Communication with delirious patients should include simple language expressed in a clearly audible and slow-paced voice. The use of orienting techniques (e.g. calendars, night-lights, reorientation by staff) and familiarizing objects (e.g. family photographs) can make the environment easier to comprehend. Recovered delirium patients report that simple but firm communication, reality orientation, a visible clock and the presence of a relative contributed to a heightened sense of control. Engaging family members in care can also help in clarifying changes from baseline status and understanding the meaning of symptoms. Relatives must be educated about delirium and its management because ill-informed, critical or anxious caregivers can add to the patient burden. The challenges of providing an optimal care environment require a careful balance between the need to minimize risk versus the provision of individualized, patient-focused care that promotes autonomy and dignity. For example, efforts to ensure the safety of delirious patients at risk of falls and wandering can result in restrictive care practices that inhibit reorientation, mobility and self-efficacy. Less restrictive care can be facilitated by electronic alarms and pressure mats to monitor patient behaviour and alert staff when vulnerable patients are at risk of wandering or falls.

Delirium has several well-identified and consistent risk factors, which makes it a highly predictable occurrence. Studies have identified a range of patients, illness and treatment factors that can predict the likelihood of developing delirium or 'delirium readiness'. In general, delirium occurs through the interaction of predisposing factors with acute precipitating insults to produce acute brain failure or delirium. One particularly important study found that a model comprising four predisposing factors (cognitive impairment, severe illness, visual impairment and dehydration) and five precipitating factors (polypharmacy, catheterization, use of restraints, malnutrition, any iatrogenic event) predicted a 17-fold variation in the relative risk of developing delirium.

Fig. 6.2 shows a detailed list of risk factors for delirium. Certain factors are more relevant in particular settings and patient groups, but old age, preexisting cognitive problems, severe comorbid illness and psychotropic medication exposure are robust predictors of delirium risk across populations. Many risk factors are modifiable, while others can help assess the risk—benefit

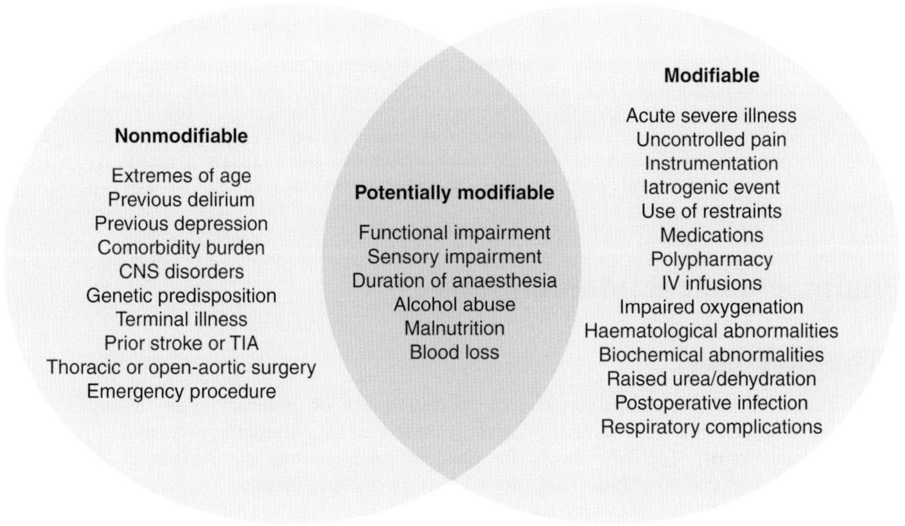

Nonmodifiable

Extremes of age
Previous delirium
Previous depression
Comorbidity burden
CNS disorders
Genetic predisposition
Terminal illness
Prior stroke or TIA
Thoracic or open-aortic surgery
Emergency procedure

Potentially modifiable

Functional impairment
Sensory impairment
Duration of anaesthesia
Alcohol abuse
Malnutrition
Blood loss

Modifiable

Acute severe illness
Uncontrolled pain
Instrumentation
Iatrogenic event
Use of restraints
Medications
Polypharmacy
IV infusions
Impaired oxygenation
Haematological abnormalities
Biochemical abnormalities
Raised urea/dehydration
Postoperative infection
Respiratory complications

Fig. 6.2   Risk factors for delirium, classed according to modifiability.

balance of surgical and other interventions in deciding upon optimal care, especially in frail, elderly patients with cognitive impairment. Intervention studies demonstrate that delirium is highly preventable by minimizing exposure to modifiable risk factors such as unnecessary polypharmacy, nonessential surgery and optimizing sensory abilities. A recent meta-analysis of 14 studies of multicomponent non-pharmacological interventions found that delirium incidence was reduced by 44%, with a significant reduction in falls and with a trend toward decreasing length of stay and avoiding institutionalization.

Clinical subtypes of delirium

Although delirium is considered as a unitary syndrome of acute generalized cognitive impairment, the presentation in terms of patterns of motor activity and arousal can vary considerably. Two principal patterns have been recognized since the time of Hippocrates: *'phrenitus'*, now termed 'hyperactive' or agitated delirium, and *'lethargus'*, now termed 'hypoactive' or somnolent delirium. In addition, a third 'mixed' subtype accounts for patients who experience elements of both increased and decreased motor activity within short time frames.

Studies comparing the clinical profiles of these presentations indicate similar levels of disturbance across neuropsychological domains, but with different patterns in terms of the underlying cause. Hyperactive presentations are more common in younger patients and substance-related delirium, while hypoactive delirium is more common in those with organ failure and preexisting dementia. Moreover, detection rates differ. Hypoactive delirium is more frequently missed or diagnosed later than hyperactive delirium. Treatment experiences vary such that patients with hyperactive or mixed features are much more likely to receive antipsychotic interventions. Adverse events vary such that hyperactive patients are more likely to fall or sabotage treatment (e.g. pull out lines), while hypoactive patients experience the adverse effects of hypostasis (pneumonia, pressure sores). Furthermore, hypoactive presentations have a poorer prognosis.

4. That evening, Marguerite's situation deteriorates as she becomes increasingly unmanageable on the ward because of agitation and restlessness. She is overtly combative with nursing staff and shouting about 'blood spiders leaking down through the roof' and a fear that the nurses are trying to poison her. She requires a full time 'special' nurse in attendance to prevent her from leaving the ward. The nursing staff ask that you review her treatment and are wondering whether she should be 'sedated'.

   10.   What pharmacological options are available and what evidence supports their use?

Pharmacological interventions

FURTHER READING

For a review of the pharmacological management of delirium, see: Meagher DJ, McLoughlin L, Leonard M, et al. (2013) What do we really know about the treatment of delirium with antipsychotics? Ten key issues for delirium pharmacotherapy. American Journal of Geriatric Psychiatry 21(12):1223–1238. doi:10.1016/j.jagp.2012.09.008

The pharmacological management of delirium in everyday practice is both controversial and highly inconsistent. Most suggested treatments derive from experiences with psychotropic agents used in the management of other neuropsychiatric conditions, particularly functional psychoses and dementia. The principal agents that have been studied include antipsychotics (both typical and atypical), benzodiazepines, procholinergics and dexmedetomidine. The best evidence is for the use of antipsychotic agents which remain the clinical standard and are the most supported in treatment guidelines.

The use of antipsychotic agents is supported by a large number of prospective studies, which suggest that approximately 75% of delirious patients who receive short-term low dosage antipsychotic treatment experience clinical response. However, because delirium is a highly fluctuating, typically multifactorial condition that frequently remits with the resolution of the primary insult, placebo-controlled studies are especially important in determining the value of interventions. However, such evidence is lacking with conflicting findings in the four existing placebo-controlled studies, which found a more rapid resolution of delirium to no benefit from and poorer survival. The National Institute for Health and Care Excellence guidelines recommend the cautious use of olanzapine or haloperidol. These interventions are justified where the patient is distressed with severe agitation or psychosis, and/or if there is a significant risk of physical harm to the patient or others, or delirium symptoms are impeding the ability to provide optimal care in terms of essential treatments.

There is a lack of high-quality evidence to demonstrate benefits from antipsychotic use in terms of medium- and longer-term outcomes. In addition, they are associated with a variety of risks, including sedation, hypotension, extrapyramidal effects, cardiotoxicity (e.g. QT interval prolongation) and an increased risk of stroke in patients with dementia. Consequently, decisions around medication use are made on a case-by-case basis with careful consideration of the balance between the likely benefits and adverse effects. In general, cardiac effects are rare when the cumulative daily dosage of intravenous haloperidol is lower than 2 mg, unless patients have additional risk factors for QTc prolongation. Other studies have highlighted how outcomes are better when the care of delirious patients is protocolized to include dose titration with regular monitoring of arousal, cardiac status and extrapyramidal symptoms (EPS). Antipsychotic treatment is more frequently used in patients with behavioural difficulties and hyperactivity because many clinicians perceive the primary therapeutic effect of neuroleptics as sedative or antipsychotic, even though a response is not closely linked to these actions.

Studies do not suggest significant differences in efficacy between haloperidol and atypical agents, but haloperidol is associated with a higher rate of EPS. Commonly used agents include risperidone (starting dose, 0.25 mg); olanzapine (starting dose, 2.5 mg); quetiapine (starting dose, 12.5 mg); or haloperidol (starting dose, 0.5 mg). Among these agents, quetiapine is relatively more sedative, while haloperidol is readily available in both oral and parenteral forms. The best practice is to 'start low and go slow', with dose titration according to response and adverse effects. Treatment is short term and typically discontinued after 3—5 days.

Evidence to support the use of other agents in delirium management is variable. Benzodiazepines are the first-line treatment in delirium because of withdrawal states or seizures but are otherwise best avoided as they can aggravate or perpetuate delirium, cloud ongoing cognitive assessment and are linked to falls, oversedation and respiratory depression. Procholinergic treatments have theoretical appeal given the link between delirium and hypocholinergic states but do not appear to be effective in the management of acute delirium episodes. Preliminary evidence suggests that dexmedetomidine, an alpha-2 adrenergic agonist, may be useful for treating delirium-related agitation.

---

5. Marguerite commences olanzapine 2.5 mg nocte and over the following 48 hours her agitation settles, and she recovers to full lucidity. The persecutory ideas abate, and she is readily able to identify the day, date, current location and can recite the months of the year in reverse without difficulty. However, upon questioning her daughter, it is apparent that she has not been functioning at her previous 'usual' self for perhaps a year or so, has stopped driving and has needed help managing the household shopping and remembering contact details and sometimes names of friends and family.
    11. What are your thoughts about this additional information?
    12. What is the nature of the relationship between delirium and dementia?

This additional information suggests that Marguerite may have some more longstanding cognitive issues that predate the recent delirious episode. It is not unusual for the first presentation of dementia to occur with an episode of delirium as diminished cognitive reserve is a major predisposing risk factor for delirium. More than 50% of cases of delirium with comorbid dementia.

More formal testing of neuropsychological status and a full dementia screen are warranted (see dementia case for workup). There are likely to be practical issues that should be considered at this point, such as day-to-day support, driving and making a will.

---

6. Three months later, Marguerite attends an outpatient clinic with her daughter to review her ongoing recovery. She reports having recurrent thoughts about her time in hospital, especially the sense of being imprisoned, and feels embarrassed by her behaviour at that time. Her daughter informs you that Marguerite has not recovered to her old self in that she often seems to miss the point in conversations, struggles to maintain focus in everyday tasks and following television programmes, and that her previous memory difficulties have worsened. In addition, her daughter is wondering how they might minimize the likelihood of Marguerite experiencing a recurrence of delirium in the future.
    13. How common are persistent difficulties after a delirious episode?
    14. What can be done to minimize any future risk of delirium?

The outcome of delirium is highly variable and ranges from a brief transient episode with full recovery to the previous level of cognitive and socioadaptive functioning to a more persistent illness with longer-term cognitive impairment and loss of functional independence. Therefore, the traditional concept of delirium as a brief, transient and highly reversible condition is no longer supported by longitudinal studies. It is estimated that delirium is associated with persistent cognitive problems, including markedly elevated rates of dementia, in around a third of elderly patients. Importantly, these difficulties often occur in patients who were assessed as cognitively intact prior to the delirium episode.

Persistent cognitive deficits may be related to previously undiagnosed dementia that progresses during and after the delirium resolution. Undetected dementia is frequent in both community-dwelling (64%) and hospitalized older people (20%). Therefore, delirium can be the beginning of a journey of cognitive decline resulting in dementia, with increasing recognition that delirium is more than a mere harbinger for dementia and maybe an aggravating or even causal factor in a more sustained cognitive disorder. Progression from an acute to chronic cognitive disorder is a recognized complication of alcohol-related neuropsychiatric disturbance where the acute cognitive disturbances of Wernicke's encephalopathy can progress to a more persistent state of cognitive impairment termed 'Korsakoff's syndrome'. Such relationships may also apply between delirium and dementia. Moreover, the occurrence of delirium is associated with a more rapid subsequent decline in cognition in patients with Alzheimer's, independent of factors such as age and previous cognitive function.

Delirium is a distressing experience for patients and their caregivers. Delirium-recovered patients may be uncomfortable discussing their delirium episodes because they equate it with being 'senile' or 'mad'. The psychological aftermath of delirium is understudied, but recent work suggests that around 50% of patients can recall the episode and that the experience of psychosis and marked agitation is especially linked to postdelirium adjustment issues. In nondemented elderly patients with delirium, it was found that more than half could recall psychotic symptoms, and many were still distressed by their recollections six months later.

Persistent psychological disturbances are a particular target for interventions that can impact upon subsequent help-seeking behaviour. Regular follow-up visits can facilitate postdelirium adjustment by allowing for discussion of the meaning of delirium and planning of how to minimize future risk (e.g. by addressing risk factors such as medication exposure and sensory impairments). In high-risk patients, *prehabilitation* prior to planned interventions (e.g. elective surgery) to minimize the risk of experiencing delirium is becoming more common. In addition, there is some evidence that low dosage antipsychotic treatments can be used as a prophylactic intervention perioperatively (e.g. low dosage risperidone or olanzapine on the day before and after surgery).

Colin

Anxiety Disorders

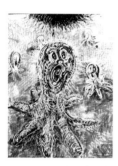

1. Describe the key clinical diagnostic features of generalized anxiety disorder (GAD), panic disorder and social phobia (social anxiety disorder), including differential diagnoses and common comorbid mental and physical disorders.
2. Briefly describe the epidemiology of the anxiety disorders, including their incidence, prevalence and gender differences.
3. Describe the key aetiological factors in the anxiety disorders and classify these in terms of the medical/biological, social and psychological factors.
4. List the main investigations involved in the assessment, diagnosis and ongoing treatment of anxiety disorders, beginning with a detailed history, mental state examination and collateral history. In addition, classify these investigations as medical/biological, social and psychological approaches.
5. Describe the main treatments for the different anxiety disorders and consider these in terms of medical/biological, social and psychological approaches.
6. Briefly describe the key prognostic factors for GAD, panic disorder and social phobia and compare them with the prognosis of other major mental health disorders.

1. Colin is a 33-year-old married man who works as a junior bank official and lives with his wife and two daughters. He was referred by his general practitioner after he presented seeking help to deal with 'stress and anxiety'. He is especially worried about an upcoming wedding in which he will be the best man for his brother and is afraid that he will not be able to deal with the responsibility of making a speech and meeting so many people.
   1. What are your initial thoughts regarding this presentation?
   2. What are the principal complaints that patients with anxiety disorders present with and how do these patterns assist the differential diagnosis?

It is not unusual for individuals with anxiety disorders to seek help many years after the onset of their problems and in the context of an acute stressor that has 'brought things to a head'. All but the most severe anxiety disorders can usually be managed through a range of adaptive responses, including many maladaptive behaviours. Speaking in public is a common fear, and it has been reported that more people fear this than death itself!

This presentation only gives a vague clue as to the nature of Colin's problems. In general, anxiety problems are considered pathological, where they can be considered beyond the usual reactions to adverse life situations and have a discernible and significant impact upon socio-adaptive functioning.

The principal patterns for anxiety symptoms include general symptoms of excessive and uncontrollable worrying about everyday life experiences and/or more specific fears relating to specific phenomena. Symptoms follow two main patterns:

1. Persistent mild-to-moderate severity in mental discomfort associated with physical symptoms of tension and 'generalized anxiety'.

2. Discrete episodes of more extreme fear associated with a sense of losing control ('panic').

The latter tends to be the more potent precipitants of help-seeking behaviour.

---

2. At the consultation, Colin describes a longstanding history of excessive worrying dating back to early adulthood. He describes problems with persistent tension, muscle aches and fatigue. He describes occasional episodes of losing control with fear—'like an explosion of anxiety'. This has occurred in stressful situations such as having to face scrutiny at work (e.g. presentations at management meetings). These episodes only occur in specific situations of perceived stress. He denies any avoidant behaviours and describes an active social life. He is worried that if things get worse, he could end up like his maternal aunt who became housebound because of 'a fear of open spaces'.

3. What are the likely diagnoses?

4. What investigations would you perform to identify/exclude any physical factors contributing to his symptoms?

5. What is a 'panic attack?'

6. What are the criteria for panic disorder and how does it compare with GAD?

7. What is agoraphobia and how does it relate to panic disorder?

The differential diagnosis for anxiety is broad and subject to a diagnostic hierarchy in which mood and other disorders take diagnostic precedence (Fig. 7.1). A primary anxiety disorder is not the favoured diagnosis if symptoms occur principally in the context of a comorbid major mental illness, such as depression or a psychotic illness. Patients with longstanding anxiety problems often

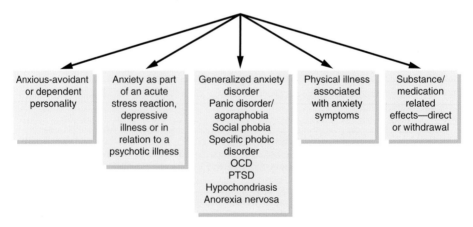

Fig. 7.1   Differential diagnosis of anxiety symptoms.

present when there has been an escalation of symptoms in the context of an emergent comorbid mood or other disorder. Comorbidities are very common among people with anxiety disorders, with 50% or more individuals typically reporting another disorder. Therefore, it is important to carefully assess the character of symptoms and their context.

Patients with premorbid anxious personality profiles are more prone to syndromal or clinical anxiety disorders, and this pattern typically presents as an acute worsening of symptoms.

Anxiety is a common feature of depressive disorders, and careful assessment for syndromal depressive illness is important. Anxiety can also be a feature of other states, such as distressing persecutory beliefs or experience of hallucinations in psychotic illness.

A range of medical conditions and substance-related circumstances can also be relevant, and a detailed medical history, physical examination and documentation of medication exposure and substance use is fundamental for identifying the causes and/or precipitating factors for anxiety. Patients with primary anxiety disorders have a three-fold greater use of medical services (e.g. 25% of cardiovascular referrals and 50% of patients assessed for irritable bowel syndrome have panic disorder).

The physical differential is broad and includes:

- Endocrine disorders (e.g. hyperthyroidism, diabetes, hypoparathyroidism or hypoglycaemia)
- Anaemia
- Cardiovascular (e.g. arrhythmias, ischaemic, congestive cardiac failure, valvular disease including mitral valve prolapse)
- Seizure-related or central nervous system (CNS) pathological condition (e.g. TLE/ vestibular nerve diseases)
- Respiratory disorders (e.g. asthma or chronic obstructive pulmonary disease)
- Gastrointestinal disorder (e.g. irritable bowel syndrome)
- Chronic pain
- Substance-related (e.g. exposure to stimulants, steroids, bronchodilators, dopaminergic agents, withdrawal from alcohol or sedative-hypnotics).
- Other conditions including porphyria, systemic lupus erythematosis (SLE), carcinoid syndrome and pheochromocytoma.

FURTHER READING

For a review of anxiety disorders and their relationship to medical conditions, see: Hoge EA, Ivkovic A, Fricchione GL. (2012) Generalized anxiety disorder: diagnosis and treatment. The British Medical Journal 345:e7500. doi:10.1136/bmj.e7500

The pattern of symptoms will direct appropriate investigations (which are often in themselves quite anxiogenic!). The investigations typically include the following: a full blood count, urea and electrolytes, thyroid function, liver function tests, an electrocardiogram, urinary drug screen and fasting blood glucose measurement. Further testing is guided by findings from the history and physical examination.

In addition, the family of anxiety disorders is broad and a clear diagnosis requires detailed consideration of the pattern of symptoms, focusing on precipitants and course. In generalized anxiety disorder (GAD), symptoms tend to be persistent and follow themes of excessive worrying about everyday circumstances, such as work, health, finances and domestic factors. In panic disorder, there is a history of panic episodes without a specific focus and associated anticipatory anxiety *(fear of the fear)* with avoidance behaviours. In agoraphobia, anxiety and panic occurs in response to circumstances that are perceived as being away from a place of safety (e.g. home) and often referred to as 'a fear of open spaces' or where ease of exit is uncertain (holidays, shopping, church, queues). In social phobia (or social anxiety disorder), anxiety relates to social situations where there is a fear of embarrassment, scrutiny or evaluation by others. Specific phobias relate to circumscribed irrational

> **BOX 7.1 ■ The diagnosis of social anxiety disorder is based upon:**
>
> 1. Persistent difficulties with fear and anxiety in social or other performance situations where the person is likely to come under scrutiny from others.
> 2. Anxiety may manifest as intense generalized anxiety and/or with panic episodes.
> 3. Anticipatory anxiety and avoidance occur when faced with the prospect of situations that are likely to provoke these responses.
> 4. The person has insight into the excessive or irrational nature of their symptoms.
> 5. These difficulties are associated with reduced functioning in social, personal or occupational activities.
> 6. The symptoms are not better explained by another mental disorder (e.g. paranoid illness), substance effects or physical illness.

fears of animals, flying, blood and insects. In posttraumatic stress disorder, anxiety relates to triggers and re-experiencing phenomena. In obsessive—compulsive disorder, anxiety relates to obsessional thoughts and compulsive behaviours, which predominate. In other disorders, anxiety occurs in relation to fears about health and well-being (hypochondriasis) and abnormal beliefs about appearance or body image (anorexia nervosa and dysmorphophobia).

FURTHER READING

For a review of social anxiety disorder, see: Leichsenring F, Leweke F. (2017) Social anxiety disorder. New England Journal of Medicine 376(23):2255—2264. doi:10.1056/NEJMcp1614701

The character of anxiety symptoms can also provide some clues. Situational factors shape clinical features; for example, shortness of breath occurs primarily with agoraphobia, while blushing, sweating and trembling are more strongly associated with social anxiety disorder. Colin's symptoms point towards a longstanding pattern of generalized anxiety punctuated by occasional panic episodes that seem to follow a pattern suggestive of social anxiety disorder (Box 7.1).

A panic attack is a discrete period of marked fear or anxiety that is associated with a variety of cognitive and physical phenomena. Panic attacks are sometimes described as an 'explosion' of panic. Panic episodes can vary considerably in frequency and duration, but are usually preceded by a prodromal period of escalating fearfulness (10 minutes or so) before the actual full-blown attack, which is usually quite brief (minutes), but occasionally, will last longer.

The symptoms of panic in the order of frequency are palpitations, pounding heart, tachycardia, sweating, trembling, shaking, dyspnoea, choking, chest pain and fear of passing out, collapsing, dying or going mad. Other features include chills or hot flushes, nausea, abdominal discomfort, dizziness or light-headedness.

Experiencing a panic episode is often described as terrifying and is associated with subsequent anticipatory anxiety regarding a recurrence. This leads to a generalization of the issue as the person tries to make sense of it; for example, if the first attack occurs in a church, the person may experience anticipatory anxiety and avoid going back to the church. The core concern is usually one of being unable to escape to safety in, for example, queues, enclosed spaces, public transport, crowds or shopping. Essentially, it is 'fear of a fear'. Furthermore, 50% of individuals with panic attacks have associated agoraphobia. Nocturnal panic attacks are unusual and suggest a physical cause. However, if they do present, they usually occur during slow-wave sleep (Box 7.2).

FURTHER READING

For a review of panic disorder, see: Katon W. (2006) Panic disorder. New England Journal of Medicine 354:2360—2367. doi:10.1056/NEJMcp052466

BOX 7.2 ■ Criteria for a panic episode:

The sudden occurrence of acute and severe anxiety that typically occurs over several minutes. The individual may experience a number of compelling physical and psychic symptoms because of psychological factors.

Possible symptoms include the following: sweating, tremor, feeling hot or chills, dizziness or a sense of feeling faint or lightheaded, shortness of breath or a sense of smothering or choking, tachycardia, palpitations, chest tightness or pain, nausea, abdominal discomfort, paraesthesia (numbness or tingling sensations), derealization, depersonalization, fear of losing control, vomiting, being incontinent or going crazy and intense fear of something bad happening or dying.

Typically, a panic episode will involve a combination of four or more of these symptoms.

Panic disorder is diagnosed when regular panic attacks cause distress and dysfunction. Previously, a minimum frequency was required, but it has been recognized that people with panic disorder can often avoid panic episodes through avoidance behaviours, and that adaptive impact is a better measure of severity than the actual frequency of episodes.

Agoraphobia is a variant of panic disorder where the focus of the fear is geographical and related to particular places or situations where 'escape to safety' is difficult, resulting in a fear of 'being trapped'. Avoidant behaviour can result in a diminished social repertoire, and in more severe cases, patients can become restricted to their homes (described by Colin in his aunt's condition as 'housebound'). The distinction between panic disorder and agoraphobia remains contentious. Many scholars, in an attempt to understand and avoid further attacks, have conceptualized agoraphobia as the attribution of panic episodes to specific places or circumstances. In 'pure' panic disorder, the cause of the attacks is less readily attributable to specific situations, and they are often reported as spontaneous or paroxysmal.

In contrast, GAD refers to less acute but more persistent anxiety and includes general anxiety, excessive worrying and apprehension that are disproportionate to circumstances. Themes include everyday matters; for example, work, finances, relationships and health. A core element is that patients with GAD struggle to control worries ('normal' worrying can be rationalized and maintained within a manageable level).

FURTHER READING

For a review of GAD, see: Gale C, Davidson O. (2007) Generalised anxiety disorder. BMJ 334 (7593):579–581. doi:10.1136/bmj.39133.559282.BE

In GAD, excessive worrying impacts the patient's quality of life and socio-adaptive functioning. For a formal diagnosis of GAD, symptoms should not be attributable to another mental disorder or caused by physical or medication/substance use (Box 7.3).

---

3. Further discussion reveals that Colin was 'always nervous as a child' and experienced an episode of depression in his early 20s during a period of unemployment, and later, had a recurrence in his late 20s during a dispute with a neighbour following an incident in which the neighbour's dog bit Colin's wife. His anxiety symptoms became much worse during these times, and he had stopped going out because of the fear of getting stressed. He reports that he has recently started to 'borrow' diazepam (Valium) tablets from his aunt when he experiences stressful situations at work but finds that these make him feel tired. He also reports having 'a few drinks' sometimes to steady himself before social

Continued on following page

(Continued)

occasions as he is very conscious of his tendency to blush, and that he has a noticeable tremor in his hands.
 8.   What is the relevance of the use of diazepam (Valium) and alcohol in the manner described?
 9.   What do we know about the cause and pathophysiology of anxiety disorders?
 10. What is their relationship to other mental health problems, such as mood disorders?

BOX 7.3 ■ Diagnosis of GAD

1. Excessive and persistent sense of worry and apprehension that is associated with psychic discomfort and physical symptoms that are of a generalized nature.
2. Typical symptoms include feeling on edge, restless, distracted, irritable, anxious or unable to relax, impaired concentration, fatigue, generalized muscle tension and disturbed sleeping patterns.
3. Symptoms that cause significant distress and/or impairment in the functioning of social, interpersonal and occupational activities.
4. Symptoms are not better explained by substance use, medical illness or another functional psychiatric disorder (e.g. another anxiety disorder, depressive illness, schizophrenia, schizoaffective disorder).

Substance misuse is common in patients with anxiety disorders and often reflects efforts to manage symptoms through self-medication. Both alcohol and benzodiazepines have rapid anxiolytic effects that make them attractive for the acute management of anxiety but are associated with a variety of adverse effects (sedation, poor coordination, disinhibition and dependency potential) and also tend to result in worsening 'rebound' anxiety as their effects wear off. The use of these agents to deal with specific situations of social discomfort emphasizes the socio-phobic element of his difficulties.

Given the prominent physical symptoms with a substantial situational context, it is hardly surprising that both genetic and environmental factors are implicated in the causation of anxiety disorders. The considerable comorbidity between different anxiety disorders is associated with many similarities in relation to perceived causation. The heritability of anxiety disorders has been estimated between 30% and 50%. Although twin studies and family clustering support some specificity for specific disorders, studies also indicate a more generalized vulnerability towards anxiety disorder with the specific pattern of symptoms shaped by environmental factors. Recent work has identified that a genomic duplication (DUP25) on chromosome 15 that occurs in 7% of the normal population is present in more than 90% of patients with panic disorder.

From a psychological perspective, there are many similar themes about the genesis of anxiety disorders (e.g. they are more common in patients with 'anxious' personality profiles). They are thought to reflect adverse development experiences relating to abnormal attachment characterized by overprotective and/or emotionally cold parenting by anxiety-prone parents. They are also linked to early loss and traumatic experiences that impact a person's perception of the world as a predictably safe place.

There are some differences in the dominant themes of each disorder. The theme of lack of control and a propensity to view ambiguous situations as threatening is particularly linked to GAD and is thought to underpin the excessive and generalized fearfulness of everyday experiences. For conditions that include panic attacks (panic disorder, agoraphobia and socio-phobia), a combination of biological vulnerability towards an extreme physiological anxiety response (panic) is coupled with situational factors through classical conditioning. Then, this relationship is maintained by operant conditioning through avoidance behaviours.

There remains considerable debate about the relative importance of biological propensity versus environmental precipitants that underpin the primary approach to treatment (to pharmacologically reduce biological panic attack propensity versus addressing psychological aspects of the episodes). In reality, most patients have a longstanding illness at the time of presentation, and therefore, it is necessary to address the biology of anxiety and situational factors that serve to maintain illness. For specific phobias, there is much emphasis placed upon 'preparedness', while most foci for phobias have some potential danger and the propensity to develop a fear may be based upon an evolutionarily imprinted survival instinct (e.g. spiders or wild animals).

FURTHER READING

For a detailed review of neurobiological anxiety disorder studies, see: Martin EI, Ressler KJ, Binder E, Nemeroff CB. 2009 The neurobiology of anxiety disorders: Brain imaging, genetics, and psychoneuroendocrinology. Psychiatric Clinics of North America 32(3):549–575. doi:10.1016/j.psc.2009.05.004

The neurobiology of anxiety disorders indicates much overlap. However, there are also specific findings in specific anxiety disorders. In general, studies have focused on exploring the autonomic nervous system reactivity and neuroendocrine stress response, serotonergic and other neurochemical systems, γ-aminobutyric acid (GABA)ergic mechanisms based on the impact of benzodiazepines, and disturbances of brain regions/circuitry that are linked to emotional processing and the fear response.

Studies indicate disturbed functioning of autonomic reactivity (e.g. abnormal galvanic skin response) and the hypothalamic, pituitary, adrenal stress axis, but with increased reactivity (e.g. firing at locus coeruleus in response to anxiogenic agents such as yohimbine) in panic disorder, but normal baseline measures and diminished reactivity in GAD.

Moreover, 30% of patients with GAD are nonsuppressors on the dexamethasone suppression test, which highlights its biological overlap with mood disorders. The effectiveness of serotonergic agents in anxiety disorders has encouraged studies on the serotonergic parameters. These have indicated diminished 5HT receptors and transporter binding on positron emission tomography in panic disorder and reduced serotonergic function (cerebrospinal fluid/platelet binding) in GAD.

GABAergic function is suggested by the link to the mechanism of action of benzodiazepines, which have a specific binding site at GABA-A receptors and enhance GABAergic inhibition in the CNS. In addition, GABA antagonists are anxiogenic (e.g. flumazenil).

Other studies have explored brain structures that are known to mediate emotional responses to stress and threats. These studies suggest overactivity of the so-called fear/anxiety circuit that includes the amygdala, hippocampus, periaqueductal grey, locus coeruleus, thalamus, cingulate and orbitofrontal areas. Neuroimaging studies have demonstrated increased right amygdala volume in GAD.

In terms of epidemiology, the lifetime risk of panic disorder is 4%, having a panic attack is 8%, GAD is 3%—4%, specific phobias is 10% and social anxiety disorder is approximately 2%—13% (depending on the particular study and diagnostic criteria used). The epidemiology of anxiety disorders highlights their considerable overlap with other anxiety disorders, depressive illness and substance abuse disorders. For example, comorbidity rates for panic disorder include two-thirds with depression, one-third with substance abuse disorder and half with social phobia.

---

4. Colin is keen to '*get something to help with the wedding in 4 weeks*'. He also explains that he would like to engage with 'any treatment that might help' as he feels that these problems have been restricting his career progress. As an example, he explains that he constantly worries about small events at work (and at home) and tends to avoid situations that might involve being scrutinized by others. He has

Continued on following page

(Continued)

avoided taking on roles of responsibility even though he enjoys his work and would like to contribute more to the strategic side of the business.

11. What treatment options are there for the short- and long-term management of his problems?
12. What are the pros and cons of using benzodiazepines as a treatment?
13. How can we decide upon the appropriateness of pharmacological and psychological treatments?

The management of anxiety disorders has two principal elements: (1) to reduce the propensity for ongoing anxiety/panic, and (2) to address and minimize any comorbid problems and maladaptive coping mechanisms, such as avoidance behaviours and substance misuse. This requires a detailed assessment of the scope and evolution of difficulties and often requires sustained therapeutic input to allow for combined pharmacological and psychological interventions.

In the short term, it is important to explore and clarify the nature of any symptoms. An explanation of how physical symptoms related to stress can often prevent a spiral of increasing psychological distress and somatization in response to physical symptoms occurring in response to psychological stress. Many patients find simple interventions around anxiety management and relaxation training allow them to gain better control over their symptoms.

Most pharmacological interventions have a delayed onset of action of between 2 and 4 weeks, and thus, the short-term use of benzodiazepines can allow symptom control in the early stages of treatment. Many patients report that having access to a remedy for anxiety (e.g. benzodiazepine) in itself reduces the fear of losing control and reduces the need to use such an option, although the use of benzodiazepines on an as-needed basis has been linked to a greater risk of subsequent dependency. Of note, benzodiazepines are only licensed for short-term use in anxiety disorders because of their adverse effects that include sedation, slurred speech, ataxia, cognitive dulling, potentiation and cross-tolerance with alcohol, dependence and recreational abuse potential. Use of benzodiazepines may also interfere with the benefits of psychological interventions. Benzodiazepines should be generally avoided in patients with a history of dependence (e.g. alcohol) or those who have particular demands (e.g. working with heavy or complex machinery, driving) for optimal alertness, and those with a history of aggression or impulsivity. Long-term use in maintenance therapy should be reserved for more severe and intractable cases in which other pharmacological and psychological interventions have not been successful. In Colin's case, simple educational interventions and a short course of benzodiazepines can allow for symptom control/stabilization in the short-term, including in the lead up to the wedding that has been worrying him.

For long-term management of anxiety disorders, a range of pharmacological and psychological approaches have demonstrated their efficacy, and in general, these have similar success rates with some evidence that combination therapy may be better than either alone. Most patients with moderate or severe symptoms receive both psychological and pharmacological inputs because anxiety disorders tend to run a chronic course, and achieving optimal symptom control often requires trialling a variety of interventions. The choice of treatment in individual patients is largely directed by their symptom pattern, treatment preferences, pattern of engagement with different interventions (e.g. attendance at psychological therapy sessions and medication compliance) and concerns regarding potential adverse effects with medications.

Cognitive behavioural approaches have demonstrated effectiveness for anxiety disorders. The content and focus of sessions differ according to the pattern of anxiety (generalized versus panic) and the actual focus of fears. In GAD, cognitive behavioural therapy (CBT) typically includes elements such as psychoeducation, symptom monitoring, relaxation training, symptom exposure and cognitive restructuring. A typical course spans 12–16 sessions. In panic disorder and agoraphobia, the principal psychological treatments include CBT (as above-mentioned, but also with habituation to fearful cues) and exposure (controlled *in vivo* exposure to panicogenic situations) or both. In cognitive restructuring, patients are assisted in identifying negative automatic thoughts and to challenge these misinterpretations and de-catastrophize by graded exposure. In socio-phobia, exposure is an important aspect of therapy, which involves graded exposure to anxiety-provoking situations until these are gradually mastered. Group approaches are favoured, along with social skills training. Confronting avoidances and cognitive restructuring to promote focusing externally rather than internally in social situations are also common elements.

There is evidence to support the use of serotonin specific reuptake inhibitors (SSRIs), serotonin and noradrenaline reuptake inhibitors, monoamine oxidase inhibitors, azapirones, pregabalin and older agents, such as imipramine and trazodone, in the treatment of anxiety disorders. The use of other agents, such as beta-adrenergic blockers, is less well-supported but preferred by some clinicians. These various approaches appear to have similar effectiveness (although well-designed comparison studies are lacking) and, hence, treatment choice is primarily determined by tolerability issues.

FURTHER READING

Look up the National Institute for Health and Care Excellence guidelines for the management of anxiety disorders in adults: NICE (National Institute for Health and Care Excellence). (2011) Generalised anxiety disorder and panic disorder in adults: management, CG113. Available at: http://guidance.nice.org.uk/CG113

Consequently, SSRIs are the preferred first-line treatment and have demonstrated efficacy across the anxiety disorder spectrum. The typical onset of action is 2—4 weeks. If using antidepressant agents, especially SSRIs, one needs to be aware of the potential for hyperstimulation in the early stages of treatment, which is linked to early treatment drop out. This can be minimized by gradual dose escalation.

The azapirones (e.g. buspirone) are indicated as second-line therapy and lack the sedative effects of benzodiazepines, have reduced dependency potential and do not potentiate the effects of alcohol. The onset of action is 2—4 weeks.

Pregabalin is a GABA analogue that is classed as an antiepileptic agent. Long-term trials have shown continued effectiveness in anxiety disorders without the development of tolerance. Unlike benzodiazepines, it has a beneficial effect on sleep and sleep architecture, produces less severe cognitive and psychomotor impairment and has a low potential for abuse and dependence. Therefore, it may be preferred over benzodiazepine. It is increasingly considered as a first-line treatment option.

As pharmacological and psychological interventions have similar effectiveness, the choice of treatment is guided by patient preference, adverse effects profile, previous response and adherence. Ultimately, the patient should dictate treatment because there is evidence that they are more likely to respond (possibly because of better adherence) to the treatment they most believe in.

---

5. Colin successfully manages the wedding without using benzodiazepines as after a discussion he recognizes the dangers of their sedative and potentially disinhibiting effects. He subsequently undergoes a trial of escitalopram and engages with a course of CBT. He also attends the local mindfulness group. Over the following six months, his symptoms settle, and he reports getting on much better in his work and personal life. He takes up squash to engage in regular exercise and minimizes his intake of alcohol without totally discontinuing it. He contacts the service to request that his general practitioner manage his care. Two years later, he is re-referred for assessment with an acute exacerbation of symptoms.

14. What are the principal diagnostic considerations at this point?

Several possible factors may be relevant to this recurrence of symptoms. Typically, symptoms will be related to a specific stressor or circumstance. However, it is important to consider the relationship between cause and effect (put another way, some events are independent of the illness process, whereas others are dependent upon it).

Colin's previous history of depression makes this an important differential, and careful assessment for depressive symptoms is required. Issues of ongoing treatment compliance and adherence to lifestyle practices (e.g. exercise and substance avoidance) need to be explored. It is important to consider the possibility of a physical illness underpinning his symptoms, even where such possibilities were previously ruled out.

---

6. It emerges that Colin had discontinued his medication 6 months ago and gradually stopped engaging in social situations. He had become more preoccupied with the hassles of life, leading up to a panic attack just before the re-referral. He agrees to recommence medication and attend 'top-up' sessions with a psychologist. Colin's condition again settles. He later attends with his wife wondering if he should again try to go for a period medication-free, as in retrospect he relates his relapse to some work stresses rather than discontinuing medications or other anxio-protective activities (e.g. regular exercise).

15. What is the likely outcome of discontinuing medication?

16. What is the prognosis for major anxiety disorders?

Once symptoms have stabilized the issue of optimal maintenance therapy often arises. The course of anxiety disorders is variable, but for many, the condition is persistent, and the focus of ongoing treatment is to achieve optimal symptom control and maximize socio-adaptive functioning. Patients in whom symptom control has been achieved with medication, symptom recurrence is very common on discontinuation. Evidence suggests that psychological interventions are associated with more enduring benefits, including reduced symptom propensity beyond the initial period following exposure (thus, contrasting with the chemical effect of pharmacological interventions). Therefore, treatment may be sequenced to use medications for stabilization, followed by psychological approaches for more enduring symptom control, and thus, enabling the reduction or discontinuation of the medications prescribed.

Overall, the prognosis of anxiety disorders is quite variable. The majority of patients gain good symptom control and functional recovery. However, 50% have persisting anxiety symptoms. A better outcome is associated with less severe symptoms, absence of comorbid disorders (personality, other anxiety disorders or substance abuse), 'good' or robust premorbid personality, strong social capital and active engagement with treatment.

CHAPTER 8

Norma

Perinatal Mental Illness

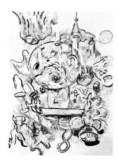

1. Describe the prevalence of perinatal psychiatric disorders.
2. Explain the principles that guide the differential diagnosis of postnatal mental disturbance.
3. Recognize how baby blues, postnatal depression and postpartum psychosis can be distinguished.
4. Recognize the relative risks posed by perinatal psychiatric disorders.
5. Outline the management of postpartum psychiatric disorder.
6. Appreciate the merits of providing care in mother and baby units.
7. Discuss the prognosis of postnatal depression and postpartum psychosis.

1. Norma is a 24-year-old woman who is referred by her general practitioner for an assessment of low mood. She has a history of a depressive episode two years ago, which responded to a serotonin and noradrenaline reuptake inhibitor after a failed trial of a serotonin-specific reuptake inhibitor. She is 14 weeks pregnant with the child of her boyfriend of 18 months, Clive. Norma reports some low mood, 'but not as severe as her previous depressive episode' and confides that she is worried about her future and whether the unplanned pregnancy might affect her relationship with Clive. She reports anergia, intermittent anxiety and loss of libido, but no other major depressive symptoms. Clive, who has accompanied her, tells you that he is pleased with the pregnancy and hopes that they might get married when he finds regular work.

   1. What are your immediate thoughts about this presentation?
   2. What intervention would you advise?

It is not uncommon for patients with less serious symptoms to be referred during pregnancy, especially where there is a history of previous psychiatric problems. The previous episode appears consistent with a depressive episode of moderate to severe intensity, which required a second trial of antidepressant treatment before it resolved. The symptoms described here seem more consistent with adjustment difficulties and are not uncommon in first and unplanned pregnancies. However, it is still important to carefully probe for the full range of depressive symptoms, including loss of interest, feelings of hopelessness, sleep disturbances, fatigue and low energy. Addressing issues of psychological and social support, and ongoing monitoring of progress can often suffice for this type of presentation, which includes adjustment difficulties.

The duration of antidepressant therapy should be clarified. For a first episode, it would be usual to continue treatment for six months after symptom resolution and monitor for recurrence thereafter.

FURTHER READING

For a review of antidepressant use in the perinatal period, see: Molenaar NM, Kamperman AM, Boyce P, Bergink V. (2018) Guidelines on treatment of perinatal depression with antidepressants: An international review. Australian and New Zealand Journal of Psychiatry 52(4): 320–327. doi:10.1177/0004867418762057

The use of antidepressant treatment during pregnancy is generally safe but warrants careful consideration of the necessity for pharmacological intervention. It is important to recognize that untreated depression can impact self-care and seeking help regarding prenatal care. Experiencing major depression during pregnancy is associated with an increased risk of premature birth and low birth weight, while unstable depression during pregnancy increases the risk of postpartum depression, early termination of breastfeeding and impacts upon mother–infant bonding. Serotonin-specific reuptake inhibitors (fluoxetine, citalopram and sertraline) are generally considered safe in pregnancy, while paroxetine has been linked to a small increase in congenital heart defects. Serotonin and noradrenaline reuptake inhibitors (duloxetine and venlafaxine) are also thought to be appropriate, but with the caveat that they may be associated with an increased risk of postpartum haemorrhage.

---

2. Norma attends several supportive sessions with the community mental health nurse and agrees to link in with her general practitioner and a public health nurse. The symptoms settle over 2–3 weeks and she gives birth to a healthy baby boy one week after the expected date of delivery. Two days postpartum, she is noted to be emotionally labile with periods of irritability and tearfulness. The staff at the maternity hospital contact you for advice.
   3. What are the possible causes of her symptoms?
   4. How common are psychological disturbances after childbirth and what is their typical timeframe for occurrence?

The postpartum period is a time of profound emotional significance and physical challenge. Recovering from difficult or prolonged labour, initiating breastfeeding, the emotional significance of bringing new life into the world, the full realization of the practical significance of a new family member, trying to fit sleeping patterns with that of a new-born baby and the challenges of re-establishing day-to-day life can all contribute to psychological distress.

Most mothers (perhaps 75%) experience a period of emotional lability (tearfulness, sensitivity) without features of the full clinical syndrome of depression. This is often referred to as 'baby blues'. It typically occurs 2–3 days postpartum and lasts for 2–3 days. It is temporally linked to postpartum hormonal changes (reductions in oestrogen, progesterone and prolactin).

Postnatal depression occurs in 10%–15% of mothers. The onset is typically later than the baby blues and peaks at three weeks postpartum; however, it may be delayed in onset for months. In general, any depressive episode occurring within one year of childbirth is considered postnatal (Fig. 8.1). Characteristic themes include feelings of guilt regarding perceived inadequacy as a mother, concerns about the baby's well-being and obsessional fears that the baby might come to

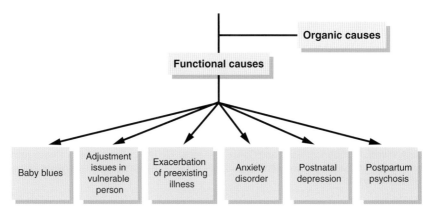

Fig. 8.1 Differential diagnosis of postnatal mental disturbance.

harm. The postnatal period is characterized by considerable disruption to biological functions such that many of the features of the so-called 'somatic syndrome' are difficult to assess (e.g. disturbed sleep, anergia, loss of libido). Careful assessment of the patient's cognitive 'set' (i.e. their perspective of the world and how they relate to it), is a key element for accurately identifying clinical depression. This includes exploring for the cognitive triad of depressive illness, which is reflected in negative thoughts about one's self, the world and the future.

Postpartum anxiety disorders occur in 10%—20% of women and are usually recurrences of pre-existing disorders. Around 10% of cases represent first episodes and can include specific themes around reactions to childbirth or worries regarding the well-being of their child or the responsibilities of motherhood. Obsessional symptoms can pose challenges in clarifying issues of risk where themes of harm to the baby are present. A key issue in distinguishing obsessional symptoms is clarifying how they are perceived by the individual and whether they are ego—dystonic and if they have been acted upon in any way (for more discussion, see Chapter 9).

Postpartum psychosis occurs in 1 in 1000 births. Onset is usually within one month of childbirth and peaks at two weeks postpartum. It is characterized by a pleomorphic clinical picture that includes elements of mood disturbance, paranoid psychosis and organic brain disturbance. The latter element includes apparent confusion and perplexity. The majority of the cases are biologically linked to bipolar affective illness in relation to both dominant acute psychopathological conditions (i.e. there are prominent affective symptoms present), illness course and genetics (many patients are subsequently diagnosed as having a bipolar illness with further episodes occurring outside of the perinatal period).

---

3. Norma's mental state settles over 2—3 days, and she is discharged home. Ten days postpartum you receive a call from her general practitioner who reports that Clive has contacted him to report that 'Norma is not herself' and 'seems obsessed with the baby, insisting on staying with him at all times', and that he awoke the previous night to find her standing over the baby, tearful, and saying that the baby was 'not right'. They agree to attend for an assessment that afternoon.
    5. What are the possible diagnoses?
    6. What additional information would you seek?
    7. How does postnatal depression compare with depressive illness occurring at other times?

This presentation is concerning, particularly because of the unusual ideas about the baby. Although these ideas may reflect obsessional worries underpinned by depressive illness, they may also represent the emergence of more abnormal ideas in-keeping with a psychotic process. It will be important to clarify the actual health and well-being of the baby and the precise nature of these ideas and any associated thoughts or impulses regarding how Norma feels the baby should be managed. It will be necessary to clarify Norma's attitude towards the baby and identify thoughts that might indicate that the baby is at any risk.

FURTHER READING

For a review of the management of mental health disorders relating to childbirth and its aftermath, see the National Institute for Health and Care Excellence (NICE) guidelines: NICE (National Institute for Health and Care Excellence). (2014) Antenatal and postnatal mental health: clinical management and service guidance, CG192. Available at: https://www.nice.org.uk/guidance/cg192

Remember that obsessional thoughts are ego-dystonic, while delusional ideas are associated with a morbid process that includes diminished insight and reality testing. While both can be distressing, obsessional thoughts are typically perceived as being less acceptable to the individual or are perceived as alien or foolish (i.e. are ego-dystonic). Arrangements for ongoing support and supervision of Norma and the baby will need to be carefully explored with her partner and other relevant family or friends.

Postnatal depression is largely similar to depression occurring at other times but does pose challenges in accurately assessing for somatic disturbances that are related to a depressive process rather than the considerable challenges of adjusting to motherhood. The negative cognitive distortions of postnatal depression typically include themes of being an inadequate mother or feeling overwhelmed and unable to cope. In addition, the emotional intensity of such a significant life event can aggravate interpersonal relationships and rekindle feelings of resentment or frustration with key relatives, including those that relate to one's own mother.

From a therapeutic perspective, these considerations are pertinent to the provision of psychological support. Pharmacological management is generally similar to depressive illness with the additional considerations of the potential for psychotropics to be transferred to the baby via breastfeeding and the need to minimize any adverse effects that might impact upon the mother's capacity to engage with and care for her baby. In general, sertraline and paroxetine are found in lower concentrations in breast milk than fluoxetine and venlafaxine.

FURTHER READING

For a review of psychotropics and breast-feeding, see: Larsen ER, Damkier P, Pedersen LH, et al. (2015) Use of psychotropic drugs during pregnancy and breast-feeding. Acta Psychiatrica Scandinavica 132(S445):1–28.

---

4. At the assessment, Norma explains that she has been worrying about her baby's health because a friend's baby died from sudden infant death syndrome. Probing for abnormal beliefs about the baby does not indicate any evidence of psychosis, and Norma denies any thoughts of harming herself or the baby. She describes feeling 'overwhelmed' and 'guilty about being hopeless as a mother'. Since hospital discharge, she has not been sleeping (even when the baby is asleep), has barely eaten and has little interest in things. She has been discouraging family and friends from visiting because she says that she does not want them to see her not coping.

8. How would you manage this presentation?

This presentation is much more suggestive of postpartum depression than the previous features of adjustment/baby blues. The character (range and severity) and the persistence of symptoms are indicative of a depressive illness with a distorted cognitive set (negative self-regard and guilt) and biological disturbance (insomnia, anorexia and anergia). Of note, the assessment does not indicate severe depressive illness with psychosis. This should be clarified along with a formal risk assessment focusing upon the welfare and safety of both Norma and her baby.

Given Norma's previous history and current presentation, it would be appropriate to commence antidepressant therapy. Venlafaxine has previously been used successfully, and therefore, is an obvious first choice agent to prescribe.

A key consideration is to explore the current levels of support for Norma in her efforts to manage the demands of motherhood. Optimizing support levels, with clear guidance as to how any further deterioration should be managed can be discussed with her partner and other relevant family and/or friends. Efficient communication with her GP and the public health nurse can allow for the identification of available support and assist in the ongoing assessment of how well she is adjusting.

5. Norma commences venlafaxine and returns home with a plan for ongoing support and review from the community mental health nurse, along with a scheduled appointment in a week. However, two days later, she is brought to an accident and emergency clinic having been found at the local shopping centre in a confused and agitated state, refusing to talk or let anybody see her baby whom she had covered with a blanket. In the clinic, she confides to the crisis nurse that she is worried that her baby may be 'bad inside', and that 'it was wrong to bring him into the world'. Upon direct questioning, she says that she knows this because her Aunt Phyllis (deceased) has been whispering it to her.

   9. What is this presentation indicative of?
   10. What is your immediate treatment plan?
   11. How would you manage Norma's access to her baby?

The presentation is now much more florid and includes overt psychosis with probable delusions and hallucinations. These features are probably mood-congruent as they include depressive themes. Therefore, this presentation is indicative of postpartum psychosis.

These experiences are also being acted upon (covering the baby up), which gives cause for concern and confers a need to ensure the safety of Norma and her baby while ongoing assessment and treatment occur. The demands of such observation (continuous monitoring by a skilled mental health professional) suggest that inpatient care is the most appropriate option. Although Norma is floridly psychotic, she may still retain the capacity to accept suggested help voluntarily and this can be explored with her. The input of her partner can be of considerable assistance in making such decisions.

Acute psychiatric admission facilities are often not appropriate places for a baby to be cared for and the availability of a specialized mother and baby unit should be explored as such facilities can potentially allow for minimal disruption of normal contacts with the baby and also facilitate the development of parenting skills. However, the benefits may be minimal during the acute/florid phase of the illness. As Norma recovers, a specialized unit will allow for careful supervision as Norma adjusts to increasing periods of access to her baby.

FURTHER READING

For a review of postpartum psychosis, see: Bergink V, Rasgon N, Wisner KL. (2016) Postpartum psychosis: Madness, mania and melancholia in motherhood. American Journal of Psychiatry 173(12):1179–1188. doi:10.1176/appi.ajp.2016.16040454

Norma's presentation indicates the need for antipsychotic treatment. An atypical antipsychotic agent given orally would be the preferred treatment. This will usually be added to the antidepressant therapy in cases that include symptoms of psychotic depression. Access to her baby should be restricted to carefully supervised periods until her abnormal ideas have abated.

6. Twenty-four hours after (voluntary) admission Norma becomes acutely agitated, demanding to leave the hospital with her baby. She is aggressive to nursing staff and shouts that they 'are in league with the cult', 'taking children away to abuse them'. You are asked to assess the situation and review Norma's treatment plan.
    12. Is a change to her current treatment warranted?
    13. Is involuntary treatment an option?
    14. How effective is electroconvulsive therapy for postpartum psychosis?

The use of involuntary procedures for the treatment of mental disorders is based upon the recognition that mental disorders can differ from other illness in respect of the capacity of sufferers to recognize that they are unwell and/or might benefit from treatment. This is assessed as part of the mental state examination under insight. Not all patients with diminished insight warrant involuntary treatment but such procedures are appropriate (and legislated for) where the patient's illness poses a significant risk to self or others (the interpretation of significance can vary) and/or they are unlikely to recover without treatment, and that treatment is likely to be of discernible benefit. This latter criterion is sometimes considered according to whether involuntary approaches are the only realistic means of providing necessary care.

Norma's current mental state would suggest that she is unwell to the extent that she lacks insight and is preoccupied with, and acting upon, delusional ideas in a way that would place both herself and baby at risk and would not be consistent with optimal care. In many cases, patients can be persuaded of the wisdom of accepting ongoing care voluntarily (although voluntarily accepting care requires that the patient can give such a commitment). However, involuntary procedures are required in approximately 5%–10% of admissions.

In addition to addressing whether appropriate treatment can be continued voluntarily, Norma's agitation will need to be addressed through psychological support, reassurance and possibly sedative medications. The sedative action of antipsychotic agents can be increased and/or the addition of a short course of benzodiazepines may be warranted. Treatment may need to be given as a dispersible antipsychotic agent or intramuscularly. Lorazepam is the preferred benzodiazepine for intramuscular administration because it has more predictable bioavailability when given by this route. It is important to remember that intramuscular administration results in approximately twice as much active agent becoming bioavailable and dosages should be adjusted accordingly. It may be necessary to initiate 1:1 nursing observation to allow for more intensive monitoring of Norma's mental state, provision of ongoing psychological support and to minimize any risk of Norma absconding from the unit.

Electroconvulsive therapy (ECT) is an option that can allow for rapid treatment of psychotic depression and is advocated by many as an effective treatment for postpartum psychosis. Most likely, the effectiveness reflects the general impact of ECT upon more severe affective psychosis rather than a specific effect for postpartum psychosis. The seriousness of many cases of postpartum psychosis is such that rapid intervention is particularly desirable. ECT is indicated for patients who do not respond to or cannot tolerate pharmacological interventions and those with symptoms that require rapid treatment because of concerns over safety and/or self-care.

7. Norma is scheduled for biweekly, high-dosage unilateral electroconvulsive therapy. Her mental state settles over the next 10 days or so, but treatment is continued for six applications. Her mood improves, and the psychotic symptoms cease such that her contacts with the baby are gradually increased. She begins to ask about reinitiating breastfeeding. She is distressed by what she can recall about events and is keen to know more about the cause. Norma and her partner schedule a meeting

with you prior to discharge to discuss an ongoing management plan and are concerned about the likelihood of recurrence of her symptoms in the future (including if she decides to have another child).

15. How frequently should electroconvulsive therapy be administered, at what dosage/location and how long should a course be continued?
16. How would you explain her illness to her in terms of diagnosis?
17. How should the immediate posthospital period be managed and how can the risk of further illness be minimized?

ECT remains a controversial treatment in psychiatry that is indicated for depressive illness that is particularly severe (e.g. treatment-resistant) and/or requires urgent intervention because of concerns about risk or ability to self-care. The continued controversy around ECT reflects concerns regarding the association between ECT and cognitive impairments that include persistent problems with retrograde amnesia and autobiographical memory loss. Cognitive problems are much less frequent with modern brief-pulse low energy stimulation as opposed to older ECT machines, which used sine-wave stimulation. In addition, evidence over the past decade has emphasized how unilateral ECT (both electrodes placed on the nondominant side of the brain) is associated with less cognitive effects. However, high-dosage treatment is needed to achieve similar efficacy to the more traditional bilateral ECT. Bilateral ECT is still preferred where effectiveness or speed of the effect is a primary concern. Dosing is dictated according to the seizure threshold (ST). Historically, a fixed starting dose of 200—225 mC was often applied. However, more recently it has been recognized that there are considerable variations in ST and that the use of low dosages at the commencement of ECT can establish the actual ST and help guide dosing during therapy (typically 50%—100% increase on ST for bilateral ECT with 100%—200% for unilateral ECT). There is a lack of precision regarding the optimal number of treatments, but typically 6—12 applications are given on a twice weekly frequency. The actual procedure of ECT itself is extremely safe (mortality 2/100,000, which is in-keeping with anaesthetic mortality).

FURTHER READING

For a review of ECT, see the NICE practice guidelines: NICE (National Institute for Health and Care Excellence). (2003) Guidance on the use of electroconvulsive therapy, TA59. Available at: https://www.nice.org.uk/guidance/ta59

The precise mechanism of action of ECT is not known. However, it does impact considerably upon a variety of neurotransmitter systems (especially monoamines), elevates neurotrophin release (e.g. brain-derived neurotrophic factor) and activates the neuroendocrine stress-axis, both of which are implicated in mood disorders.

Postpartum psychosis frequently reflects an underlying bipolar affective disorder with some studies suggesting that as many as 95% of sufferers are diagnosed with a bipolar illness at five-year follow-up. In other cases, unipolar depression and schizophrenia may be the underlying conditions. This distinction is important in planning for optimal ongoing management both in general and during future childbirth. Maintenance treatment with mood-stabilizing pharmacotherapy is particularly relevant where a bipolar illness is the underlying diagnosis, while antidepressant and/or antipsychotic therapy is indicated for the other circumstances.

Once Norma's mental state has stabilized, a careful plan for postdischarge care is needed that includes regular contact (e.g. day hospital, outpatients) to facilitate readjustment and allow for the ongoing monitoring of her mental state. Sleep loss is a major precipitant of mania such that optimizing the quality of sleep is a key consideration. Partner/family support with night-time feeding is immensely helpful. Community-based supports (e.g. public health nurse, mother and baby groups) can be particularly helpful components of a comprehensive ongoing care plan. It is important to ensure that all these parties collaborate so that any emerging difficulties are quickly recognized and responded to.

The risk of recurrence of postpartum psychosis is substantial, both in terms of further postpartum episodes and episodes not directly related to pregnancy and childbirth. The risk of recurrence of postpartum psychosis is estimated at 50% with higher rates where prophylactic treatment is not used.

CHAPTER 9

Kathleen

Obsessive–Compulsive Disorder

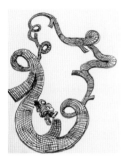

LEARNING OBJECTIVES

1. Describe the key clinical diagnostic features of obsessive–compulsive disorder (OCD) and list some important differential diagnoses along with common comorbid disorders.
2. Briefly describe the epidemiology of OCD, including the incidence, prevalence and gender differences.
3. Describe the postulated cause for OCD and consider this in terms of medical/biological, social and psychological factors.
4. List the main investigations involved in the assessment, diagnosis and ongoing treatment of OCD, beginning with a detailed history, mental state examination and collateral history. Furthermore, consider these investigations as medical/biological, social and psychological in nature.
5. Describe the main treatments for OCD and consider these in terms of medical/biological, social and psychological approaches.
6. Briefly describe the key prognostic factors for OCD and compare its prognosis to other major mental disorders.

1. The first patient at your afternoon outpatient clinic is Kathleen, a 46-year-old married mother of three, who was referred for urgent consultation by a local general practitioner. Before she enters, the clinic secretary tells you that she arrived before lunch and has asked about her appointment time on 5–6 occasions since arriving. The general practitioner referral is brief, indicating that she is not known to him, but attended earlier that morning with her husband in a distressed state having revealed to him the previous day that she has been having thoughts about harming their children. Of note, her mother,

Continued on following page

(Continued)

who had lived with the family for some years, died four months previously and Kathleen reports feeling 'down' ever since. Although she had reassured the general practitioner that she would never actually harm her children, he felt it prudent that she receives expert review as soon as possible.

1. What are your immediate thoughts about this presentation?
2. What is filicide and how common is it?

This urgent referral raises immediate concerns regarding the potential risk of serious harm to this woman's children. Of note, she appears to be actively seeking help. The context of recent significant loss (bereavement) and reports of low mood warrants careful consideration.

FURTHER READING

For a detailed review of filicide, see: Resnick PJ. (2016) Filicide in the United States. Indian Journal of Psychiatry 58(Suppl 2):S203–S209. doi:10.4103/0019-5545.196845

Filicide, or the deliberate killing of one's own child, is an uncommon event and is associated with serious parental psychiatric illness, especially psychotic depression and schizophrenia. It is estimated that about 2.5% of all homicide arrests in the United States are for parents who have killed their children.

2. At the consultation, Kathleen is initially very tearful and difficult to engage. She explains that she has been feeling very low since her mother's death. She feels physically and emotionally exhausted, and she is sleeping poorly. She has constantly been checking on the children as she has had a 'bad feeling' that something untoward could happen to them. In the past week, she has taken to visiting the school during break times to check on their safety.

3. What additional information about her symptoms would you seek?

Kathleen describes symptoms of disturbed mood and a preoccupation with the safety of her children. In addition to assessing for depressive symptoms, the nature of her preoccupations should be carefully examined. Her attitude towards the thoughts—why she thinks the children might be in danger and the extent to which she can objectively appreciate the risk—must be probed. The initial report indicates that she had been having thoughts that she could harm her children, and this should be explored carefully. The extremely distressing nature of these thoughts also raises concerns as to Kathleen's risk to herself.

3. Kathleen reports a range of depressive symptoms, including initial and middle insomnia, anergia, poor appetite with a 7-kg weight loss (she has dropped a dress size), loss of interest in her usual activities, social withdrawal and loss of libido. She reports feeling 'disgusted' and 'repulsed by' the thoughts that harm might come to her children, including worries that she could be responsible for their harm by not caring for them properly or inadvertently feeding them contaminated food.

She reports feeling afraid that having lost her mother, she needs to take special care of her remaining family. She reports that she feels she could have done more to care for her mother, who lived with the family during a prolonged illness but is unable to identify any specific thing that she might have done differently.

She admits to considering ending it all with an overdose as she feels useless and a burden on her family. It emerges that she has always been quite a particular person, being extremely house-proud and 'a stickler for punctuality'. She typically spends considerable amounts of time cleaning and polishing as she has always worried about 'dirt'. She keeps a variety of disinfectants in the house. These preoccupations have worsened considerably over the past few months to the point whereby Kathleen has been struggling to find time to cook as she is so busy cleaning and checking on her children's well-being.

4. What are the features of obsessional thoughts and compulsive behaviour and how can you probe for them?

5. What are the common themes for obsessional and compulsive phenomena?
6. How do they differ from other preoccupations, such as phobic, hypochondriacal or dysmorphophobic ideas?
7. What is the differential diagnosis and what is the relationship between obsessive–compulsive disorder and other conditions, such as mood and anxiety disorders, psychotic illness and organic conditions?

Obsessions are recurrent, intrusive and distressing thoughts, images or impulses. Obsessional thoughts differ from other preoccupations by their intrusiveness, distressing effect, ego-dystonic nature (i.e. out of keeping with the person's core beliefs and perspective—'not my own real thoughts'); importantly, the individual experiencing them recognizes the abnormal and unreasonable nature of the thoughts. This can vary from regarding the thoughts as 'silly', 'foolish' or 'crazy', to simply perceiving them as abnormal by their excessive nature.

Compulsive behaviours are repetitive actions that are seemingly with purpose that the person feels a compulsion to perform. Resisting carrying out these acts is anxiety-provoking. Compulsive behaviours are commonly linked to obsessional thoughts.

A key characteristic of obsessive and compulsive symptoms is their severity and functional impact. These symptoms are excessive, in frequency or intensity, cause significant distress and interfere with one's ability to function in day-to-day life. This latter criterion distinguishes true compulsions from other repetitive 'pleasurable' activities, such as substance use or gambling.

FURTHER READING

For a clinical review of OCD, see: Veale D, Roberts A. (2014) Obsessive-compulsive disorder. The British Medical Journal 348:g2183. doi:10.1136/bmj.g2183

Common themes for symptoms of obsessive–compulsive disorder (OCD) include checking, washing, contamination, obsessional doubts (approximately 50%), counting, symmetry and aggressive or religious themes (approximately one-third). Moreover, 75% of the patients have both obsessions and compulsions.

Obsessional thoughts differ from phobic ideas in both theme and pattern. The focus in phobias is upon harm to oneself, whereas, with obsessional thoughts, it is typically a fear of causing harm to others. Phobias are associated with avoidance behaviour rather than compulsive actions. In hypochondriasis, the focus is usually limited to personal ill-health rather than the broader themes of obsessions and compulsions. Similarly, in dysmorphophobia, the focus is upon the sufferer's appearance. Anorexia nervosa is characterized by distorted body image with the preoccupation and behaviour focusing upon weight control. In hypochondriasis, anorexia and dysmorphobia, the thoughts are not clearly ego-dystonic. Although the latter conditions are classically restricted to themes of ill-health, distorted body image and imagined ugliness, it is unusual for some other obsessional features to be present in individuals with these conditions.

The differential diagnosis of this presentation includes a range of 'functional' and organic causes (Fig. 9.1). Any symptoms that occur in the context of a depressive episode may be secondary either as a component of depression or as an aggravation of premorbid tendencies. Depressive episodes can be associated with an exaggeration of usual 'premorbid' personality traits. However, in Kathleen's case, there is a longstanding history of obsessive–compulsive behaviour that is beyond that which could be attributed to simple obsessional personality traits, because of its intensity and impact upon her everyday functioning.

OCD is a condition that has been historically underappreciated as many sufferers work around their symptoms rather than seeking help. Consequently, prevalence estimates in the general population have been revised up to 2% from a historical (under-reported) estimated frequency of <0.5%.

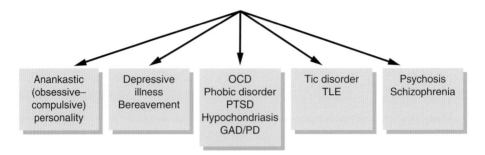

Fig. 9.1 Differential diagnosis of abnormal thoughts/preoccupations, anxiety and mood disturbance.

BOX 9.1 ■ The diagnosis of OCD is based upon:

1. Experiencing obsessional thoughts, that is, recurrent thoughts, urges, or impulses that are intrusive and unwanted, anxiogenic in nature, ego-dystonic and associated with resistance anxiety and in many cases compulsive behaviour, and/or
2. compulsive behaviour, that is, repetitive goal-directed behaviours (e.g. hand washing, ordering, checking, performing rituals) or mental actions (e.g. praying, counting, reciting words) that are excessive and/or without practical purpose and that are frequently directly related to obsessional thoughts or impulses as a means of reducing or neutralizing them.
3. The person has insight into the excessive or irrational nature of their symptoms.
4. These difficulties are time-consuming and associated with reduced functioning in social, personal or occupational activities.
5. The symptoms are not better explained by another mental disorder (e.g. paranoid illness, depressive illness, body dysmorphic disorder, eating disorder), substance effects, gambling or other pleasurable or ego-syntonic impulse disorder, anankastic personality or physical illness.

The most likely formulation in Kathleen's case is that the emergence of clinical depression in the context of a major loss event has aggravated the underlying and longstanding OCD. Of note, two-thirds of the patients with OCD experience major depression at some point. The criteria for OCD are listed in Box 9.1.

The bereavement is a significant element of the presentation and is a significant temporal precipitating factor. Although the time frame is consistent with 'normal' grieving, the emergence of clinical depression and some abnormal guilt feelings indicate possible abnormal grief. Additional features to assess for include the extent to which Kathleen has adjusted to the death, including elements of denial or 'mummification' (maintaining the person's existence by holding on to their possessions or keeping space for them).

Other anxiety disorders can be identified according to the pattern of symptoms (see above for distinction from hypochondriasis and phobias). Patients with OCD can experience generalized anxiety and even panic episodes. However, the clinical picture is dominated by obsessions and compulsive behaviours with anxiogenic intrusiveness and resistance, which can be reduced over the short term by compulsive behaviour.

Key considerations in assessing a person presenting with unusual thoughts that have an obsessional theme are listed below.

- What is the character of the thoughts in terms of intrusiveness, sense of compulsion, sense of ego-syntonicity and impact upon the person in terms of anxiety?
- What is the focus of the thoughts?
- What behaviours are associated with the thoughts?

- What is it that the person most fears?
- How does the person view the thoughts in terms of personal ownership of the content and rationality?

OCD is typically considered a neurotic condition, wherein insight is maintained. The symptoms contrast with psychosis in that they are part of normal experience but excessive. We can often empathize with neurotic symptoms as they are part of the normal human experience. In more severe OCD, the disturbances can be so overwhelming and bizarre that it can be difficult to distinguish from psychosis. The early or prodromal phase of schizophrenia can sometimes be characterized by obsessional or compulsive symptoms prior to the emergence of full psychosis. The relationship can be further clouded by the frequency of comorbid OCD in chronic schizophrenia, which has been estimated to be diagnosable in up to 25% of cases and is associated with poorer prognosis.

Other evidence linking OCD to specific neurological conditions emphasizes the relevance of particular brain regions in OCD. Symptoms of OCD are common in tic disorders (especially Tourette's syndrome), Sydenham's chorea (an autoimmune condition occurring with rheumatic fever) and postencephalitic damage. These conditions are all characterized by disturbance of basal ganglia function and its interaction with the thalamus and prefrontal cortex. Occasionally, the seizures that can occur in temporal lobe epilepsy can involve intrusive thoughts, feelings or images that mimic OCD.

---

4. Kathleen indicates that she found her mother's death difficult but attended the funeral and has disposed of most of her possessions and renovated the room where her mother resided. She attends the grave regularly and finds this comforting. She does not report any personal health concerns or phobic symptoms. A consultation with her husband reveals that he is very supportive and appreciates that her symptoms reflect an illness that will require ongoing treatment and support. They agree to undertake a trial of antidepressant medication (fluoxetine, 20 mg) and for Kathleen to engage with a key worker in the multidisciplinary team for support and anxiety management. Over the next month, her mood, sleeping pattern, appetite and energy improve, but she continues to experience obsessional thoughts (principally about cleaning and less so in relation to the children's safety). She remains socially withdrawn, spending 3–4 hours per day cleaning the home.

    8. What is the diagnostic significance of these developments?
    9. What do we know about the pathophysiology of obsessive–compulsive disorder?
   10. What treatment strategies would you now consider?

The persistence of OCD symptoms, despite the significant improvement in the depressive illness, support the above-mentioned formulation, i.e. this is a case of depressive illness that has accentuated underlying OCD.

Studies of the pathophysiology of OCD have implicated neurochemical and structural abnormalities. Dysregulation of serotonergic mechanisms is the principal neurochemical disturbance supported by findings of hypersensitivity of postsynaptic 5-Hydroxytryptamine (5-HT) receptors and elevated cerebrospinal fluid levels of 5-Hydroxyindoleacetic acid (a serotonin metabolite) and platelet 5-HT transporters. In addition, metergoline (5-HT receptor antagonist), meta-chlorophenylpiperazine (a non-selective 5-HT–receptor agonist) and sumatriptan (5-HT$_{1D}$ and 5-HT$_{1B}$ agonist) can aggravate symptoms in patients with OCD. Elevated dopaminergic activity is suggested by the association with tic disorders, the effectiveness of dopamine blockade in their treatment and elevated sulphotransferase activity (an enzyme involved in dopamine catabolism).

FURTHER READING

For a review of the neurobiology of OCD, see: Nakao T, Okada K, Kanba S. (2014) Neurobiological model of obsessive–compulsive disorder: Evidence from recent neuropsychological and neuroimaging findings. Psychiatry and Clinical Neuroscience 68(8):587–605. doi: 10.1111/pcn.12195

Neuroimaging studies indicate a bilateral reduction in the caudate nucleus size, as well as elevated blood flow and metabolism in the basal ganglia, cingulum and orbitofrontal regions that normalize with successful treatment. Neurosurgical treatment is occasionally used (as a last resort) for OCD and focuses upon tracts that relate to the cingulum.

Genetic studies indicate an elevated frequency of OCD in first-degree relatives of sufferers (35%) and higher concordance in monozygotic than dizygotic twins (50%−80% versus 25%, respectively). Candidate genes include those involved in serotonergic metabolism (e.g. 5-HT transporter genes).

The distressing and disabling nature of OCD means that supportive inputs are an important element in assisting sufferers and their families to deal with the condition. Psychological theories of OCD suggest that the onset of obsessions occurs through association with an anxiety-provoking stimulus by classical conditioning with reinforcement of the anxiolytic effect of compulsive behaviours through operant means.

Psychological treatments are effective in two-thirds of cases and tend to focus on cognitive and behavioural elements. These include 'thought stopping' techniques for obsessions, response prevention for compulsions and exposure therapy for both. The abnormalities of cerebral blood flow/metabolism in OCD can be reversed with successful psychological interventions.

Serotonin specific reuptake inhibitors (SSRIs) are considered the first line in the pharmacotherapy of OCD and are often used at higher doses than for simple mood disorders (e.g. fluoxetine, 40−60 mg daily). The onset of their therapeutic effect can be considerably delayed and may not appear for 2−3 months in some cases. Clomipramine is an older tricyclic agent with prominent serotonergic activity that was the favoured treatment prior to the emergence of the better-tolerated SSRIs. However, it is still sometimes used as an alternative where SSRIs are found to be ineffective. Various evidence exists for the use of other strategies, such as monoamine oxidase inhibitors, buspirone and antipsychotics.

Psychosurgery is very occasionally used (cingulotomy), but only in the most severely disabling and intractable cases.

FURTHER READING

For a review of the treatment of OCD, see: Hirshtritt ME, Bloch MH, Mathews CA. (2017) Obsessive−compulsive disorder advances in diagnosis and treatment. JAMA 317(13): 1358−1367. doi:10.1001/jama.2017.2200

Treatment of OCD is similar to depression, in that it includes antidepressant agents but differs, in that the most effective agents are those with serotonergic activity and the optimal therapeutic dose is often greater than that required to treat depressive illness. Therefore, an increase in the dose of fluoxetine is warranted for Kathleen.

5. Kathleen is commenced on a higher dose of fluoxetine (40 mg per day) and engages with the psychologist for cognitive behavioural therapy, which focuses upon thought-stopping and response prevention. Her symptoms settle considerably, but at a review three months later, she indicates that she would like to consider further treatment options to try and minimize or completely stop her obsessive−compulsive disorder symptoms. Of note, her mood is good, and she no longer is experiencing worries about her children's safety. She remains preoccupied regarding issues of contamination and continues to spend 1−2 hours per day cleaning. She has decided that she would like to get out more and, if possible, return to work as a secretary in a local legal firm where she was employed until the birth of her third child.

11. What would you tell Kathleen about possible treatment options?
12. What is the natural course and prognosis of obsessive−compulsive disorder?

A further increase in fluoxetine or switching to clomipramine could further improve her symptoms. Equally, a review of therapeutic approaches used during the cognitive behavioural therapy may reveal additional strategies. There is a lack of evidence to support other strategies. The relative balance between the risk of adverse effects from treatments versus how disabling her present symptoms are, should be considered. OCD is typically a chronic condition such that full symptom resolution may not be possible for all sufferers. More extreme interventions, such as psychosurgery, are clearly not warranted in her case.

OCD is often of sudden onset, typically during the early 20s, and maybe chronic or phasic in course. Typically, 25% of patients with OCD experience major improvement with treatment, while 50% show a moderate improvement. In the remaining 25%, the course is chronic and worsens over time. A better prognosis is linked to well-adjusted premorbid status, higher socio-adaptive functioning (e.g. married, working), a clear precipitating event, episodic course, greater ego-dystonicity of symptoms and female sex. Poorer outcomes occur where the onset is early, there are comorbidities, such as a tic disorder, depressive illness or premorbid anankastic personality, less resistance to compulsive behaviours, bizarre compulsions or where symmetry is a prominent theme.

---

6. Kathleen agrees to an increase in the dose of fluoxetine to 60 mg per day. At subsequent reviews, her symptoms further settle, and she returns to work. Her general practitioner assumes responsibility for her ongoing treatment. Two years later, Kathleen is re-referred because of a marked worsening of her symptoms such that she has been struggling to attend work on time because of compulsive cleaning. She reports getting up early to start her 'chores' but finds it difficult to leave them aside to go to work. Family life is also suffering as she has been finding it hard to keep up with preparing her children for school. She confides that she decided to try and wean herself off the fluoxetine and had discontinued it eight weeks previously.

13. What are the main diagnostic considerations?

Key here will be to identify the extent to which this episode includes major disturbance of mood or if Kathleen's symptoms are mostly limited to OCD. Precipitating life events and ongoing stressors may need to be addressed. Relapse is extremely high in OCD with discontinuation of medication (estimated at 90% within two months). Studies suggest that the dose that is effective for acute treatment is likely to be the required dose for maintenance or 'the dose that makes you well, keeps you well'.

CHAPTER 10

Walter

Treatment-resistant Depression

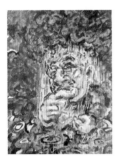

1. List the symptoms of depressive illness and understand how an episode can be graded in terms of severity.
2. Define treatment-resistant depression (TRD).
3. To understand the principles of pharmacological management of depressive illness, including TRD.
4. To understand the role of nonpharmacological approaches in the treatment of depression.
5. Describe the role of electroconvulsive therapy (ECT) in the management of depression.
6. List the side-effects of ECT.

1. Walter, a single 35-year-old farmer who lives alone, presents to his general practitioner accompanied by his sister. He reports a history of sleep disturbance with early morning awakening, poor energy, weight loss of 6 kg over the previous month or so, poor concentration and low mood. These symptoms have been present for the past six weeks and are getting worse. Walter has ongoing financial problems, having borrowed a large amount of money for new farm machinery. He is having difficulty managing the farm currently.
    1. What are your initial thoughts regarding this presentation?
    2. What are the principal complaints that patients with depressive disorders present with and what are the criteria for diagnosing mild, moderate and severe depressive illness?
    3. What further questions would you ask Walter?

Walter appears to have a depressive disorder of moderate severity. The International Classification of Diseases-10 details three severity levels of depression, including mild, moderate and severe depressive disorder. Core or 'typical' symptoms include the following: (1) depressed mood, (2) loss of interest and (3) reduced energy leading to increased fatigability. Other common symptoms are as follows:

- Reduced concentration
- Disturbed sleep
- Disturbed appetite
- Reduced self-esteem and self-confidence
- Ideas of guilt and worthlessness
- Bleak and pessimistic views of the future
- Ideas or acts of self-harm or suicide.

Classification of mild depressive disorder requires at least two of the typical symptoms, with two of the other symptoms listed above. Moderate depressive disorder requires at least two typical symptoms with at least three and preferably four of the other symptoms. In moderate depressive disorder, there is often difficulty managing social, work or domestic duties. Severe depressive disorder manifests with all three typical symptoms plus at least four other symptoms. Besides, severe agitation or retardation is often present. Psychotic symptoms may or may not be present, but when manifested, the severity of illness is inevitably considered to be severe. Delusions with guilt or nihilistic themes (sin, illness, death or imminent disaster) may be present and second person auditory hallucinations of accusatory voices or olfactory hallucinations of decomposing filth may occur. Delusions or hallucinations may be specified as mood-congruent or incongruent depending on the extent to which they can be understood in terms of the prevailing mood.

The so-called 'clinical depression' or 'biological depression' is characterized by the presence of symptoms that indicate a disturbance of body physiology and include disturbances to sleep, appetite, motor activity, energy and libido.

Probing regarding anxiety (both generalized anxiety and panic attacks), any exacerbation of preexisting phobic, obsessional symptoms or hypochondriacal preoccupations are mandatory. Excessive consumption of alcohol or self-medication can occur. It is important to document whether Walter has had a previous hypomanic or manic episode as he could potentially have a bipolar disorder with a current depressive episode.

---

2. Further questioning finds that Walter has been drinking three pints of beer at home each night for the past six weeks. He explains that 'it's the only way that I can get to sleep'. Further questioning reveals he has recently been complaining of upper gastrointestinal pain. He does not have a compulsion to drink, there is no evidence of a withdrawal state or tolerance and he is keen to stop drinking. There are no other associated comorbid obsessional or hypochondriacal preoccupations. He has not experienced symptoms suggestive of either a manic or hypomanic episode in the past, and this is his first depressive episode.

  4. List the Diagnostic and Statistical Manual of Mental Disorders-5 criteria for alcohol use disorder.
  5. How are units of alcohol calculated?
  6. What is the significance of Walter not having either a manic or hypomanic episode?

Alcohol misuse is characterized by excessive intake despite a desire or good reason to stop (e.g. ill physical effects or negative social impact). More severe alcohol misuse disorder is characterized by a pattern of increasing psychological and physical dependence whereby alcohol use increasingly occludes other activities and/or is prioritized in day-to-day patterns, and the person starts to experience greater tolerance to the effects of alcohol with withdrawal upon cessation of use (Box 10.1).

Units are a simple way of expressing the quantity of pure alcohol in a drink. One unit equals 10 mL or 8 g of pure alcohol, which is the amount of alcohol the average adult can typically process

---

BOX 10.1 ■ **Alcohol use disorders are diagnosed according to:**

1. Excessive intake of alcohol.
2. A strong desire to consume alcohol (craving).
3. Inability to control alcohol intake, even with efforts to do so.
4. Excessive time spent around alcohol use, both in terms of consumption and recovery from its effects.
5. Interference with social or occupational functioning, with evidence of increasing primacy of alcohol over other activities.
6. Continued use despite adverse effects that may be social, psychological or physical in nature.
7. Evidence of physical addiction with increasing tolerance to acute effects.
8. Evidence of physical addiction with symptoms of withdrawal upon cessation of use.

The severity of alcohol use disorder is graded as mild, moderate and severe according to the number of the above features that are evident.

---

in one hour. The strength of an alcoholic beverage is indicated by the alcohol by volume (ABV), which is the amount of pure alcohol as a percentage of the total volume of the drink. The ABV is specified on all alcoholic beverages. The number of units of alcohol in a drink can be calculated by multiplying the total volume of a drink (in mL) by its ABV (measured as a percentage) and dividing the result by 1000. The following equation shows how to calculate the number of units of alcohol in a bottle of medium strength wine:

$$\text{strength (ABV)} \times \text{volume(mL)} \div 1000 = \text{units}$$
$$13\% \times 750 \text{ mL}/1000 = 9.75 \text{ units}$$

To calculate your alcohol intake in units, visit: https://alcoholchange.org.uk/alcohol-facts/inter-active-tools/unit-calculator.

Briefly, low-strength beer has just over two units of alcohol per pint, while a strong beer (e.g. 5.5%) has three units of alcohol per pint. A typical bottle of wine has 8–11 units, while fortified wines (e.g. sherry or port) have 15–20 units of alcohol per bottle and spirits have 30 or more units of alcohol per bottle.

Establishing whether manic, mixed or hypomanic symptoms exist is important as this suggests a bipolar type illness, which has important implications for management. Antidepressant medications should be prescribed with caution in such individuals, and always in conjunction with a medication with mood-stabilizing effects due to the risk of a shift to mania.

---

3. Walter commences venlafaxine. Initially, he is prescribed 75 mg per day, which is titrated over a week to 150 mg daily. He is reviewed after a fortnight, and at that time, he admits to experiencing thoughts of self-harm with urges to commit suicide. However, he insists that he would not act on these thoughts because he is very close to his sister and her family. His dose of venlafaxine is increased to 225 mg daily as an outpatient.

Four weeks later he has failed to improve with worsening agitation, persisting thoughts of self-harm and almost total neglect of his farm. He is admitted, at which point, his dosage of venlafaxine is increased to 300 mg daily.

  7. What are the indications to admit an individual?

Indications for psychiatric admission include: (a) a high risk of suicide or harm to others in those with a mental disorder; (b) worsening psychotic symptoms; (c) severe agitation or retardation with a risk of malnutrition and death; or (d) need for medical care/investigations.

4. One month after admission to the local psychiatric hospital, Walter has failed to improve and has lost 19 kg in weight since his depressive illness began. He is complaining of poor memory and concentration, is constantly pacing and is very distressed. He is no longer able to guarantee his safety. A discussion ensues with the consultant psychiatrist regarding augmenting his antidepressant.
    8. What is treatment-resistant depression (refractory depression)?
    9. What do you know about augmenting antidepressants and other treatment modalities?

FURTHER READING

For a review of TRD and its management, see: McIntyre R, Filteau M-J, Martin L, et al. (2014) Treatment-resistant depression: definitions, review of the evidence, and algorithmic approach. Journal of Affective Disorders 156:1–7. doi:10.1016/j.jad.2013.10.043

An estimated 30%–40% of patients do not adequately benefit from initial antidepressant treatment. Treatment-resistant depression (TRD) is a term used to describe cases of major depressive disorder that do not respond adequately to appropriate courses (adequate in dosage and duration) of at least two antidepressants. Some patients are mistakenly labelled as being treatment resistant, when in fact, they are misdiagnosed or inadequately treated (e.g. because of poor adherence). The patient should be reassessed regarding personality factors, significant relationship difficulties and medications or substances known to be associated with depression for cases of persistent depression.

There is a lack of consensus regarding the optimal treatment of TRD with a variety of potential interventions that include high dosage antidepressant therapy, combination antidepressant therapy, augmentation with antipsychotic or mood-stabilizing agents, thyroid supplementation, use of dopamine agonists, psychostimulants, dexamethasone or pindolol, ECT, light therapy, sleep deprivation therapy and ketamine.

Results of the sequenced treatment alternatives to relieve depression ($STAR^*D$) programme have helped to improve the evidence for the management of TRD. All patients ($N = 2786$) were initially prescribed citalopram (level 1) with nonresponders progressing to level 2. At this stage of the trial, patients were switched to a variety of treatments, including bupropion, venlafaxine or sertraline. Alternatively, bupropion or buspirone was added to citalopram.

FURTHER READING

For a discussion on the treatment of refractory depression, see: Taylor DM, Paton C, Kapur S. (2015) The Maudsley Prescribing Guidelines in Psychiatry, 12th edition. Hoboken, NJ: Wiley-Blackwell.

For those who failed to respond during level 2 interventions, level 3 of $STAR^*D$ included augmentation of antidepressant medication with lithium or triiodothyronine. A switch to mirtazapine or nortriptyline comprised the other treatment arms at this stage of the trial. Augmenting with lithium is well supported by the literature and appears to be effective in approximately 50% of cases. There are several disadvantages to using lithium, including tolerability and toxicity issues and the need for frequent blood monitoring. (See Chapter 15 for further details on lithium therapy.) Augmentation with triiodothyronine is generally well-tolerated, and its use is borne out by $STAR^*D$. Nonresponders at this stage entered level 4 of the trial and were prescribed tranylcypromine, a monoamine oxidase inhibitor, or a combination of venlafaxine and mirtazapine (the so-called California rocket fuel because of its theoretical potential to enhance monoamine activity). Approximately half of the participants in the $STAR^*D$ study became symptom-free after two treatment levels. For all four treatment levels, almost 70% of those who did not withdraw from the study became symptom-free. A key observation in the *STAR*D* trial was that no single intervention emerged as markedly superior but that further trials were associated with small but accruing benefit in terms of response rates. This emphasizes the need in real-world practice to tailor treatment to the individual needs and preferences of patients.

Antipsychotic medications, such as olanzapine, quetiapine, risperidone and aripiprazole, have also been used successfully to augment antidepressants in treatment-resistant cases. The use of olanzapine with fluoxetine, for example, appears to display some benefits. The major disadvantage of using olanzapine is the risk of weight gain.

There has been increasing evidence that quetiapine is efficacious as an antidepressant in the acute and maintenance treatment of major depressive disorder. Its effect may be mediated by its low D2 receptor occupancy, serotonin 5-Hydroxytryptamine (5-HT)2 A, 5-HT2C antagonism and 5-HT1A partial agonist and noradrenaline reuptake inhibition. The Food and Drug Administration (FDA) review of quetiapine for treating major depressive disorder (April 2009) concluded that although quetiapine would not replace serotonin specific reuptake inhibitors (SSRI)/serotonin-norepinephrine reuptake inhibitor antidepressants within the treatment cascade, it was a valuable additional treatment option for patients not indicated for first-line therapies. In addition, its efficacy is well established in the acute and maintenance treatment of bipolar depression. The major limitations of use in major depressive disorder related to the potential for sedation, weight gain and disturbed lipid/glucose metabolism.

Agomelatine (M1/M2 melatonin agonist and 5-HT2C antagonist) and vortioxetine (a combined SSRI and serotonin receptor modulator) are relatively new antidepressants that appear to be effective in severe depression and also in the prevention of depressive relapse.

FURTHER READING

For a review of psychological approaches to TRD, see: Ijaz S, Davies P, Williams CJ, et al. (2018) Psychological therapies for treatment-resistant depression in adults. Cochrane Database of Systematic Reviews 5(5):CD010558. doi:10.1002/14651858.CD010558.pub2

Where depressive symptoms do not respond to pharmacological interventions, augmenting with psychological interventions such as cognitive behavioural therapy (CBT) may be successful. Emerging evidence supports the use of psychotherapy for moderate-to-severe TRD. An expanded role for CBT and interpersonal therapy to reduce depressive relapse in recurrent and chronic depression is supported by good evidence.

Nonpharmacological approaches, such as vagus nerve stimulation and repetitive transcranial magnetic stimulation, have shown positive results in some studies. The United States FDA has approved vagus nerve stimulation as an adjunctive therapy. However, benefits are only evident after prolonged use. In this procedure, the vagus nerve is stimulated periodically via an incision on the left neck; a stimulator electrode is cuffed around the nerve and leads are tunnelled subcutaneously to the left chest wall. Anecdotal adverse events include glottis spasm and hoarseness.

Repetitive transcranial magnetic stimulation works as a neuro-stimulator and neuro-modulator at the same time. It has been proposed that this technology can modify the functionality of the brain circuits involved in the pathophysiology of mental illness, especially depressive disorder. Evidence to date suggests that it is more effective in less severe depressive illness, and as such, its role in TRD is limited.

Ketamine has emerged as another potential option with growing popularity, particularly with the advent of intranasal delivery methods. Ketamine is an N-methyl-D-aspartate antagonist that has been used as a dissociative anaesthetic and for managing perioperative pain. It became popular in the 1990s as a 'club drug' being used recreationally as a dissociative agent ('Special K'). In depression, it acts as a euphoriant and has a rapid onset. However, its effects upon mood are transient and short-lived. Therefore, continuation therapy is often needed. To date, there is a lack of evidence of its efficacy from well-designed trials, but it represents an attractive therapeutic option.

Psychosurgery has been very occasionally used for chronic and treatment-refractory depressive illness, but it is not a realistic option for the vast majority of people with a depressive illness.

---

5. Walter declines pharmaceutical intervention, and his sister is keen for him to try electroconvulsive therapy as she has heard it can provide rapid relief to his symptoms. Walter is willing to consider this therapeutic option, and although he has a severe depressive illness, his consultant psychiatrist deems he can consent.
   10. What do you know about electroconvulsive therapy and what are its indications?
   11. What would you tell his sister regarding its efficacy?

ECT is an option for severe, life-threatening depression when a rapid response is required and/or when other treatments have failed. Indications for ECT are as follows: (1) severe biological features; (2) marked psychomotor retardation; (3) high risk of self-harm self or others; and (4) markedly diminished self-care, such as food or fluid refusal.

The National Institute for Health and Care Excellence guidelines (which have remained unchanged for many years) for ECT suggest the following: (a) obtaining valid informed consent without pressure or coercion; (b) reminding the person of their right to withdraw consent at any point; and (c) adhering to recognized guidelines about consent and involving advocates or carers. One must ensure the patient is cognizant of the risks associated with a general anaesthetic, medical comorbidities and potential adverse events, including cognitive impairment and the risks associated with not receiving ECT (i.e. continued severe depression). The mechanism of action of ECT is poorly understood, but it has demonstrated significant effects upon monoamine levels and promoting the release of neurotrophins, such as brain-derived neurotrophic factor.

During ECT, a small amount of electrical current is passed between two electrodes placed on the skull that induce a seizure. The duration of the seizure is thought to be a key indicator of the effectiveness of ECT. The so-called sham ECT in which the patient receives an anaesthetic, but no electrical stimulus, is not an effective intervention indicating that the electrical dosage is key to the effectiveness of ECT. Unilateral electrode placement involves placing both electrodes on the same side of the head. This is associated with less memory impairment but at equivalent electrical dosages is less effective than bilateral ECT where the electrodes are placed at either side of the head. ECT is usually given two or three times weekly for a total of 6–12 treatments. Potential side-effects include headache, nausea and vomiting, muscle stiffness and memory problems, particularly short-term memory problems. ECT remains one of the safest procedures given under general anaesthetic with a mortality of 1 in 50,000.

ECT is thought to be more effective than pharmacotherapy in the short term, and limited evidence suggests it is more effective than repetitive transcranial magnetic stimulation. Tricyclic antidepressants (TCAs) may improve the antidepressant effect of ECT during treatment. The rate of relapse in people who have responded to ECT can be reduced through the continuation of TCA combined with lithium.

---

6. After six sessions of electroconvulsive therapy, Walter is much improved. He is eating normally, his agitation is much less disabling and is no longer experiencing suicidal thoughts. However, he does complain of memory loss. He continues on venlafaxine 300 mg daily and after two weeks is discharged home. Furthermore, arrangements are made for him to be followed up at his local day hospital.
   12. What do we know about memory loss post electroconvulsive therapy?

FURTHER READING

For a review of ECT as a treatment, including its effects upon memory, see: Weiner RD, Reti IM. (2017) Key updates in the clinical application of electroconvulsive therapy. International Review of Psychiatry 29(2):54—62. doi:10.1080/09540261.2017.1309362

Although the modern application of ECT is considered a highly effective and generally safe intervention for severe depression, ECT remains a highly controversial treatment largely because of its reported potential to cause cognitive impairment and memory loss. This is the subject of much debate because ECT frequently causes amnesia around the time of administration and many (29%—55%) patients also report longer-term memory difficulties, in some cases persisting for years after ECT and including both retrograde and anterograde memory loss. Of note, patients with severe depression often have significant cognitive impairment during the depressive episode, which confounds efforts to attribute cognitive effects to treatment. There is a disparity between subjective memory loss reported by patients and the degree of memory impairment identified with objective testing, which suggests that significant memory loss beyond retrograde amnesia for the period when ECT was administered is uncommon or rare. Either way, if ECT is used it is important to note that cognitive effects are more severe with bilateral electrode placement, high dosage treatment, frequent (> 3 times per week) administration, multiple treatments (e.g. more than the typical 8—10 treatments in a typical course), administration while receiving lithium carbonate or anticholinergic agents and in those with pre-existing neurological diseases, such as Alzheimer's or Parkinson's disease.

CHAPTER 11

Emma

Eating Disorders

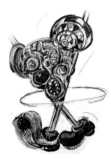

LEARNING OBJECTIVES

1. Define the main categories and key clinical diagnostic features of eating disorders.
2. Describe the epidemiology (incidence and prevalence) of common eating disorders.
3. Explain how body mass index is calculated and what are the accepted ranges for low pathological weight, overweight and obesity.
4. Describe how to assess patients with anorexia nervosa.
5. Describe the postulated biopsychosocial factors associated with eating disorders.
6. Outline the main biopsychosocial treatment strategies, including circumstances for involuntary care.
7. Describe the prognosis of eating disorders.

1. A 22-year-old single woman is referred to your psychiatric service for assessment. The referral letter is from a local general practitioner and reads as follows:

Dr J. Murphy, Majorville, Limerick
Psychiatric Clinic
Day Hospital
Long Street
Limerick
Re: Emma Kelly, The Park, Rathloe, Limerick
Dear doctor,
Please see the above named 22-year-old woman. She is the daughter of a GP colleague. She is in her final year of Dentistry at University College Dublin. Her Dad is worried about her, saying that she has been very stressed for the past two years, but this is now starting to get extreme. He feels she should never have studied Dentistry and that the course is too demanding for her.

Continued on following page

(Continued)

Emma reported to me that she is ok and felt her father 'was fussing;' she admits to having trouble concentrating on her studies and missing home. On presentation, she was very thin and scored three on the SCOFF questionnaire. Please review from a psychiatric viewpoint and advise.

Yours sincerely,

Dr Joe Murphy.

MICGP

You arrange to see the patient at your next outpatient clinic. She presents alone. She is pleasant and cooperative with the interview. Her only complaint is that of 'stress' relating to her course. She says that she has difficulty keeping up with the course and misses her parents since she moved to Dublin. She comes home every weekend and seems to be constantly studying. You notice that she appears younger than her years and is underweight, wearing baggy clothes. Her affect is bright and reactive and her mood is euthymic.

1. What is the Sick, Control, One, Fat, Food (SCOFF) questionnaire the general practitioner referred to and what is its significance?
2. You suspect an eating disorder. What further questions would you ask?

The Sick, Control, One, Fat, Food questionnaire (Box 11.1) is a primary care screening tool for eating disorders such as anorexia nervosa and bulimia nervosa. It consists of five questions. Two or more 'yes' answers indicate that further assessment is warranted. It has been shown to have high specificity of typically 80%−90% but variable sensitivity.

This detailed assessment should address each of the following areas:

1. Whether there is an underlying physical disorder.
2. Current, lowest-ever and highest-ever weights.
3. Eating pattern for a typical day and whether this varies from day to day.
4. Whether there is a history of dieting.
5. Whether there is an avoidance of certain foods or fluid restriction and any associated compensatory behaviours, such as fasting or excessive exercise.
6. If binging is present, what does it consist of and how often it occurs. The patient's feelings before, during and after the binge should be explored.
7. Whether purging behaviour, including the use of laxatives, diuretics, enemas or self-induced vomiting is present.
8. Exploration of how the patient views their own body (body image), including what they perceive as their ideal weight and how this relates to body mass index (BMI) ranges.
9. Whether amenorrhoea or a disrupted menstrual cycle is present.

A full mental state examination needs to be conducted to explore for any associated psycho-pathological condition, with an emphasis on depression, psychosis, obsessive−compulsive disorder and personality traits.

BOX 11.1 ■ The SCOFF care screening tool

[S] Do you make yourself **S**ick because you feel uncomfortably full?

[C] Do you worry you have lost **C**ontrol over how much you eat?

[O] Have you recently lost more than **O**ne stone in a 3-month period?

[F] Do you believe yourself to be **F**at when others say you are too thin?

[F] Would you say that **F**ood dominates your life?

2. It transpires that Emma has no significant depressive symptoms or evidence of psychosis. Her past medical history is unremarkable. On detailed questioning, she reveals that she is very unhappy with her body shape and weight. She reveals that she has always felt like this, but more so in recent years. She has two older sisters; although they are close, they are also very competitive. She sometimes feels that she is the 'failure' of her family as both her sisters are studying medicine. She says that she weighs herself at least daily and that her ideal weight is 'less than seven stone'. You strongly suspect anorexia nervosa. Before establishing the diagnosis, you double-check the Diagnostic and Statistical Manual of Mental Disorders-5 diagnostic criteria and satisfy yourself that it is not a different eating disorder. You obtain Emma's consent to conduct a physical examination.

  3. What are the diagnostic criteria for anorexia nervosa and bulimia nervosa?
  4. How would you explain the diagnoses of anorexia nervosa and bulimia nervosa to a colleague?
  5. How would you calculate body mass index and what is its significance?

Physical causes of weight loss, such as Crohn's disease, malabsorption syndrome, diabetes mellitus or any chronic debilitating diseases, must be ruled out. Substance misuse, for example, amphetamines, can also result in significant weight loss.

Patients with anorexia nervosa have a body weight 15% or more below their expected weight, or a BMI of 17.5 or less. They have an overwhelming idea that they are 'fat'. Moreover, they fear weight gain and often go to extremes to maintain a very low body weight. They highly value weight and shape in terms of their self-worth and may try to lose weight in a variety of ways, including food restriction, over-exercise, and purging with self-induced vomiting, laxatives, diuretics and slimming medication. They may elect to stand or move rather than sit to burn more calories. Self-loathing is often described, and weight loss can make them 'feel better about themselves'. They have difficulty escaping the cascade of obsessive behaviour that leads them to lose weight with a cycle of weighing, mirror-gazing and target weight setting. In addition to these obsessional symptoms, they may present depressive symptoms or features of a personality disorder.

Bulimia nervosa is characterized by the failure to control the urge to binge (eating a large quantity of food that is considered excessive by most people within a short period of time) and an intense preoccupation with eating. It can be challenging to diagnose as binge eating, purging and overvalued ideas involving shape and weight can occur in all eating disorders. In the individuals who are underweight and exhibit bulimic behaviours, the current classification systems would favour the diagnosis of anorexia nervosa. There is often a history of an earlier episode of anorexia nervosa in this group. In bulimia nervosa, treatment is often delayed. This is, in part, explained by the stigma of self-induced vomiting and purging. Furthermore, treatment rates have been reported to be as low as 10%. Patients usually have normal weight but can be overweight. Patients may present medically with complications such as hypokalaemia, cardiac arrhythmias, menstrual irregularities and metabolic alkalosis. In clinical practice, comorbid depression and substance abuse are common in patients.

BMI is a weight to height ratio, expressed as kg/m^2. The healthy BMI range is 18.5–24.9. A BMI below 18.5 is considered underweight, a BMI of 25–29.9 is considered overweight, and a value over 30 is considered obese. A BMI less than 17.5 in adults (or 85% of the expected weight in children) is suggestive of anorexia nervosa.

3. You arrange to meet Emma's parents to discuss her presentation. Her father is unaware of her concerns regarding her weight and body image, putting everything down to stress. Emma's mother reports *'The girls have always been such high achievers, such perfectionists. I always thought that Emma was the fussiest of them all regarding her eating and her figure. Even from an early age, she was very particular about what she would eat'.* Emma's father, Dr Kelly, becomes visibly upset as the interview

Continued on following page

(Continued)

progresses. *'She wasn't abused or neglected in any way. We treated all of the girls the same way. Maybe I was a bit demanding, but I only wanted them to work hard so they could get the best out of their education'*. Looking toward his wife, he queried, *'I think that as a child Emma spent too much time with her maternal aunt'*. He went on to explain that Emma's aunt has bulimia nervosa.

6. What is the epidemiology of anorexia and bulimia nervosa?
7. What are the key aetiological factors in anorexia and bulimia nervosa?

BOX 11.2 ■ Diagnoses of eating disorders:

Diagnosis of anorexia nervosa

1. Low weight because of caloric restriction and/or consumption (that can include dietary restriction, exercise, use of laxatives). Body weight is 15% or more below the expected value (body mass index ≤ 17.5).
2. Morbid fear of gaining weight or becoming fat.
3. Disturbed body image in respect of the perception of one's weight or shape with an excessive preoccupation on body weight and diminished recognition of the seriousness of low body weight.

Diagnosis of bulimia nervosa

1. Recurrent episodes of binge eating that involve a loss of control over intake typically over a short space of time.
2. Compensatory behaviour aimed at preventing weight gain (self-induced vomiting; prolonged fasting, laxative or diuretic use, excessive exercise).
3. Disturbed body image with regard to excessive self-evaluation according to body shape and weight.
4. The disturbance is not associated with the weight loss characteristic of anorexia nervosa.

There are several known aetiological factors, both genetic and environmental, which contribute to the development of eating disorders. See Box 11.2 for diagnoses of eating disorders.

Genetic factors

The familial nature of anorexia nervosa is well established. There is a significantly greater lifetime prevalence of anorexia nervosa (3%–12%) in first-degree relatives of patients than in the relatives of controls (0–4%), i.e. the relatives of those with anorexia nervosa are 11 times more likely to have anorexia than the relatives of controls. Similarly, for bulimia nervosa, the risk in first-degree relatives of patients is estimated to be between 4 and 10 times greater than that in the relatives of controls.

Cross-transmission occurs as relatives of individuals with an eating disorder have an increased risk of developing either anorexia or bulimia nervosa. As suggested, genetic influences may increase with age, mediated by the ovarian steroids in 'switching on' genes of possible significance during puberty.

The estimated heritability for eating disorders is between 48% and 83%. Twin studies suggest an anorexia-like phenotype rate of 48%–74%. The genetic risk for developing eating disorders appears to be shared with other disorders. Family and twin studies have shown independent familial transmission of obsessive–compulsive disorder and both eating disorders. Furthermore, increased rates of obsessive–compulsive personality disorder in the relatives of anorexia probands have been reported. It is estimated that about a third of the genetic risk for eating disorders, depression, anxiety and addictive disorders is shared.

Multiple genes have been implicated in the development of eating disorders, including those regulating weight, appetite, temperament and personality traits. *5-HT2A* and brain-derived neurotrophic factor genes have been proposed as susceptible genes for anorexia nervosa. Studies of dopamine-linked genes have also shown an association, with evidence supporting the role of the catechol-O-methyltransferase gene.

Genome-wide linkage analysis has implicated linkage regions on chromosomes 1 and 3 for both anorexia and bulimia nervosa, as well as certain regions of chromosome 4 for anorexia nervosa and that of chromosome 10 for bulimia nervosa.

Biological factors

> **FURTHER READING**
>
> **For a good overview of eating disorders, see:** Treasure J, Claudino AM, Zucker N. (2010) Eating disorders. The Lancet 375(9714):583–593. doi:10.1016/S0140-6736(09)61748-7

Neuroimaging in patients with anorexia or bulimia nervosa shows brain atrophy, widening of the sulci and enlarged ventricles, which largely resolve on recovery. Functional imaging shows increased activation in the orbitofrontal cortex and anterior cingulate region in response to food cues.

Hypercortisolaemia persists after recovery from anorexia nervosa and might be a risk factor for the disorder.

Personality traits

Perfectionistic traits are often prominent, and negative self-evaluation and extreme compliance are recognized risk factors. Negative emotionality and high levels of stress reactivity can persist after recovery. An avoidant coping style is also recognized in individuals with anorexia nervosa.

Perinatal and childhood risk factors

Complications during pregnancy and prematurity are associated with an increased risk of anorexia and bulimia nervosa. Various childhood environmental factors, including enmeshment, rigidity, lack of conflict resolution, abuse and the death of a close relative, have been reported to increase risk.

Risk factors for psychiatric disorders, including exposure to parental psychiatric disorders such as depression or alcohol and substance abuse during childhood, contribute to the risk of developing bulimia nervosa.

Cultural factors

There is an emphasis placed on excessive thinness in Western society. The perceived pressure to be thin, modelling of body image, thin-ideal internalization (a belief that slimness is desirable) and self-reported dieting have all been identified as risk factors. Studies have reported that critical comments from family about weight, shape and eating, and family and personal history of obesity are associated with the development of eating disorders.

Historically, eating disorders were thought to be almost exclusively a female illness, but eating disorders are increasingly recognized in males. Approximately 10% of those who receive treatment are males; however, compared with females, the detection rates are impacted by lower help-seeking in males and poorer recognition in males by clinicians. One study of third level students found that the one in three students who had a positive screening for an eating disorder was male. A higher risk is reported in males who are involved in activities that require them to monitor and control their weight, such as jockeying, gymnastics, swimming, dancing, wrestling, rowing and running.

Pubertal factors

Body fat rises from 8% in middle childhood to 22% after puberty. Post-pubertal girls have more weight and shape issues than pre-pubertal girls. It has been suggested that anorexia may be a means of preventing the physical transition into womanhood in terms of changing body shape and menstruation.

In 1873, Lasegue first described anorexia nervosa. In contrast, bulimia nervosa was first described by Russell as recently as 1979. In young women in the West, the average prevalence rates of anorexia nervosa are 0.3% and it is the most common cause of weight loss in this population group. The incidence of anorexia nervosa in the general population is eight cases per 100,000 per year. The incidence increased over the past century until the 1970s and is now stable. Bulimia nervosa is more prevalent, and the typical age of onset is later. Prevalence rates of 1% and incidence rates of 12 cases per 100,000 have been reported for bulimia nervosa. These rates have levelled off more recently, after increasing sharply in the first decade after its introduction into the DSM-III in 1980. The female-to-male ratio in both conditions is approximately 10:1.

---

4. It is now three months after the initial assessment, and Dr Kelly and his wife present to your clinic. They are increasingly concerned about Emma; *'We know there is significant mortality associated with her condition. She's less than six stone now I'd say, although she's very good at hiding it. She told me last night that she thinks a lot about death and that sometimes she sees no point in going on. I worry that she might do something to harm herself. What are her most recent blood tests showing? Do we need to get her into hospital for a while? She's doing her finals in a few months, but she could defer them until next year'.*

    8. What findings might you expect on physical examination?
    9. What are the main clinical effects of anorexia nervosa?
   10. List the potentially life-threatening clinical effects.
   11. What are the criteria for hospital admission (medical or psychiatric) in anorexia nervosa?

Findings on physical examination may include cold extremities, peripheral cyanosis, dental caries, parotid swelling, dry skin, hair and nails, fine lanugo hair and/or an orange tinge to the skin. Hypotension and bradycardia leading to dizziness are common. Proximal muscle weakness and peripheral neuropathy may occur.

Anorexia nervosa can result in disruptions across multiple organ systems. Such damage may not be fully reversible. Potential issues include the following:

Gastrointestinal: delayed gastric emptying, constipation and bloating

Haematological: leukopenia, thrombocytopenia and anaemia

Endocrinological and metabolic: hyponatremia, hypokalaemia, altered thyroid function, hypercholesterolemia, osteoporosis, reduced luteinizing hormone (LH), follicle-stimulating hormone (FSH), oestrogen and progesterone, arrested puberty, amenorrhea, reduced libido and fertility

Cardiovascular: cardiomyopathy prolonged QT, mitral valve prolapse, arrhythmia or heart failure

Neurological: peripheral neuropathy, pseudoatrophy of the brain with sulcal widening and cerebral atrophy (which corrects with weight gain)

Dermatological: brittle hair, lanugo (fine downy) body hair

Renal: renal calculi, acute renal failure.

Anorexia and bulimia nervosa are associated with depression, anxiety, other mood disorders, personality disorders, obsessive—compulsive disorders and alcohol and substance misuse. There is a significantly increased risk of suicide. The standardized mortality ratio (SMR) is estimated to be 5.0 for lifetime anorexia nervosa and 2.3 for bulimia nervosa with no history of anorexia nervosa. The SMR is the risk of death as compared to a general population of similar sex and age characteristics.

The criteria for hospital admission include the following:

- Very rapid or excessive weight loss
- Failure to engage in outpatient treatment such that the patient poses a significant medical or psychiatric risk
- Severe electrolyte imbalance, hypoglycaemia, syncope, severe bradycardia, hypotension or electrocardiogram (ECG) changes and renal impairment, or a marked reduction in platelet count or white blood cell count
- Risk of suicide
- Lack of social or family support.

---

5. You arrange for Emma to be admitted to the Department of Psychiatry at the University Hospital Limerick because of her mother's concern regarding the potential risk of self-harm. She is accompanied by her mother and her aunt, Polly. You perform a physical examination and record Emma's height and weight to calculate her body mass index. You are significantly concerned as her body mass index is calculated to be 13. You organize for baseline investigations and contact your medical colleagues to alert them to the situation, asking them to book a bed for Emma.

    12. What blood tests and other investigations will you perform and what results do you expect, given her very low weight?

The following investigations are recommended: full blood count, urea and electrolytes, including phosphate, liver function tests, albumin, creatine kinase, glucose, thyroid function tests, FSH and LH. An ECG may identify a prolonged QT interval, which is especially important if the patient has low potassium because of excessive vomiting, or laxative and diuretic misuse.

Given Emma's current weight, it is likely that she will display significant electrolyte imbalances, such as hypokalaemia, hyponatremia, hypocalcaemia, hypophosphatemia, hypomagnesaemia and/or hypochloraemia. Raised urea and creatinine could indicate dehydration.

Leukopenia, thrombocytopenia and anaemia may also be present. Her haemoglobin may be elevated because of dehydration. Glucose may be low, and cholesterol elevated secondary to low T3. Sex hormone levels would typically be reduced and growth hormone and cortisol raised. The ECG should be reviewed for evidence of QT prolongation, which can lead to fatal arrhythmias.

---

6. Emma's blood results indicate combined hypokalaemia (2.5 mmol/L) and hyponatremia (125 mEq/L). Since her arrival in the ward 3 h ago, she has refused to eat or drink anything despite encouragement. You explain to Emma that she is to be transferred to the medical ward for nasogastric feeding. She has been assigned a 24-h 'special' nurse from the psychiatric service.

    13. What will your advice be to the 24-h 'special' nurse?
    14. What are the key legal and ethical issues involved here?
    15. What are the dangers of feeding in anorexia nervosa?

At this stage, 24-h direct nursing observation is important to provide psychological support and to closely supervise the patient so that they do not sabotage weight gain by excessive movement or purging behaviour. This includes closely observing all behaviours, including use of toilet and bathing facilities. It is not unusual for bed-confined patients with anorexia to try to exercise under the bedsheets covertly.

Detention and treatment under the Mental Health Act may be used in the case of anorexia nervosa when there is a serious threat to health, and when compulsory feeding is necessary to treat both the physical complications and the underlying mental disorder. The issue of insight is complex, but it is accepted that the body image distortion and associated dangerous weight-reducing behaviours indicate a lack of insight, which can justify involuntary treatment. Generally, patients with a BMI of less than 15 are likely to experience demonstrably impaired cognition, which also impacts judgement. Treatment should be subjected to regular, multidisciplinary review, and discontinued as soon as is practicable.

Hospital refeeding can be useful in adolescents in whom lengthy periods of low weight can adversely affect growth and development, but this should be an intervention of last resort. Caution must be exercised as refeeding can expose the patient to infections and potentially lead to 'refeeding syndrome'. This is a potentially life-threatening condition that can lead to sudden cardiac death. Refeeding syndrome is caused by sudden shifts in electrolyte levels (especially hypophosphataemia) that occur as the body adjusts from metabolizing fat back to predominantly metabolizing carbohydrates as an energy source. The highest risk is in the first two weeks, often in the first few days. Excessive bloating and peripheral oedema are often the first signs of refeeding syndrome. Other features include lethargy, confusion, seizures and cardiac arrhythmias. Electrolyte imbalances should be corrected before feeding starts to minimize the risk, and electrolytes repeated every three days initially. Daily calorie intake should be increased slowly under the close supervision of a dietician until a steady weight gain of 0.5−1 kg per week is attained.

---

7. With nasogastric feeding and bed rest, Emma's body mass index gradually increases to 14 over the subsequent five weeks. She is transferred back to the Department of Psychiatry and discharged home after a further four weeks of inpatient treatment.
  16. What are the main treatment strategies that you would employ during this phase?
  17. How might this compare with the treatment of bulimia nervosa?
  18. What is Emma's prognosis and how would this compare with the prognosis of those with bulimia without anorexia?

A multidisciplinary approach is important, including medical, nutritional, social and psychological components, which can be delivered to the patient individually or with the family in the case of adolescents.

FURTHER READING

For a review of treatment options in anorexia nervosa, see: Zipfel S, Giel KE, Bulik CM, et al. (2015) Anorexia nervosa: aetiology, assessment, and treatment. Lancet Psychiatry 2 (12):1099−1111. doi:10.1016/S2215-0366(15)00356-9

A previous Cochrane review did not recommend any particular psychological treatment for adults with anorexia nervosa. Cognitive behavioural therapy (CBT), interpersonal psychotherapy, cognitive analytical therapy, psychodynamic and behavioural therapies have all shown weak evidence for treating anorexia nervosa. Moreover, no psychotherapeutic treatment has shown to have greater success than any of the above options. For adolescents with anorexia nervosa, family psychotherapy practised according to the Maudsley method is recommended for a period of 6 months or longer.

To date, no strong evidence supports drug treatment in the management of anorexia nervosa either in the acute phase or subsequently. Use of serotonin specific reuptake inhibitors (SSRIs), including fluoxetine and tricyclic antidepressants, provide weak evidence only. The role of atypical antipsychotics has recently been considered in the management of anorexia nervosa. Initial studies report a decrease in obsessive symptoms and increased weight gain; however, larger trials are necessary to explore the benefits further.

FURTHER READING

For a review of bulimia nervosa, see: Hail L, Le Grange D. (2018) Bulimia nervosa in adolescents: prevalence and treatment challenges. Adolescent Health, Medicine and Therapeutics 9:11—16. doi:10.2147/AHMT.S135326

Few people with bulimia nervosa seek help. One study reported that just 10% seek treatment. Both CBT and antidepressants reduce binge eating and purging, as well as improve depressive symptoms. CBT is considered as the first-line treatment for bulimia nervosa, with binge remission rates of 30%—40% reported. It is considered to be as effective for eating disorders not otherwise specified as it is for bulimia nervosa. The National Institute for Health and Care Excellence recommends a typical course of CBT involving 16—20 sessions over 4—5 months.

Antidepressants and CBT are considered equally effective, and the addition of tricyclic agents or fluoxetine to CBT is not more effective than CBT alone. Interpersonal therapy is also shown to be efficacious, but symptoms respond more slowly than with CBT. Dialectical behavioural therapy is being explored as an alternative psychotherapeutic modality in the treatment of bulimia nervosa.

Evidence for pharmacotherapy in bulimia nervosa is robust, but with better evidence for short-term rather than long-term efficacy. Moreover, most studies have been conducted in adults rather than adolescents and children. SSRI (especially, high dose fluoxetine [60 mg daily]) has the best evidence for improving impulse control and the tendency for binging.

A longer duration of illness chronicity is associated with a poorer prognosis in patients with anorexia nervosa. On average, it takes 5—6 years from diagnosis to recovery. However, up to 30% of the patients do not recover. A young age at onset and short duration of illness is associated with a good outcome in anorexia nervosa. Physical and psychiatric comorbidity is associated with a poor outcome. Requirement for hospitalization, especially on a compulsory basis, is associated with poor longer-term outcomes.

In contrast to anorexia nervosa, the longer the illness duration in bulimia nervosa, the greater the chance of recovery. A German study reported that only one-third of patients with bulimia nervosa admitted to hospital had an eating disorder 12 years later.

John

Polysubstance Misuse

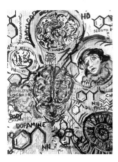

1. Discuss typical presentations of substance use disorders in general medical and psychiatric clinical settings.
2. Obtain a thorough substance use history.
3. Know the clinical features of intoxication with common substances.
4. Recognize the clinical signs and recommend management strategies for substance withdrawal.
5. Discuss the epidemiology, course of illness and the medical and psychosocial complications of common substance use disorders.
6. Discuss management strategies for substance abuse and dependence.
7. Discuss the characteristic presenting features and approach to managing drug-seeking patients.
8. Be aware of current guidelines for safe prescribing of substances of potential abuse (benzodiazepines).

1. You are surprised to meet Gillian, a 48-year-old married mother of two at your local wine bar. You know her because she has attended your service with a diagnosis of bipolar affective disorder that has been stable for years. She asks for an 'off-the-record' consultation and turns out to be quite concerned about her 17-year-old son, John, who recently performed very well in his Leaving Certificate examination and has taken a year out, intending to study English at university next year. Gillian has developed an interest in psychology over the years and is now concerned that John may be experiencing 'symptoms of schizophrenia'. In support of this possibility, she describes how he stays in his bedroom for long hours during the day reading on his own, often with incense burning, while listening to electronic music.

Continued on following page

(Continued)

Recently, John appears to have little interest in meeting his friends from school and stays up late at night on his computer, eating junk food. When he does venture downstairs, John talks in a disjointed manner about philosophy, obscure music and literature. He occasionally sees his friend William who is at a university in London but returns home sporadically. When he visits William, John tends to return looking 'vague' with red, watery eyes and can be quite forgetful. He has put on about a stone in weight. He does not drink alcohol and is quite dismissive of peers who do.

1. What are your immediate thoughts about this presentation?
2. How would you address Gillian's concerns?

This collateral history points to social withdrawal, deterioration in general functioning, cognitive disturbance and possible thought disorder. As such, Gillian's concerns about an underlying psychiatric disorder are understandable. However, the presentation is more consistent with cannabis use.

FURTHER READING

For a review of the evidence linking cannabis use to mental disturbance, see: Ksir C, Hart CL. (2016) Cannabis and psychosis: a critical overview of the relationship. Current Psychiatry Reports 18(2):12. doi:10.1007/s11920-015-0657-y

Cannabis is the most popular illegal recreational drug worldwide. According to the World Health Organization, 2.5% of the world's population smoke cannabis. John is demonstrating some of its psychoactive effects, which include an induced state of relaxation and (to a minor degree) euphoria, creating a capacity for philosophical thinking (including areas such as introspection and metacognition) and in many instances, inducing anxiety, paranoia ('the fear') and hunger cravings ('the munchies'). These effects normally subside a few hours after consumption.

Although over 100 cannabinoids contribute to the psychopharmacological effects of cannabis, there are two main constituents. The primary psychoactive ingredients of cannabis are tetrahydrocannabinol (THC) and cannabidiol (CBD). The ratios of these and other cannabinoids vary considerably in preparations of cannabis. The endogenous cannabinoid system consists of two types of G-protein-coupled receptors: cannabinoid-1 (CB1) and cannabinoid-2 receptors. CB1 receptors are the most abundant in the brain and are highly concentrated in neural circuits putatively implicated in psychosis. Specific regions of concentration include the hippocampus, prefrontal cortex, anterior cingulate, basal ganglia and cerebellum.

Cannabinoids produce an increase in dopaminergic activity in the mesolimbic reward pathway, a tract that is associated with the addictive effects of most drugs of abuse. The increased dopaminergic activity elicited by the cannabinoids may underpin the increase in positive psychotic symptoms induced by THC. Recurrent cannabis use produces prolonged and excessive stimulation of the CB1 receptor, with subsequent disruption to the function of the endocannabinoid system. Recent research has suggested that cannabinoids and their receptors have a role in the pathophysiology of schizophrenia. It has been proposed that this CB1 receptor overstimulation may be a contributing factor in triggering THC-induced psychosis.

Psychosis

You may be able to allay some of Gillian's concerns as it does not appear that John is acutely psychotic. Nonetheless, many studies have explored the link between cannabis and psychosis.

Recent meta-analyses have demonstrated an increased risk of psychosis in cannabis users than nonusers, with odds ratios approaching six in heavy cannabis users.

However, these studies have been criticized, particularly regarding controlling confounding factors such as noncannabis drug use, a family history of psychosis and unmeasured vulnerability to psychosis.

The extent to which cannabis use might interact with the clinical course of schizophrenia remains unclear. Findings suggest that patients with schizophrenia who use cannabis experience increased severity of psychotic symptoms, are more likely to have relapses, have a greater likelihood of re-hospitalization and experience a poorer therapeutic response to antipsychotic medication than patients who are cannabis-naive. Furthermore, preonset cannabis use may trigger an earlier age of onset of psychosis, which is of critical importance given the negative prognostic features associated with earlier onset.

Individuals whose presentation has clearly been precipitated by cannabis use may constitute a clinically distinct subgroup of patients with psychotic disorders. In this respect, cannabis use may trigger the onset of psychosis in vulnerable individuals in whom a psychotic disorder may not have developed otherwise. Therefore, these patients may have a better prognosis, exhibit fewer negative symptoms, have better social skills and have an enhanced treatment response than nonusers.

---

2. Gillian returns to the clinic a few days later for her own routine appointment, with a gift of your favourite brandy to thank you for your previous input. She confronted John after she saw a box 'absolutely full of cannabis leaves'. When she questioned John about this, he was amused and pointed out that the box was full of tobacco and dried 'useless leaves', differentiating these from some 'buds', which he was happy to show his mother.

He admitted to frequent cannabis use but only over the last year and that he preferred to smoke 'resin' to the 'skunk' that his friend William had brought from London. He said that resin had a more relaxant effect but admitted to feeling 'totally wired' since smoking the skunk. He appeared surprised that this did not reassure Gillian.

3. What factors increase the risk for cannabis-induced psychosis?
4. What is the significance of the family history of psychiatric illness?

Certain risk factors have been reported to interact with cannabis use to increase the vulnerability to developing psychosis. Psychosis is associated with early use, greater frequency of use and consumption of high potency cannabis in those with a genetic predisposition to psychotic illness.

Early cannabis exposure

The association between the amount of cannabis use and development of psychosis was first observed in a Swedish conscript cohort study (after a 15-year follow-up) that demonstrated that cannabis use on more than 50 occasions led to a six-fold increase in the risk of schizophrenia. However, it is unclear whether the psychotic symptoms pre-dated the cannabis use.

Further clarification was provided by the Dunedin Multidisciplinary Health and Development Study. This was a prospective, longitudinal study of adolescent cannabis use, considering psychotic symptoms that occurred before cannabis use. Data were compiled from a large birth cohort consisting of 1037 individuals. Information about psychotic symptoms was obtained at age 11 years, and drug use was self-reported at ages 15 and 18 years. Psychotic symptoms were measured using a standardized interview schedule at age 26 years. The results showed that those who had used cannabis by ages 15 and 18 years had more psychotic symptoms than controls. Specifically, cannabis use by the age of 15 years predicted psychosis with an odds ratio of 4.5. Cannabis use by the age of 18 years also predicted psychosis; however, with a lower odds ratio of 1.65.

BOX 12.1 ■ Cannabis, how to ask:

How many joints/spliffs would you smoke in a day? Maximum?
Do you smoke, grass, hash, skunk, oil?
Note: Typically, there is around 0.25 mg to 1 g of cannabis in each joint/spliff.

These findings may be explained in terms of neuroplastic change. Adolescence represents a sensitive period of neurodevelopment, with the brain being more vulnerable to the effects of cannabis as dopamine receptors are 'pruned'. Alternatively, the heightened risk may simply be a consequence of greater cumulative cannabis use in those using cannabis at an earlier age.

These theories are not mutually exclusive, and the latter explanation is consistent with data revealing a dose−response effect. Risk of psychotic symptoms is increased by approximately six times in those who used cannabis frequently. An alternative theory is that the social implications of early age cannabis smoking may increase the possibility of psychotic illness.

Strength of preparation

The strength of cannabis is thought to influence the possibility of later psychosis (Box 12.1). This is primarily thought to be because of higher concentrations of THC. However, the role of CBD has been of recent interest. Cannabis resin has equal concentrations (4%) of THC and CBD, 'grass' or 'weed' is estimated to have average CBD and THC concentrations of 2% and 9%, respectively, and high potency preparations contain THC concentrations as high as 18% but negligible CBD levels.

The fact that the two constituents have different properties may explain the manifestation of different psychological symptoms among users. CBD appears to have anxiolytic properties and may attenuate the higher anxiety levels caused by THC alone. Indeed, recent studies suggest that CBD may potentially have antipsychotic properties along with neutral or even pro-cognitive effects and there is increasing support for legal preparations of cannabis for medical use.

Genetic factors

Gillian's concern that John may have an increased risk of psychosis given her own history of major psychiatric illness, has some foundation. The Dunedin study investigated whether specific genes increase the risks associated with early cannabis use. The study examined the role of the catechol-O-methyltransferase gene, which is involved in the metabolism of dopamine and has frequently been recognized in genetic studies of schizophrenia. A functional polymorphism of this gene, Val158Met, slows the breakdown of dopamine, which potentially increases the risk of psychosis. The results of the study showed that the presence of valine polymorphism was not significant unless coupled with adolescent cannabis use. Individuals with Val/Val or Val/Met genotypes and adolescent cannabis use were at increased risk of developing adult psychosis, while individuals with Met/Met genotypes were not. These findings implicate genetic factors as important contributors to the link between cannabis and psychosis.

---

3. While browsing in the supermarket, you again bump into Gillian. She is pleased to tell you that John has gone to university, has a large group of friends and is proceeding well with his studies. He had come home from university on the previous evening and subsequently went out to a club with his friends. Gillian was pleased to note that when he arrived home, he did not have an alcoholic fetor. However, he was speaking very fast (repeatedly going off in difficult-to-follow tangents) and was

extremely affectionate. He was shivering and appeared to have lost his jacket. However, when Gillian asked him about this, he told her that he had given his jacket to a stranger who looked cold. He said that he had also tried to give someone his shoes, but they had refused to take them.

When Gillian woke up, John was still awake and was 'quite all over the place'. He appeared happy one moment and then frightened and 'on edge' the next moment. He said that 'something strange is going on' and asked if she could 'see the music everywhere'. He asked Gillian for some diazepam that she was prescribed for intermittent anxiety.

Gillian reluctantly agreed to this and John slept for the rest of the morning.

5. How would you describe John's symptoms in terms of psychopathology?
6. What similarities/differences are there between John's symptoms and 'functional' psychosis?
7. What do you think about the use of benzodiazepines in this case?

Hallucinogenics

Again, Gillian is concerned about the possibility of John's genetic predisposition to psychotic illness and would have reason to believe that he may be experiencing a psychotic episode with a delusional atmosphere, pressured speech, formal thought disorder and perceptual disturbance (synaesthesia; see below). These symptoms seem to have come on more rapidly than is typical with 'functional' psychiatric illness and appear consistent with intoxication. However, they are not the typical effects of one recreational drug but demonstrate some of the features of both amphetamine and hallucinogenic use. This scenario is not unusual, given that drug manufacturers often combine hallucinogenic drugs with amphetamine-based products and (despite current attempts by the web community to clarify matters) the purity of a substance sold is unknown to the typical user.

Lysergic Acid Diethylamide (LSD)

The effects of LSD are similar to that of other hallucinogens such as psilocybin ('magic mushrooms'). The drug acts as a partial receptor agonist of multiple 5HT receptors and is particularly concentrated in the prefrontal cortex and limbic system of users. LSD may cause a wide range of psychological and physical effects, some of which are consistent with John's symptoms. LSD's psychological effects (colloquially called a 'trip') vary greatly from person to person, depending on factors such as previous experiences, state of mind and environment and dosage strength. John appears to be experiencing perceptual distortions and changes in auditory and visual perception are typical. Unlike the perceptual disturbance seen in functional psychosis, visual disturbances are common and may include illusions of movement, coloured patterns (typically geometric), trails from moving objects (sometimes referred to as 'tracers'), an intensification of visual imagery and (rarely) frank hallucinations.

The auditory sensory distortions induced by hallucinogens also have different properties to those seen in functional psychotic illness. The auditory effects of LSD may include echo-like distortions of sounds, changes in the ability to discern concurrent auditory stimuli and a general intensification of the experience of music. John is experiencing synaesthesia, which is frequently associated with LSD use where a stimulus typically appreciated by one sensory modality is experienced in another ('seeing the music').

With its strong capacity to induce introspection and metacognitive processes, LSD can lead to profound mystical experiences with users reporting a loss of identity with their ego and a sense of dissolution between themselves and the outside world. Unsurprisingly, such effects may, at times, become deeply unpleasant and frightening for users. John is displaying emotional lability, features of panic and at times, appears 'frightened'. The individual credited with discovering LSD, Albert Hoffman, reported such features of a 'bad trip' after his initial pleasant experiences with the drug (Box 12.2).

'Flashbacks' are a reported psychological phenomenon in which an individual experiences an episode of LSD's effects long after the drug has worn off, typically in the days after using LSD.

BOX 12.2 ■ **Hoffman's experiences on an LSD 'bad trip'**

'Extraordinary shapes with an intense, kaleidoscopic play of colours'.

'The lady next door was no longer Ms R but rather a malevolent, insidious witch with a coloured mask...a demon had invaded my body mind and soul'.

In some rare cases flashbacks may be protracted, but they are generally short-lived and milder than the actual LSD 'trip'. Flashbacks can incorporate both positive and negative aspects of LSD trips and are often elicited by triggers such as alcohol or cannabis use, stress, caffeine or sleepiness. Although flashbacks themselves are not recognized as a medical syndrome, DSM-5 recognizes the syndrome of hallucinogen persisting perceptual disorder in which LSD-like visual changes are not temporary and brief, as they are in flashbacks, but instead are persistent and cause clinically significant impairment or distress.

3,4-Methylenedioxy-N-hydroxy-N-methylamphetamine (MDMA)

Several features of John's presentation are consistent with MDMA or 'ecstasy' intoxication. MDMA can induce euphoria, a sense of intimacy with others and diminished anxiety. There is an intensification of bodily senses and, classically, a substantial enhancement of the appreciation of music quality. The ability to normally discuss anxiety-provoking topics with marked ease initially raised expectations that MDMA could be utilized for psychotherapeutic purposes.

The primary effects attributable to MDMA consumption are predictable and relatively consistent among users. In general, users report feeling its effects 45 minutes to an hour after consumption, hitting a peak at approximately 3 hours, reaching a plateau that lasts about 2–3 hours, followed by a 'come-down' of a few hours. After the drug has run its course, many users report fatigue, although more long-lasting effects are recognized such as diminished mental capacity, light sensitivity, paranoia and impaired cognitive ability.

MDMA increases prefrontal activity and decreases amygdala activity, which may improve emotional regulation and decrease avoidance behaviour. There is also increased noradrenaline release and raised cortisol levels, which may facilitate a sense of emotional connectedness. (See Box 12.3 for routine assessment questions on MDMA use.)

Adverse effects of the drug include difficulty concentrating, bruxism, lack of appetite, dry mouth and the syndrome of inappropriate antidiuretic hormone secretion, which may lead to hyponatraemia and seizures. An overdose of MDMA may lead to serotonin syndrome symptoms and a hypertensive crisis.

BOX 12.3 ■ **3,4-Methylenedioxy-N-hydroxy-N-methylamphetamine/lysergic acid diethylamide—how to ask?**

How much acid do you take each time (swallow or keep under the tongue)?
Were they in the form of blotting paper or sugar crystals?
How many Es or ecstasy tablets do you take each time?
Do you ever snort MDMA?
How often would you take them in a week?
When did you last take them?

A self-limiting period of depressed mood, frequently observed a few days after MDMA consumption, is sometimes referred to as 'Tuesday blues', possibly caused by depleted serotonin levels following weekend drug use.

Several studies indicate that repeated recreational users of MDMA have increased rates of depression and anxiety, even after cessation of drug use. A meta-analysis of the published literature on memory effects found that ecstasy users may suffer short-term and long-term verbal memory impairment, with 70%—80% of ecstasy users displaying impairments. Others have reported the possibility of executive functioning impairment and neurotoxicity. Reassuringly, other studies have suggested that any potential brain damage may be at least partially reversible following prolonged abstinence from MDMA.

Benzodiazepines

Gillian reluctantly provided John with a dose of diazepam to alleviate his anxiety. Benzodiazepines enhance the effect of the neurotransmitter γ-Aminobutyric acid resulting in sedative, hypnotic, anxiolytic, anticonvulsant and muscle relaxant effects, all of which may be of help to John in this acute state.

Benzodiazepines are generally viewed as safe and effective for short-term use, although cognitive impairment and paradoxical effects, such as aggression or behavioural disinhibition, occasionally occur. These effects may be accentuated with concomitant drug use; therefore, Gillian's actions were not without risk.

High dose use of benzodiazepines can produce acute toxicity which can include drowsiness, slurring of speech, confusion, weakness, poor coordination, respiratory depression and even coma. The effects of benzodiazepines are significantly augmented by concurrent use of alcohol or other sedative agents.

Benzodiazepines may lead to physical and psychological dependence with sustained use. Dependence can result in withdrawal symptoms (anxiety, tremor and confusion) and progress to seizures, especially if stopped abruptly. The symptoms of withdrawal usually develop anywhere from 2—4 days after last use to up to two weeks, although they can appear earlier with shorter-acting agents.

FURTHER READING

For a review of benzodiazepine misuse, see: Lader M. (2014) Benzodiazepine harm: how can it be reduced? British Journal of Clinical Pharmacology 77(2):295—301. doi:10.1111/j.1365-2125.2012.04418.x

---

The prevalence of benzodiazepine use in the general population is 5%. Usage increases with age and females are prescribed benzodiazepines twice as often as males. Roughly one-quarter of the individuals receiving benzodiazepines are long-term users, a high proportion of whom become dependent.

Benzodiazepine abuse most commonly occurs in conjunction with other drugs. Benzodiazepines are typically secondary drugs of abuse for most individuals, with opioids and alcohol most commonly being the primary substance of abuse. In such cases, benzodiazepines are commonly used to enhance the euphoric effects of other drugs, reduce the unwanted side-effects of drugs (e.g. insomnia because of stimulant use) or alleviate withdrawal symptoms.

---

4. Several years later, Gillian brings John into your clinic. He is working in a highly paid editing position for a national newspaper in the United Kingdom. Gillian had seen you in recent weeks, and although she did not feel John was ill, she had remarked that he was restless, working excessively, had become unpleasant and arrogant in his demeanour and 'self-obsessed'.

Continued on following page

(Continued)

He is currently home in Ireland on sick leave from his work. He presents in a markedly distressed state, appears disorientated, perplexed and cannot sit still. He scratches at his skin and says that there are insects crawling underneath it. When you examine him, he has mild damage to his nasal septum, tachycardia, and tells you that he has been experiencing intermittent central chest pain. He says that his bag with his medication was left on the plane and needs you to help him.

8. What is the most likely cause for this presentation?
9. How would you proceed (in terms of psychiatric and medical management)?

John is again presenting with neuropsychiatric symptoms, appearing delirious and agitated. This time, the most likely explanation is one of cocaine withdrawal with a list of differentials, including amphetamine abuse.

Cocaine

Cocaine is a powerful nervous system stimulant that increases alertness, feelings of well-being and euphoria, energy and motor activity, feelings of competence (note John's newfound arrogance) and sexuality. Athletic performance may be enhanced in sports where sustained attention and endurance is required.

Anxiety, paranoia and restlessness are also frequent. The drug is most commonly 'snorted' (Box 12.4), with almost immediate effects, which can last up to one hour at a time. In the acute setting, cocaine misuse doubles the risk of both haemorrhagic and ischaemic cardiovascular events; therefore, John's chest pain should be investigated urgently. Chronic intranasal usage can degrade the nasal septum.

Occasional cocaine use does not typically lead to physical or psychological dependence, and physical withdrawal is not dangerous. Nonetheless, physiological changes caused by cocaine withdrawal include vivid and unpleasant dreams, insomnia or hypersomnia, increased appetite and psychomotor retardation or agitation.

Dependency after habitual usage appears to be mediated by homeostatic dysregulation of normal dopaminergic signalling via the downregulation of dopamine receptors. The decreased dopaminergic signalling after chronic cocaine use may contribute to depressed mood and sensitize brain reward circuits to the reinforcing effects of cocaine (as normal dopaminergic function only returns with repeated drug intake). This sensitization contributes to the addictive properties of the drug.

Cocaine has the potential to induce temporary psychosis, with more than half of the cocaine abusers reporting some psychotic symptoms at some point. Typical symptoms experienced by cocaine users include delusions that they are being followed and that their drug use is being watched, occasionally accompanied by hallucinations which support the delusional beliefs. John is displaying the symptom of formication ('cocaine bugs'). Cocaine-induced psychosis leads to sensitization toward the psychotic effects of the drug and therefore psychosis tends to become more severe with repeated use.

BOX 12.4 ■ Cocaine—how to ask?

Ask whether it is powder coke or crack cocaine
How many lines do you snort (powder)? Maximum?
How many rocks would you smoke (crack cocaine)? Maximum?
Do you ever inject cocaine?
When did you last use?

It is of note that the cocaine epidemic that occurred in the United States in the 1980s had an important impact on our understanding of drug misuse. The traditional notion that drug use is initially driven by the reward of pleasurable effects and that continued use is to avoid unpleasant withdrawal effects applies quite well to opiate use, but this has been augmented by the concept of drug-seeking behaviour (i.e. the capacity of a substance to drive behaviour, often despite negative effects) and not necessarily primarily by physical dependence.

Amphetamines

Amphetamine and methamphetamine may prolong wakefulness, increase focus and feelings of energy and decrease fatigue. They may produce euphoria, induce anorexia and be used to treat narcolepsy and attention-deficit/hyperactivity disorder. Adverse effects include anxiety, aggression, paranoia, hyperactivity, reduced appetite, tachycardia, increased breathing rate, dilated pupils, increased blood pressure, headache, insomnia and arrhythmia.

Amphetamines inhibit dopamine reuptake by interacting with the dopamine transporter, thereby increasing the concentration of dopamine in the synaptic cleft.

The dopamine hypothesis continues to dominate psychosis research, and amphetamines are known to induce psychosis, typically when chronically abused or in high dosages. Therefore, unsurprisingly the symptoms of acute amphetamine psychosis are very similar to that of the acute phase of 'functional' psychoses. However in amphetamine psychosis visual hallucinations are more common and thought disorder is rare. Amphetamine psychosis may be solely due to drug use or it may be that drug usage unmasks an underlying vulnerability to psychosis. There is some evidence that vulnerability to amphetamine psychosis and schizophrenia may be genetically related. Relatives of methamphetamine users with a history of amphetamine psychosis are five times more likely to have been diagnosed with schizophrenia than relatives of methamphetamine users without a history of amphetamine psychosis. The disorders may be distinguished by a typically rapid resolution of symptoms in amphetamine psychosis, while schizophrenia is more likely to follow a chronic course.

Treatment approaches

Before treatment is considered, a thorough substance use history should be established using empathic, nonjudgemental interviewing techniques. Past and recent abuse should be determined (amount and frequency) along with features indicating dependence, complications, past treatment history, readiness to change, the patient's support network and socio-forensic issues.

Several psychological strategies may be employed to facilitate abstinence from substance use

Motivational interviewing is a brief psychological intervention that aims to strengthen the motivation to change, utilizing a cost—benefit analysis. Therapists aim to guide individuals through contemplative and precontemplative stages to make their own decision about whether they wish to change.

Cognitive behavioural therapy (CBT) may strengthen the motivation to abstain from addictive substances or activities. Typically, CBT entails around three months of treatment for addictions, but shorter treatment programmes may also be helpful, including brief, computer-based CBT interventions.

Other strategies include contingency management (a form of behavioural therapy, based on operant conditioning), mindfulness-based relapse prevention (integrating mindfulness meditation with standard relapse prevention practices) and harm reduction (maximizing positive change by reducing harm to addicted persons without insisting upon abstinence). Social and family-based interventions are necessary components of successful approaches.

5. Several years later, you meet John by chance at a farmer's market where you are viewing a micro-brewery beer stall. You note that he is smoking a rolled-up cigarette with a distinctive odour and looks a little dishevelled. However, he is charming and affable in manner. He tells you that he has had the first draft of a novel considered for publication and is married with two daughters named Sylvia and Adrienne. He has had no other contact with the mental health services and indeed is in all-round good health. He thanks you for your previous interaction with him and tells you that he would never consider 'synthetic class As' again but has positive views on the legalization of cannabis. He says his mother is well but does voice his concern over her ongoing treatment with lithium, which he thinks will 'dry out her kidneys'. As you leave the market for your local pub, you note the large bag of organic fruit and vegetables in John's hand and his patient attentiveness to his children.

  10. What is the prognosis for cannabis use over time?
  11. What are the arguments for the legalization of cannabis?

Cannabis has a lower rate of dependence than both nicotine and alcohol, with around 9% of users reaching criteria for dependency. It is clear that cannabis is safely enjoyed by the vast majority of users and is perhaps comparable with alcohol in that the risk of its use is associated with younger age, increased frequency of use and increased potency of the product. It is of note that several recent presidents of the United States have admitted to cannabis use. As such, there has been considerable debate around the potential legalization of the substance. Advocates of the approach claim that there would be no discernible upswing in the prevalence of mental ill-health and cite the evidence for the use of cannabis in specific medical illnesses. In general, psychiatrists would observe that the fact that cannabis affects individuals differently does not alter the systematic harm it causes. There is clear evidence for its role in the development of psychotic illness and it has associations with anxiety and depression. Nonetheless, the question of legalization (or decriminalization) should perhaps be considered separately, as it is complicated by other areas (including civil liberties, individual choice and opportunity costs).

John's narrative demonstrates the 'gateway' theory that cannabis use can lead to exposure and the use of 'harder' drugs later in life. Although there is evidence for this theory, there are several confounding factors. For example some individuals are willing to experiment with any substance and the 'gateway' drugs are merely the ones that are accessible at an earlier age.

Furthermore, the pattern of drug use is constantly evolving. For instance, individuals may use ecstasy or amphetamines as their first drug and subsequently become exposed to harder opiate-derived drugs to help with the symptoms of acute withdrawal. The 'reverse gateway' phenomenon should also be highlighted where, for example, cannabis users may become subsequently addicted to nicotine.

Finally, these narratives have not focussed on the recent phenomenon of the head shop. Such outlets have provided several synthetic drugs that have been sold under the guise of nondrug products, such as bath salts. These drugs include synthetic cathinone (mephedrone), synthetic cannabinoids (spice) and synthetic cocaine (dimethocaine).

Where head shops have been successfully targeted with legal intervention, drug distribution has evolved through the internet. The 'darknet' market, along with the use of cryptocurrencies, has changed the format of drug dealing, facilitating the purchase of drugs in large quantities at relatively low risk to the individuals involved. More positive web developments include sites that educate users around the substances they are taking and disseminate information on contaminated drug batches in the community.

Natasha

Medically Unexplained Symptoms

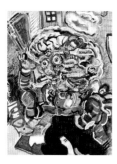

1. Consider the differential diagnoses of patients presenting with medically unexplained symptoms (MUPS).
2. Recognize how to distinguish different symptom patterns, including somatization, hypochondriasis, conversion and body image distortions.
3. Differentiate factitious disorder from malingering.
4. Understand the concept of primary and secondary gain.
5. Consider the biopsychosocial underpinnings of MUPS.
6. Outline a general approach to patients with MUPS.
7. Consider the prevalence and health care costs of MUPS.
8. Understand what we know about the neurobiology of these syndromes.
9. Detail the prognosis of these disorders.
10. Understand the clinical relevance of fibromyalgia as a syndrome, including its prevalence, postulated causes and treatment.

1. Natasha, a 23-year-old single mother, presents with generalized aches, anergia and feeling bloated. She has attended 29 times in the 12 months since joining the practice. During this time, she has presented with back pain, irregular periods, headaches, nausea and tiredness. She has documented mild asthma and irritable bowel disease, but an extensive investigation has not identified causes for most of her ailments. She has a history of a similar pattern of engagement with her previous general practitioners.
   1. What are your initial thoughts regarding this presentation?

This presentation is the latest in a sequence involving repeated help-seeking for symptoms that relate to multiple organ systems and for which physical investigations have failed to identify a simple or effective explanation. While some multisystem conditions can present with a wide range of complaints, the presence of multiple unexplained physical symptoms with such intense help-seeking is highly suggestive of a significant psychological element to this illness. At the very least, the psychological impact of having to cope with this level of morbidity can serve as a starting point for exploring the psychological elements of the presentation.

Of note, a variety of terms are used to describe such symptoms, including 'medically unexplained', 'somatoform' and 'functional' symptoms and syndromes. Isolated unexplained symptoms are common in the general population and often transient, while more persistent, disabling symptoms that involve multiple systems and intense help-seeking are strongly linked to psychiatric illness including mood, anxiety and somatoform disorders.

---

2. At interview, Natasha appears distressed and preoccupied with her symptoms and their impact upon her ability to function. She is keen to describe the symptoms in detail so that you might grasp their precise character. When questioned about mood and psychological well-being, she responds that she feels depressed because of these symptoms and their effect on her lifestyle. She requests a referral to 'the new gastro doctor' whom she has learned has joined the consultant staff at the local hospital, stating 'maybe he can get to the bottom of my problems'.

   2. What factors influence the character of functional symptoms in any individual case?
   3. What are the possible diagnoses for somatic symptoms occurring in the context of psychological illness and what are their key features?
   4. What do you make of Natasha's attribution of the direction of causation for physical versus mental distress?
   5. Should you refer her to the newly appointed consultant in gastrointestinal medicine for an opinion?

The pattern of functional symptoms in an individual reflects the combined role of physiological and psychosocial elements in shaping the character of symptoms. Symptom profile is influenced by the following: (1) previous medical experiences and beliefs (e.g. pseudoseizures commonly occur in patients with 'true' epilepsy) and symptoms often reflect an exaggeration or excessive focus/awareness of existing problems; (2) personality; (3) social circumstances, as symptoms often worsen at times of psychosocial adversity; and (4) prevailing mental state (symptoms often worsen at times of mental stress and/or overt episodes of mood disorder).

The differential diagnosis of medically unexplained symptoms (MUPS) is broad and ranges from single brief symptoms that occur as adjustment-like reactions through to persistent and intense help-seeking for multiple symptoms that are largely unexplained despite extensive investigations, often repeated by a variety of healthcare professionals and which are seriously functionally disabling (Fig. 13.1).

It is not unusual to experience transient unexplained somatic symptoms at times of stress and most commonly, these symptoms settle without the need for major investigation or repeated help.

During a depressive episode, certain patients, especially the elderly, experience somatic disturbances. The presence of concomitant disturbances of mood, cognition and vegetative function,

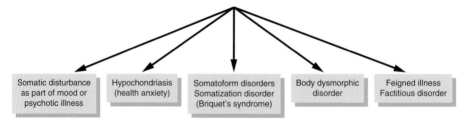

Fig. 13.1   Differential diagnosis of medically unexplained somatic symptoms.

especially preceding somatic complaints, point towards a possible mood disorder. For example, in one international study of over a thousand patients with major depression, 69% reported only somatic symptoms when visiting their primary care physician.

Similarly, both generalized anxiety and panic disorder can include a range of physical symptoms, but again, these occur in the particular context of the psychic discomfort and course of these disorders. Patients with schizophrenia may similarly complain of multiple aches and pains. However, in such cases one finds not only symptoms typical of schizophrenia but also often bizarre and implausible complaints.

In hypochondriasis (sometimes called 'illness anxiety disorder' or 'illness phobia'), the patient is not so much concerned with the illness and its symptoms, but rather with the concept of having a disease that may be terrible and as yet undiagnosed. The focus is upon medical reassurance that they are healthy. In contrast, for patients with somatization disorder, the focus is often upon undergoing diagnostic measures and receiving symptomatic treatments.

In conversion disorder, the number of symptoms is small, often only one, and is generally referable to only one organ system, typically the central nervous system (e.g. blindness or hemiplegia). In psychogenic pain disorder, the perception of pain is the dominant feature. In contrast, patients with somatization disorder present with a multitude of symptoms that range widely over many different organ systems.

Malingerers and those with factitious illness typically also lack the number and range of symptoms presented by patients with somatization disorder, and the focus is upon primary or secondary gain, respectively.

Primary and secondary (morbid) gain are concepts that are used in medicine to describe the unconscious psychological motivations that underpin symptoms, especially those that are unexplained medically. Primary gain is most typically demonstrated in conversion disorder, where, for example, a neurological presentation allows a patient to escape the stress of directly addressing a circumstance that they are in. An example of this is unexplained hemiplegia in a mother who cannot cope with excessive multifunctioning demands of work and providing for the extended family or a person who becomes blind after witnessing a murder. The 'gain' may not be particularly evident to an outside observer. Secondary gain has an external motivator, e.g. being unwell results in missing work, avoiding military duty or jail or obtaining compensation. When the action is conscious, deliberate and contrived, resulting in a tangible benefit for the person, it is considered malingering.

A variety of multisystem diseases (e.g. systemic lupus erythematosus, multiple sclerosis, sarcoidosis) may produce many symptoms and thus mimic somatization disorder. Indeed, some patients with these disorders may become quite embittered and demanding after a succession of physicians have all failed to uncover the underlying disease. Thus, a thorough patient examination and laboratory follow-up are always indicated before diagnosing somatization disorder.

Natasha's attribution of primary versus secondary significance of symptoms lies at the core of somatization disorder, whereby physical issues are emphasized as the primary concern. Addressing this is key to effectively managing patients with somatization disorder. Interestingly, Natasha does recognize the relevance of psychological elements, and this can be a good starting point in the so-called 'reattribution' of primary significance that in turn can allow for a shift in the emphasis of diagnosis and management, during which the emotional and psychosocial factors can be the major focus.

Referral for further (repeat) tests by a new clinician is unlikely to be helpful diagnostically and will serve to reinforce the dysfunctional pattern of symptom management, whereby identifying a physical cause has dominated management to the detriment of dealing with the primary factors that underpin symptoms. It could be argued that a referral might confirm the need to focus upon non-physical elements (e.g. the new consultant may review notes and suggest that further investigation is not warranted at the current time) and can help to build a sense of confidence that you are taking the possibility of a physical cause seriously. However, it is often the case that tests are repeated, thus distracting from the psychological factors. The patient must not perceive that they are being refused appropriate help or prevented from undergoing useful investigations. Focusing upon what is likely to help (given previous experiences) can help to make the case against further physical investigations ('what if they are also negative—is that likely to improve things for you?').

---

3. You suggest to Natasha that further investigations are unlikely to identify treatable reasons for her ongoing symptoms and suggest that a more productive focus might be to consider working on enhancing her ability to deal with the psychological and functional impact of her difficulties. You schedule for her to link in with the practice nurse for support sessions and to explore coping strategies to enhance her day-to-day quality of life. You bring her case to the weekly team meeting to discuss her ongoing management. A colleague who has just joined the practice comments that 'is there any point to this? We should be focusing our energies on helping people who are really sick'.

    6.   What are the principles of managing patients with persistent medically unexplained symptoms?

    7.   How would you respond to your colleague's comments?

The management of patients with MUPS needs to focus on promoting overall functionality rather than seeking a 'miracle' cure. A key aspect involves encouraging patients to recognize the significance of psychological distress as an element of the problem and focusing on therapeutic efforts upon addressing psychological issues. There tends to be a phase of negotiation where the focus upon seeking physical explanations or performing diagnostic tests may need to be gradually de-emphasized. This can allow for the therapeutic relationship to be founded upon the understanding that the symptoms are being taken seriously and that an emerging physical pathological condition will not be missed. Quick fixes are rarely effective and are frequently associated with an escalating frequency of consultations.

FURTHER READING

For a detailed description of how to approach the management of patients with medically unexplained symptoms, see: Smith RC, Lein C, Collins C, et al. (2003) Treating patients with medically unexplained symptoms in primary care. Journal of General Internal Medicine 18(6):478–489.

It is important to make consultations more meaningful and, initially, this can involve greater time and attention being focused upon these patients, while the gradual de-medicalization of symptoms should ultimately reduce the intensity of reliance upon services for solutions.

In the initial phase, this involves a detailed patient-centred assessment. This involves a detailed analysis of their symptoms, the possible causes, patient worries regarding their possible cause, their impact upon day-to-day functioning, their association with socio-environmental factors (without implying causality) and patient expectations and hopes for the treatment.

It is important to provide reassurance regarding diagnosis, and that these symptoms are serious by virtue of their impact upon daily functioning rather than because they represent an acute threat to physical integrity. The value of previous investigations in clarifying that an ominous cause has not been identified should be discussed.

Patients also require further reassurance that specific medical or surgical interventions or further investigations are not needed at present but that they will be available if needed at any time. Failure to convince patients that they will receive optimal ongoing physical care frequently provokes 'doctor-shopping'.

It should be emphasized that the patient's problems/symptoms are real, and if necessary, that they are not 'just a psych case'. Sometimes, this requires exploring the connectedness of bodily systems and clarifying that through connections between central and peripheral nervous systems and hormonal factors that the brain and body are intrinsically linked and that the traditional dualist view of physical versus psychological origins of illness is no longer accepted and considered grossly over-simplistic. Conditions such as phantom-limb syndrome can emphasize the relevance of the central nervous system to our perception and interpretation of peripheral pathological conditions.

It is important to (sometimes gradually) acknowledge that stress, depression and anxiety are part of the problem and that their reduction can help with overall symptom severity. This phase should focus upon normalizing psychological elements and the beginning of a process of reattribution of symptoms. At subsequent consultations, it is important to facilitate the discussion of psychological aspects of the presentation, if needed by showing preferential interest in these elements. For example, when faced with physical complaints, one might enquire 'how did that make you feel?'

It is important to be aware of the possibility of substance misuse and that the use of narcotics and tranquillizers aggravate the problem.

Where possible, it is important to aim for symptom control/enhanced function rather than cure.

It can be useful to negotiate a plan for care, frequency of attendance and who is best suited to providing support. Establishing a link with a key person (e.g. a nurse practitioner) can allow for consistency in communication and also serves to de-medicalize the care process. It is important to recognize the likelihood of future problems and plan for how to deal with symptom worsening if it occurs as these are key points at which patients can lapse into a cycle of unwarranted investigations.

The observations of your colleague raise some interesting issues about the phenomenon of somatization as an illness and the role of healthcare services in providing for the physical and emotional needs of the population. Somatization can be viewed as the physical expression of emotional distress, heightened awareness of bodily sensations, a presentation of occult psychiatric disorder or as a component of the spectrum of symptoms that occur in psychiatric syndromes. The impact at a personal and service level mandates consideration since the distress and functional loss associated with such symptoms are undeniably real, while patients with these presentations account for disproportionate service utilization.

More specifically, in community surveys, 10% of people report at least one medically unexplained symptom in the previous year. Patients with unexplained physical symptoms account for 50% more consultations, 50% greater healthcare costs and 33% more hospitalizations than other service attenders. They occur in 15%—30% of all primary care consultations and up to 65% of attendances at specialist outpatient clinics (estimated average of 52%). It is also relevant that the tendency for increased investigations is driven primarily by doctors rather than patients. Finally, the impact of these problems is emphasized by the observation that individuals with MUPS have twice the standardized mortality ratio for mortality from cancer, accidents and suicide.

---

4. Natasha presents again with a worsening of her back pain and intermittent 'tummy cramps'. She appears irritable and says that she is angry because she feels that you are not taking her problems seriously and 'think it's all in my head'. It emerges that she has made an appointment to see a specialist privately but is feeling guilty and depressed because the cost of this assessment will have to be taken from her usual household budget and this means that her eldest son will not be able to attend a multisport summer camp.
  8. How would you respond to her accusations about your apparent beliefs and management of her problems?
  9. What would you advise regarding the private consultation?

It is important to avoid reducing symptoms down to the outdated and unhelpful dichotomy of physical vs mental, and inevitably real vs unreal. This represents a good opportunity to reinforce key elements of the management plan by emphasizing that: (1) the symptoms are real, as is the associated distress; (2) simple medical explanations do not suffice and equally, neither does a simple psychological explanation; (3) symptoms reflect physiological disruption but socio/emotional factors aggravate this, and it is this combination that ultimately determines symptom severity; and (4) solutions must holistically address all of these factors.

In dealing with the planned private consultation, it will be important to explore the pros and cons of further investment in investigations/diagnostics than an approach that focuses upon optimizing functionality. It would be important to emphasize the relationship between psychological well-being (including mood) and symptom severity such that there is a strong possibility that this consultation will not identify clear physical causes for her symptoms, and if anything, may aggravate symptoms by increasing her sense of frustration and negative self-regard.

---

5. Natasha decides to cancel the appointment with the private consultant and agrees to engage with the practice nurse for one-on-one sessions. She misses two scheduled appointments for medical review and discontinues visiting the practice nurse after one visit. Two months later she re-attends complaining that she has stopped going out because of panic attacks. She also describes having no interest in things and a sense of pointlessness.
    10. What additional symptoms should you assess for?
    11. What are the common comorbidities that occur in somatization disorder?

It would be important to explore for symptoms of depression and characterize the pattern of panic episodes and their impact, including dysfunctional coping strategies.

Two-thirds of patients with somatization disorder will experience an additional psychiatric disorder at some point (Fig. 13.2). Most commonly, these involve depression and/or anxiety, but

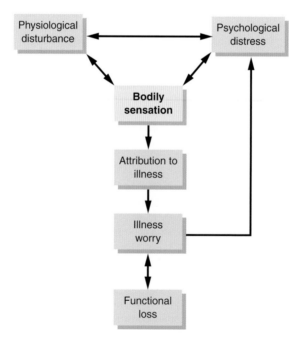

Fig. 13.2 A model of the factors involved in the cycle of somatization.

substance misuse is also a common complication. In hypochondriasis, over a one-year follow-up, 50% of patients also meet the criteria for an anxiety or depressive disorder.

---

6. Natasha responds to treatment and notes that her physical symptoms seem less bothersome now that her mood and anxiety levels are better. She believes that she may have 'finally been cured'. She is keen to understand what the causes of her condition are.

    12. What is the prognosis for somatization disorder?

    13. What is known about the pathophysiology of somatoform disorders?

FURTHER READING

For a review of prognosis in patients with somatization disorder and hypochondria, see:
Olde-Hartmann TC, Borghuis MS, Lucassen PL, et al. (2009) Medically unexplained symptoms, somatisation disorder and hypochondriasis: course and prognosis. A systematic review. Journal of Psychosomatic Research 66(5):363–377. doi:10.1016/j.jpsychores.2008.09.018

Most patients who present with unexplained medical symptoms find that they resolve over a short period. The prevalence of actual somatization disorder is estimated at 0.5% of the population. Risk factors include lower educational achievement, female sex, ethnic minorities and lower socio-economic status.

Most patients (approximately 75%) improve over time, while between 10%–30% have persistent or worsening symptoms. Persistence is associated with a greater number of symptoms, greater functional impairment at presentation and higher incidence of comorbid depressive or anxiety disorder. Prognosis appears somewhat less favourable for patients with hypochondriasis.

The perception of physical symptoms results from a complex interaction of somatic, psychological and environmental factors. This perception process involves a primary sensory event. Other biological systems or psychosocial influences can modulate factors that either trigger, amplify or attenuate this perception process. In many cases, a vicious cycle of escalating distress with associated physical symptoms that are attributed to serious physical pathologic conditions occurs, thus provoking further psychological distress and perpetuation of the distress cycle.

Neuroimaging studies of patients with somatoform disorder have an overall pattern of increased activation in the limbic and sensory cortex in response to unpleasant stimuli. This observation is supported by the electrophysiological literature in which painful somatic symptoms have been associated with increased sensory evoked potentials in response to aversive stimuli. Increased activity in limbic areas is consistent with a cognitive model of somatoform disorders which predicts a heightened emotional salience of noxious stimuli.

Therefore, neuroimaging data provides support for the contention that medically unexplained pain may reflect abnormalities in the higher-order modulation of perception. The strong association with depressive disorder suggests shared pathophysiological mechanisms but, interestingly, patients with depression, who often report somatic complaints, do not seem to show increased activity in these regions during the administration of painful stimuli suggesting that somatoform pain disorders may be differentiated from depression. In addition, functional neuroimaging has revealed selective decreases in the activity of frontal and subcortical circuits involved in motor control during hysterical paralysis, decreases in somatosensory cortices during hysterical anaesthesia or decreases in the visual cortex during hysterical blindness.

Both noradrenergic and serotonergic pathways are implicated in emotional regulation and pain perception, while immune activation via proinflammatory processes can modify symptom perception thresholds and can induce fatigue and asthenia. Stress and its psychobiological regulation via the hypothalamic, pituitary, adrenal axis also modulate this process. All these biological systems are subject to genetic factors.

---

7. Natasha makes good progress over the following six months and stays in regular contact with the practice nurse. However, her frequency of attendance again increases after the sudden death of her mother. She says that she is coping well mentally with the loss. She has again been experiencing abdominal discomfort and reports muscular aches and pains. She has been researching these symptoms on the internet and is wondering if she 'might have had fibromyalgia all along'.

    14. What is the longer-term likelihood of major physical illness in patients with medically unexplained symptoms?

    15. What is fibromyalgia and what is its relationship to mental health disorders?

FURTHER READING

For a systematic review of follow-up studies of patients with medically unexplained symptoms, see: Stone J, Smyth R, Carson A, et al. (2005) Systematic review of misdiagnosis of conversion symptoms and "hysteria". The British Medical Journal 331(7523):989. doi:10.1136/bmj. 38628.466898.55

Similar to the general population, patients diagnosed with somatoform disorders can develop a major physical illness. Although this is at a higher frequency than that observed in the general population, rates of misdiagnosis are reassuringly low (2%–10%).

Early studies suggested that more than 50% of patients admitted for investigation of neurological symptoms had clear neuropsychiatric diagnoses at follow-up. However, more recent work has suggested that in fact this figure is considerably lower with a rate of only 5%.

FURTHER READING

For a state-of-the-art review of fibromyalgia, see: Clauw DJ. (2014) Fibromyalgia a clinical review. Journal of the American Medical Association 311(15):1547–1555. doi:10.1001/jama. 2014.3266

Fibromyalgia is a chronic musculoskeletal disorder that is characterized by widespread pain (both sides of the body, above and below the waist and in the axial skeleton). It often includes other clinical manifestations, such as sleep disturbance, fatigue, irritable bowel syndrome, cognitive difficulties, headache and mood disorders. It is more common in females and affects approximately 2%–7% of people in industrialized societies.

Fibromyalgia can be viewed as a disorder of pain amplification because of the increased sensitivity of the pain system. Management of simple fibromyalgia involves education regarding the nature of the problem, an exercise programme and advice on stress management. A key aspect of managing fibromyalgia is in patient education. This includes providing advice regarding symptoms and their origin; for example, the symptoms are real, not because of damage or inflammation of tissues and that lifestyle management is central. A key issue for many sufferers is to have their symptoms taken seriously as a 'real' illness. Studies have demonstrated how fibromyalgia is a 'centralized pain state' whereby patients experience elevated levels of pain in respect of that expected from the nociceptive input. Moreover, the person's control setting for experiencing pain is altered. Magnetic resonance imaging studies indicate activation of areas associated with pain processing when confronted with mild pressure or heat. Educational strategies should address misunderstandings and common myths about fibromyalgia; for example, exercise does not 'injure' tissue or worsen symptoms, but such activities and exercises are beneficial.

A range of medical treatments, including antidepressants, opioids, nonsteroidal anti-inflammatory drugs, sedatives, muscle relaxants and antiepileptics have been used to treat fibromyalgia. Nonpharmacological interventions, including exercise, physical therapy, massage, acupuncture and cognitive behavioural therapy, can all be helpful. Few of these approaches have been demonstrated to have clear-cut benefits in randomized controlled trials. However, preliminary work indicates that serotonin specific reuptake inhibitors and duloxetine (which are used by a number of clinics and rheumatologists and have a noradrenergic impact on pain) are associated with symptom improvement that is relatively independent of effects upon mood. The multifaceted nature of fibromyalgia suggests that multimodal individualized treatment programmes are required to achieve optimal outcomes.

CHAPTER 14

Michael

Attention Deficit Hyperactivity Disorder

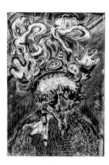

1. Understand the differential diagnosis of a child presenting with disturbed behaviour and academic difficulties.
2. List the key features of attention deficit hyperactivity disorder (ADHD).
3. Outline genetic and environmental aetiological factors in ADHD.
4. Describe the process by which a diagnosis of ADHD can be established.
5. Understand the importance of a biopsychosocial approach to the management of ADHD listing the common nonpharmacological and pharmacological treatment options.
6. List the side-effects of commonly used ADHD medications and understand the importance of physical monitoring and follow-up.
7. Understand the prognosis and the potential comorbidities associated with ADHD.
8. Recognize the increasing relevance of ADHD in adulthood as a diagnostic entity.

1. You are a non-consultant hospital doctor working in child and adolescent psychiatry. At the recent multidisciplinary referral intake meeting, you agreed to assess Michael, a 10-year-old boy, who was referred by his general practitioner. The referral letter states that Michael is overactive, disruptive, constantly talking and refuses to do his homework. His mother, Rose, is very concerned at his behavioural and academic difficulties. The letter goes on to say that the school principal is considering suspending Michael from school if his behaviour does not improve.

    1. What is the differential diagnosis at this point?

Given the limited amount of information you have, the differential diagnosis (and potential comorbidities) at this point is broad and includes conditions outlined in Table 14.1.

TABLE 14.1 ■ **Differential Diagnosis in a Child Presenting with Disruptive Behaviour and Academic Difficulties**

Diagnosis	Description
Attention deficit hyperactivity disorder (ADHD)	ADHD is a neurodevelopmental disorder. It is characterized by problems with attention, excessive activity or difficulty controlling behaviour that is not appropriate for a person's age.
Oppositional defiant disorder (ODD)	This is characterized by a pattern of hostility, angry/irritable mood and argumentative/defiant behaviour. Unlike children with conduct disorder, children with ODD are typically not aggressive towards people or animals, do not destroy property and do not show a pattern of theft or deceit. ODD and ADHD frequently coexist.
Conduct disorder (CD)	A repetitive and persistent pattern of behaviour in which the basic rights of others or major age-appropriate norms are violated. These behaviours are often referred to as 'antisocial behaviours'.
Autistic Spectrum Disorder (ASD)	ASD encompasses a range of neurodevelopmental disorders that includes autism and related conditions. Individuals diagnosed with ASD present with problems in social communication and social interaction and restricted, repetitive patterns of behaviour, interests or activities. Symptoms are typically recognized between one and three years of age. Those with ASD may display inattention, social dysfunction and challenging behaviour, which can be mistaken for ADHD (see Chapter 16).
Intellectual disability	Individuals with intellectual disability demonstrate limitations in intellectual functioning and adaptive behaviour. Affected individuals may display ADHD-like symptoms specific to the learning environment. Children with ID are three times more likely to have ADHD than the general population.
Specific learning difficulties	Specific learning difficulties is an umbrella term used to describe a number of difficulties, including: Dyslexia—characterized by trouble with reading despite normal intelligence. Different people are affected to varying degrees. Problems may include difficulties in spelling words, reading quickly, writing words, 'sounding out' words in the head, pronouncing words when reading aloud and understanding what one reads. Dyscalculia—affected individuals have difficulty in understanding numbers, learning how to manipulate numbers, performing mathematical calculations and learning facts in mathematics. Dyspraxia—this is a form of developmental coordination disorder that affects fine and/or gross motor coordination. Dysgraphia—This is characterized by difficulty in written expression. Children may struggle with spelling and putting their thoughts on paper. Some will have trouble holding a pencil, and handwriting tends to be messy.
Tourette's/Tic disorders	Tics may be motor or vocal and represent repetitive, stereotyped, involuntary vocalizations or movements. For a diagnosis of Tourette's, the individual must have two or more motor tics and at least one vocal tic for an extended period. While ADHD is associated with fidgetiness, repetitive stereotypic movements are typically not a feature.
Sensory impairment	Children with sensory impairments may present as inattentive or disruptive.
Sensory processing disorder	Sensory processing disorder is a condition in which the person has difficulties receiving and responding to information that comes in through the senses. Typically, they have increased sensitivity to sound and touch. Poor coordination may also be evident. Sensory processing problems are commonly seen in developmental conditions like ASD.
Attachment disorder	Reactive attachment disorder may develop when the child's basic needs for comfort, affection and nurturing are not met. Those with reactive attachment disorder can be socially disinhibited, similar to those with ADHD.

(Continued)

TABLE 14.1 ■ **Differential Diagnosis in a Child Presenting with Disruptive Behaviour and Academic Difficulties—cont'd**

Diagnosis	Description
Substance misuse	Active substance use may present with features similar to ADHD, such as disinhibition and impulsivity. Evidence of ADHD symptoms prior to substance misuse is required to make a diagnosis.
Depression and anxiety disorders	Inattention, restlessness and sleep disturbance which occur in ADHD are also common to depression and anxiety disorders.

2. Before assessing Michael himself, you discuss the case with his mother, Rose, who has accompanied him to the appointment. Rose feels that Michael's behaviour has been an issue for several years. She describes his attention span as very short and reports that Michael's teachers have also commented on this. Rose reports that Michael is always 'on the go', finds it difficult to sit still and fidgets a lot with his hands or objects. She describes Michael as irritable and often impatient with his younger sister. His sleep has been poor for as long as she can remember, and he often insists on staying up past a reasonable bedtime, stating that he is not tired enough to go to bed. He does not appear to sleep during the day.

He has had letters sent home from school, reporting that he has been verbally argumentative with teachers and has displayed both verbal and physical aggression towards other students. At home, Michael is often reluctant to follow instructions or take direction from his mother and has lashed out physically on a couple of occasions when corrected for his behaviour. While frequently restless, Michael does not complain of feeling anxious or unhappy apart from occasions when he is arguing with others. He has not expressed any thoughts of self-harm to his family, and his mother reports that he does not have any history of self-harm. He does not use illicit substances or alcohol, according to his mother. He had not undergone any interventions to date.

2. Given this information, what is the most likely diagnosis and what are the diagnostic criteria for this diagnosis?
3. How would you proceed with your assessment?

Michael's symptoms are suggestive of attention deficit hyperactivity disorder (ADHD) (Box 14.1). However, it is important not to rush to this diagnosis without completing a thorough assessment as another diagnosis may be more appropriate. Further, another condition may exist comorbidly.

The core features of ADHD are inattention, overactivity and impulsivity (see Fig. 14.1). These features must be present in more than one situation or environment (e.g. home and school) for a diagnosis of ADHD to be made.

Indicators of inattention include difficulties in sustaining focus on tasks, distractibility in interpersonal interactions and difficulties with functional task completion, organizational difficulties with forgetfulness and a tendency to make errors when required to demonstrate focused attention.

Hyperactivity and impulsivity are evidenced by a tendency for restlessness and fidgeting, inability to maintain physical ease (e.g. sit down for prolonged periods), excessive physical and verbal

---

BOX 14.1 ■ The diagnosis of attention deficit hyperactivity disorder is based upon the following:

History of difficulties with:

1. significant inattention and/or
2. hyperactivity—impulsivity
3. that has a significant functional impact, e.g. educational development, social functioning
4. and is persistent over time and domain of existence (e.g. home, school, work, hobbies).

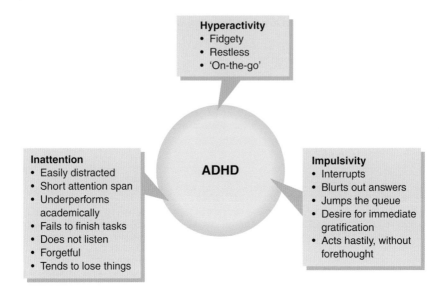

Fig. 14.1   Core features of ADHD.

activity, impatience, a tendency to respond prematurely or engage with tasks without completing them.

Assessment process

In children, ADHD is diagnosed through a careful history, examination and collateral information (from parents, teachers, coaches) and involves meeting the child, their parents or guardians together with teachers and other significant individuals in the child's life. Observing the child in his/her normal environment is important in gaining a clear picture of the dynamics at play in different situations and to understand the psychosocial context more fully (see Fig. 14.2). This information not only aids diagnosis but is also useful in devising a suitable and tailored management plan.

Details about pregnancy, perinatal issues and the child's early development are important as are early social and communication skills. Children with ADHD are more likely to have a history of being a 'fussy' infant with difficulties sleeping, feeding and persistent crying. Children with ADHD often have evidence of delayed language, social and motor development. It is important to elicit when Michael's problems were first noted and how they have progressed chronologically. In addition, you need details about Michael's physical health, significant life events, symptoms of other mental or developmental disorders (e.g. anxiety and affective disorders which are not considered in the Diagnostic and Statistical Manual of Mental Disorders (DSM)-5 diagnostic criteria but important nonetheless), family history and social circumstances. Neuropsychiatric reports on any assessments to date (e.g. psychology, speech and language) should be obtained. If not already completed, intelligence testing and testing of memory, language attention and executive function, which is perhaps not given due consideration in DSM-5, may be necessary to rule-in or rule-out relevant conditions.

The Conners Comprehensive Behaviour Rating Scale is a tool used to gain a better understanding of academic, behavioural and social issues that are seen in young children with suspected ADHD. It comes in a variety of forms (short and long, and parent, teacher and child completed versions). It includes DSM-5 symptoms of ADHD and explores for hyperactivity, behavioural difficulties at school, learning issues, language difficulties, emotional problems, aggression, compulsive behaviour and separation anxiety.

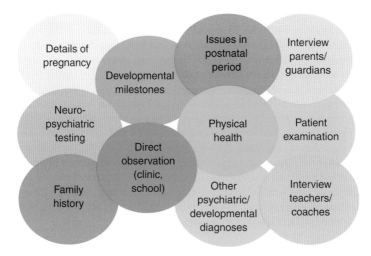

Fig. 14.2 Elements involved in the assessment of ADHD in children.

In the adult, screening questionnaires such as the adult ADHD self-report scale, which looks at current symptoms, and the Wendler Utah rating scale, which is a retrospective rating of childhood symptoms, can also aid diagnosis.

3. You proceed to ask Rose about her pregnancy with Michael. Rose reports that she was well throughout her pregnancy, did not consume alcohol or use any illicit or prescribed drugs. She is a life-long nonsmoker. She tells you that Michael was naturally delivered at full-term and was physically well in infancy. However, he was a poor sleeper and cried a lot. Rose brought Michael to his general practitioner when he was 18 months old as she felt that he was not talking and walking the same as other children of his age. When you mention motor skills and explain this term, she states that Michael was 'clumsy' as a toddler and remains so when picking up and handling objects. He does not suffer from any chronic medical conditions and is not on any regular medication. He has not undergone any surgical procedures. Michael does not appear to be experiencing an anxiety or affective disorder, from his mother's account. His appetite and oral intake are good.

There is no known family history of mental disorders or substance misuse in her own or Michael's father's family as far as she is aware. She describes other members of her extended family as 'hyper', and she was described as 'giddy' by her family during her school-going years. She reports that although bright, she struggled academically.

Rose explains that she and her partner separated two years previously after living together for 12 years. Michael's father now lives abroad. Michael has a 3-year-old sister who lives with Michael and his mother.

Rose denies significant financial difficulties and Michael's father contributes financially every week. Rose maintains an amicable relationship with Michael's dad and denies any history of major domestic disharmony when they cohabited. Michael has regular contact with his father, who is aware of his son's difficulties and his appointment with Child and Adolescent Mental Health Services and is keen to assist in the assessment process in any way he can.

4. What is the epidemiology of attention deficit hyperactivity disorder and describe its cause?

FURTHER READING

For a clear account of our understanding of attention deficit hyperactivity disorder, see:
Feldman HM, Reiff MI. (2014) Attention deficit-hyperactivity disorder in children and adolescents. New England Journal Medicine 370(9):838−846. doi:10.1056/NEJMcp1307215

The prevalence of ADHD is reported as 8%−12% worldwide. Increased prevalence in the United States being more than Europe can be accounted for by the different application of diagnostic criteria rather than the true increased prevalence in the United States. Boys are affected more than girls at a ratio of 3:1. At age 25 years, 15% of adults diagnosed with ADHD in childhood still fulfil the criteria for ADHD, while 65% show partial remission. A recent Irish study suggests the possibility of relatively higher rates of ADHD in a general adult mental health service than previously thought, with 20% of patients screening positive.

Twin, adoption and molecular genetic studies show ADHD to be highly heritable, suggesting that genetic factors account for as much as 75% of ADHD symptoms, although no single causative gene has been identified. There is a greater concordance in monozygotic twins (approximately 50%) versus dizygotic twins. Family studies indicate a 4–10-fold risk to first-degree relatives as compared to the population rate, with prevalence among first-degree relatives in the range of 20%– 50%. Dysregulation of dopamine and noradrenaline in the prefrontal cortex is implicated. Reduced frontal lobe disinhibition is supported by imaging studies, and frontal lobe hypoperfusion and lower frontal lobe metabolic rates have been noted. Environmental factors, including maternal smoking or substance misuse during pregnancy, low birthweight, prematurity and any cause of fetal hypoxia, are associated with ADHD, as is psychosocial adversity.

---

4. At school, Michael struggles to make friends. His classmates say that he is too rough, but he enjoys being on the local soccer team and gets on well with the other players, although he can be unfocused during matches. The coach feels he 'could play under-16s, he's so good' according to Michaels mother. She is delighted that he is 'good at something' as she worries that a negative school experience will damage his self-esteem. She also remarks that he is so much calmer and more placid after training sessions and matches. She becomes tearful as she explains that Michael has been 'mitching off' school and she worries that his truancy will be the final straw for the school.

It transpires that Michael did have a previous assessment by an educational psychologist attached to the National Educational Psychology Service six months previously. This assessment found that Michael's Full-scale Intelligence Quotient was 88 and that he did not have a specific learning difficulty, such as a specific reading or arithmetic disorder. However, it did state that Michael displayed symptoms and signs suggestive of attention deficit hyperactive disorder and recommended referral to child psychiatry services and the allocation of extra educational resources to assist Michael.

    5.   What kinds of difficulties might Michael be experiencing in school?
    6.   What is the difference between school refusal and truancy?

Owing to the inability to maintain attention, children with ADHD often struggle academically and may require extra educational resource input. Because of heightened activity levels, a special needs assistant (SNA) may be necessary to facilitate Michael's learning by gently drawing his attention back to his work when necessary, helping him with organization, repeating verbal instructions from the teacher and ensuring he does not distract other students. Children like Michael, can be verbally challenging to other students, appear quick to anger and can become involved in physical altercations with other pupils, so much so that disciplinary measures, such as suspension, may be considered. Teachers often report fidgeting and restlessness with an inability to relax for sustained periods and comment that the child will often blurt out incorrect answers even before the teacher has an opportunity to finish the question. SNAs have a role in reducing this behaviour by gentle redirection. Different patterns of symptoms can be prominent at different ages; for example, in adolescence, hyperactivity lessens, conflicts with parents continue and high-risk behaviours often appear. In adults, hyperactivity usually decreases significantly, while inattention and impulsivity remain.

---

5. You now meet with Michael himself. He appears restless and fidgety. He is just above average height and weight for his age, as measured on a centile chart. Michael is overfamiliar and spontaneously asks you what football club you support prior to you asking him any questions. You explain that the appointment today is for him and you ask him how he feels he is getting on in school. He states that he does

not like school as he is bored a lot of the time. He feels that the teachers do not understand him and that the other pupils do not like him. Michael does not express any animosity towards any particular individuals.

He describes his thinking as 'overloaded' at night and states that this prevents him from going to sleep. However, he admits that his sleep routine is poor and that he will often insist on staying up late to watch television programmes and play video games. He admits that he is often grumpy in school and at home, especially when he must do his homework but is generally happy and not overly anxious. He denies any recent stressors and says that he has accepted his parent's separation. He denies being bullied by or bullying others. He denies the use of illicit substances or alcohol but admits to smoking cigarettes previously on a few occasions. Michael describes being satisfied with his current home situation and that in the longer term, he would like to continue to live with his mother and to leave school as soon as he can and get a job. You go on to conduct a mental state examination.

7. Summarize the salient features you should explore for during Michael's mental state examination?

During the mental state examination, Michael may present as overfamiliar and impatient (e.g. asking repeatedly if the appointment is over so that he can go home). One would expect good eye contact. Rapport would likely be reasonable overall, but redirection and reassurance may be required. Speech may be normal in rate, rhythm and tone with slightly increased volume. Thought content might relate to unhappiness at school. Michael would likely describe himself as happy, with no anhedonia and no acts or thoughts of self-harm and not present with psychotic symptoms. His attention is reduced at interview although interestingly he can concentrate on video games for extended periods and is also able to keep his concentration during soccer matches for the most part. Michael is likely to have sufficient insight to realize he has a problem, wishes to change his behaviour but is incapable of doing so.

6. You ask Michael's mother, father and teacher to complete a screening questionnaire for attention deficit hyperactivity disorder separately (Conners parent and teacher rating scales). You arrange an appointment in the coming weeks once the questionnaires are completed and returned. In the meantime, you arrange a school visit so that you can observe Michael in the school environment and discuss his case with his teachers. Michael's mother gives her consent for this.

Michael returns to your clinic with his mother three weeks later. You speak with his mother, while Michael plays in the supervised waiting area. You state that you have assessed and rated the Conners' questionnaires and that Michael scores high in both hyperactive and inattentive parameters, and the oppositional parameter, particularly in his mother's form. You provide feedback on what you observed of Michael in the school environment and your discussion with his teacher and school principal. You explain that Michael seems to have much difficulty sitting quietly in the classroom, that he would fidget and interrupt continuously and seemed unable to stop himself despite correction from the teacher. Given this information in conjunction with collateral accounts, Michael's own account and assessment of Michael's mental state, you believe that Michael fulfils the diagnostic criteria for attention deficit hyperactivity disorder. You are happy to arrange an appointment with Michael's father to discuss your finding when he is next home. Rose enquires about treatment and asks if this is something Michael will grow out of.

8. What are the management options in treating attention deficit hyperactivity disorder?
9. What are the risks associated with not treating Michael's condition?
10. What is the natural history of attention deficit hyperactivity disorder and what are its presentations in adulthood?

Management

Parent management programmes are offered by many Child and Adolescent Mental Health Services (CAMHS) teams providing educational forums designed specifically to assist parents in supporting children with ADHD. A variety of behavioural interventions and techniques are taught to parents in a group setting. The group setting also allows parents to meet with other parents of children with

ADHD, which has a supportive and educational benefit. Children, like Michael, often benefit from psychoeducation, social skills training and impulse control interventions provided through their CAMHS team. Neurofeedback typically involves computer-based exercises in which electroencephalogram allows for monitoring of attention levels so that patients receive points when their brain activity shows positive changes. Patients are thus trained to monitor and control attention levels. Older children and adults may benefit from cognitive behavioural therapy which focuses on helping the patient to develop a more planned and reflective approach to thinking and behaving, including social interactions, problem-solving activities and academic functioning. Classroom interventions, including the aid of an SNA, are key to the successful treatment of ADHD. Children with ADHD are eligible for resource hours, and it is important to link with the school in this regard to minimize the impact on the child's education and social development. Dietary interventions, such as the minimization of additives and ensuring a diet rich in protein and vitamins, can be helpful.

FURTHER READING

For a review of the diagnosis and management of ADHD, see: NICE (National Institute for Health and Care Excellence). (2018) ADHD diagnosis and management, NG87. Available at: https://www.nice.org.uk/guidance/ng87.

When necessary, medications may be used in children over six years of age. In general, medications are divided into stimulant and nonstimulant groups. Methylphenidate, a stimulant medication, is usually recommended as first-line therapy. The effect of methylphenidate is thought to be mediated through increased dopamine and noradrenaline levels in the prefrontal cortex. It may seem paradoxical to give a hyperactive patient a stimulant. However, such a strategy is thought to reduce the patients need to self-stimulate.

People with ADHD do not usually have difficulties paying attention to video games, which provide constant visual, auditory and tactile stimulation. However, reading books and following directions are not stimulating activities. Those with ADHD may try to manage these experiences by self-stimulating through wiggling and talking. Stimulants increase both fine and gross motor control and cognitive performance and executive function. Possible side-effects of stimulant medications include nausea, abdominal pain, headache, anxiety, sleep disturbance, appetite and weight reduction and mild growth retardation. 'Drug holidays', such as at weekends or during school holidays, can be useful if weight loss is an issue. Stimulant medication can increase blood pressure and heart rate. Hence, these should be monitored at each clinic visit. Some patients can have suicidal thoughts, dysphoria, mood lability or psychosis; however, this is rare. Tics can develop with sustained use. Switching to a different medication can usually overcome these difficulties. Other stimulant medications include amphetamine, dextroamphetamine and dexmethylphenidate. One should be aware of the abuse potential when prescribing stimulant medication, and this is reflected in their categorization as a controlled drug.

Nonstimulant medications, such as atomoxetine or guanfacine, are also successfully used in the treatment of ADHD. Atomoxetine is a noradrenaline reuptake inhibitor. The more common side-effects include nausea, dry mouth, anorexia and insomnia. It may cause irritability, behavioural changes and suicidal thinking. Rarely, atomoxetine can cause liver damage. Guanfacine is another option. Its mechanism of action is via direct stimulation of postsynaptic α2A-adrenergic receptors to enhance noradrenaline neurotransmission. Common side-effects include fatigue, headache and gastrointestinal disturbance.

Risks associated with untreated ADHD

Approximately 70% of children with ADHD experience a discernible reduction in symptoms when treated with either stimulant or nonstimulant medications, provided there is adequate family and school support in place. Untreated ADHD can have serious consequences for the child's academic development, social development, self-esteem and confidence, which may limit the child's potential and present problems into adulthood. Rates of unemployment, unwanted pregnancy, substance misuse and criminal convictions are all higher in untreated ADHD. Children with untreated ADHD are at risk of developing severe behavioural problems, including conduct disorders in later childhood, manifesting in antisocial behaviour, which may persist into adulthood.

Natural history of ADHD

FURTHER READING

For a review of adult attention deficit hyperactivity disorder, see: Kooij SJ, Bejerot S, Blackwell A, et al. (2010) European consensus statement on diagnosis and treatment of adult ADHD: The European network adult ADHD. BioMed Central Psychiatry 10(1):67. doi:10.1186/1471-244X-10-67

Overall, 60% of children with ADHD display a persistence of symptoms into adulthood with significant functional impairment. Hyperactivity and impulsivity tend to decrease with age, while inattention persists. This may be associated with the maturation of the prefrontal cortex in early adulthood. In general, a diagnosis is more difficult in adults as symptoms are common to a range of psychiatric disorders, e.g. anxiety disorders and substance misuse. Recent studies suggest *de novo* ADHD may occur in adulthood, but this is by no means a universally accepted concept and contrasts with the conventional view that adults with ADHD in adulthood invariably had features as a child.

---

7. Both Michael and his mother are satisfied to proceed with a trial of stimulant medication, and you obtain written consent from Michael's mother to begin methylphenidate.
   11. What steps would you take prior to initiating stimulant medication and what ongoing monitoring is recommended?

You should give families written information on the medication you propose and obtain signed consent from the parents or guardians before initiating. Before initiation of methylphenidate, Michael's height, weight, blood pressure and pulse should be recorded together with an electrocardiography if a history of cardiac issues exists or is suspected. Slow-release formulations are available and facilitate once-daily morning-time dosing. A low starting dose (e.g. 5 mg b.i.d.) is recommended and titrated slowly upwards based on response (the generally accepted upper dose limit in adults is 60 mg per day). Children on stimulant medication should be closely monitored during dose titration and at six-monthly intervals after that. Each time the child is seen in clinic, their height, weight, blood pressure and pulse should be recorded together with a review of the child's progress from both the parents and the teachers' point of view.

The effect of stimulant medication on growth is controversial. It has been noted that children with ADHD that receive stimulant medications may experience minor reductions in growth, possibly because of effects upon appetite or through direct effects upon metabolism or growth factors. However, longitudinal studies have suggested that these children ultimately catch up and that as adults, they are no shorter or slimmer than expected. Drug holidays can assist where growth effects are noted.

---

8. You arrange follow-up for Michael in one month. When he attends, both himself and his mother feel that the situation has improved significantly and that Michael's degree of overactivity and inattention has reduced. They outline full compliance with medication as prescribed. His appetite has reduced

Continued on following page

(Continued)

slightly with 1 kg weight loss since his last visit. Since a growing child should gain weight steadily, you advise Michael's mother to try to increase his oral intake, particularly in the evening when the medication has 'worn off'. After a further month, Michael has regained the lost weight, and his mother reports that she is feeding him as you advised during the previous visit.

Reports from Michael's teacher (both verbally and written follow-up screening questionnaires) show significant improvements in behaviour and a modest academic improvement. Michael tells you that he has started to make friends. You conclude that the current dose of medication is appropriate and you congratulate Michael on doing so well.

Caroline

Bipolar Affective Disorder

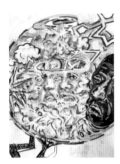

1. Outline the general criteria that are required to make a diagnosis of bipolar I and II disorder.
2. Outline the diagnostic features of a manic episode.
3. Appreciate the potential causes of a manic episode.
4. Explain what is meant by 'cyclothymic disorder' and 'bipolar disorder with rapid cycling'.
5. Describe the evidence that supports that bipolar illness is a highly genetic condition.
6. Understand the epidemiology, including prevalence, of bipolar illness?
7. Explain the role of lithium in the management of bipolar illness, with a particular focus on its use in maintenance treatment?
8. Describe the role of other mood-stabilizing agents in the management of bipolar illness.

1. Caroline is a 31-year-old supermarket manager who has been attending mental health services for almost 10 years and has an established diagnosis of bipolar I disorder. She has previously experienced several episodes of illness and undergone three previous hospitalizations with acute mania (twice) and depression (once). Her illness has been stable for the past five years since commencing lithium therapy. She is attending for a routine three-monthly review.
   1. What is the significance of the diagnosis of bipolar I disorder?
   2. What is lithium and what is the evidence for its use in bipolar illness?
   3. What is the proposed mechanism of action for lithium?

Bipolar I disorder is characterized by a clinical course that includes the occurrence of one or more manic or mixed episodes (i.e. episodes with features of low mood/irritability with elation). Usually, individuals have also had one or more major depressive episodes such that a pattern of unipolar mania is unusual, especially over longer-term follow-up. Episodes of substance-induced mood disorder (because of the direct effects of a medication, or other somatic treatments for depression, a drug of abuse or toxin exposure) or of mood disorder due to a general medical condition do not count toward a diagnosis of bipolar I disorder. In addition, the episodes are not better accounted for by schizoaffective disorder and are not superimposed on schizophrenia, schizophreniform disorder or a psychotic disorder not otherwise specified.

In contrast, the essential feature of bipolar II disorder is a clinical course that is characterized by the occurrence of one or more episodes of major depression accompanied by at least one hypomanic episode. Hypomania is less severe than mania in terms of its impact upon socioadaptive functioning, and does not include overt psychosis. Episodes of substance-induced mood disorder (because of the direct effects of a medication, or other somatic treatments for depression, a drug of abuse or toxin exposure) or of mood disorder due to a general medical condition can count toward a diagnosis of bipolar II disorder.

A further consideration is that of cyclothymia, which is chronic mood disorder widely considered to be a more chronic but milder or subthreshold form of bipolar affective disorder. It occurs in 1% of the population, but recognition rates are increasing. Cyclothymia is characterized by numerous mood swings that typically last days or weeks that involve periods of elevated mood and increased activity that do not meet the criteria for a manic episode, alternating with periods of mild or moderate symptoms of depression that do not meet the criteria for a major depressive episode. Such persons are often considered 'moody' by friends and family. This can represent a prodromal phase for full bipolar illness. Although the emotional highs and lows of cyclothymia are less extreme than those of bipolar affective disorder, the symptomatology, longitudinal course, family history and treatment response of cyclothymia are consistent with bipolar spectrum. Importantly, the frequency of bipolar illness is elevated in those with cyclothymia, and twin studies indicate high concordance in monozygotic twins.

Comparison of bipolar I and bipolar II disorder

Dividing bipolar illness into I and II has an obvious phenomenological basis, but there are pathophysiological, therapeutic and prognostic differences as well. A detailed longitudinal study of the course of bipolar illness over 20 years found the following:

- Bipolar I and II patients had similar demographics and ages of onset at the first episode.
- Bipolar I patients had more severe acute episodes.
- Both had more lifetime co-occurring substance abuse than the general population.
- Bipolar II had significantly higher lifetime prevalence of anxiety disorders, especially social and other phobias.
- Bipolar II patients experience a substantially more chronic course, with significantly more depressive episodes with shorter periods of remission between episodes.

From a genetic perspective, concordance between monozygotic twins for bipolar I disorder is 30%–90%. Other work indicates that the risk of bipolar II disorder is elevated in both bipolar I and II patients, but that the risk of bipolar I does not appear to be markedly increased in the relatives of those with bipolar II disorder.

A variety of studies have identified genetic variants that predict lithium responsiveness (Rev-erb-Alpha, BDNF and Glycogen Synthase Kinase 3-Beta). Lithium is a mood-stabilizing agent that is generally considered to be the first-line treatment for the prophylaxis of classical bipolar illness. Its use has been well studied, compared to other mood stabilizers, and is supported by multiple placebo-controlled trials that have indicated a significant preventative action versus illness relapse. It is less effective in atypical illness, such as that which involves mixed affective presentations or rapid cycling. Lithium can also be used in the management of acute mania, but has a delayed onset of action and modest sedative properties, and typically requires augmentation with other agents.

Although lithium has been in use for over 50 years and has well-established effectiveness, its mechanism of action is not well understood. Lithium is a basic element that can substitute for sodium, potassium, calcium or magnesium in cellular systems and influences neurotransmitter release, receptor upregulation and activation of second messenger systems. It has been postulated that these effects act to stabilize cell membranes, and that this is the mechanism of action in bipolar illness wherein destabilized neurotransmission and/or kindling are suggested pathophysiologies. Of note, 'kindling' in neurobiology refers to a process whereby the occurrence of an event sensitizes the brain to further similar events at a higher intensity. It is applied to epilepsy in terms of the notion that 'seizures beget more seizures'. In terms of mood disorder, it may apply in terms of having an increasing propensity for episodes as more episodes occur. Interestingly, lithium contrasts with most psychoactive agents in that it typically produces no obvious psychotropic effects in normal individuals at therapeutic concentrations.

Suggested mechanisms for the mood-stabilizing effect of lithium:

- Decreasing norepinephrine release
- Increasing serotonin synthesis
- Modulating N-methyl-D-aspartate (NMDA) receptor/nitric oxide signalling
- Neuroprotective properties acting against oxidative stress by upregulating complex I and II of the mitochondrial electron transport chain
- Altered dopamine-associated G-protein function
- Lithium competes with magnesium for binding to NMDA glutamate receptor, increasing the availability of glutamate in postsynaptic neurons
- Lithium has mixed effects on cyclic adenosine monophosphate (cAMP): it increases basal levels of cAMP but also impairs receptor coupled stimulation of cAMP production
- Effects on inositol-phosphate activity: lithium inhibits the enzyme, inositol monophosphatase, which is involved in degrading inositol monophosphate to inositol.

---

2. At review, Caroline reports a recent worsening of her mood, especially in the morning, and that she has been feeling low for most of the day. This has also been associated with sluggishness and a general lack of interest in things. She is wondering if this is related to her lithium treatment.
  4. What are the possible causes of this presentation and how can they be further explored?
  5. What are the problems that can occur with lithium therapy and how should they be monitored for?

While the occurrence of depressive illness is always a key consideration in patients with affective disorder, especially when there is evidence of lowering of mood and altered functioning of biological functions, it is also important to be aware that normal sadness or fatigue, secondary to everyday life events, occur in everyone and are not necessarily indicative of a morbid process. In addition to usual medical causes of low energy (e.g. anaemia, hypothyroidism, diabetes, chronic obstructive pulmonary disease, sleep apnoea, chronic infection, post-viral illness), the potential role of treatment effects should be considered (e.g. sedation). Hypothyroidism secondary to lithium use is common (occurring in up to one-third of users and more common in females). This is readily diagnosed and can usually be treated with thyroxine without discontinuation of lithium.

The differential diagnosis includes a depressive episode, a physical illness that is not directly related to the bipolar diagnosis or its treatment, sedative or other adverse effects of treatment (e.g. hypothyroidism) and normal sadness. Distinguishing these causes is achieved by taking a thorough history exploring the context of these difficulties in terms of onset and progression and relationship to life events and treatment exposures, ascertaining the presence of cognitive and somatic symptoms of depression, other physical symptoms that might indicate an organic cause (e.g. thinning of hair, hypersomnia, fatigue, increased sensitivity to cold, constipation, weight gain, muscle weakness) and physically examining for anaemia, goitre and bradycardia. The usual comprehensive battery of tests for fatigue, including thyroid function tests, are also indicated.

This presentation can be investigated by taking a thorough history for symptoms of clinical depression, symptoms indicative of hypothyroidism, recent physical illness and medication/drug exposure. The nature and severity of low mood and its relationship to other symptoms, such as fatigue, are important to clarify. Usual blood screening [full blood count (FBC), urea and electrolytes (U&E), liver function tests (LFT)], lithium levels and thyroid function tests, are essential tests that should be performed initially.

Prescribed substances that can cause elation

- Steroids: Cortico and anabolic compounds
- Stimulants, e.g. methylphenidate, D-amphetamine, fenfluramine
- Antidepressants [especially tricyclic antidepressants and serotonin and noradrenaline reuptake inhibitors (SNRIs)]
- Malaria treatment (mefloquine)
- Thyroxine
- Opioid analgesics
- L-Dopa and other prodopaminergic agents, such as selegiline
- Isoniazid and iproniazid.

Lithium therapy is well tolerated by many patients, but 75% will experience some adverse effects, and typically 50% of users discontinue use within 12−24 months of initiation. Problems with lithium therapy can be broadly separated into effects caused by acute toxicity and effects that occur over time with sustained use.

Lithium toxicity is typically an acute syndrome caused by elevated serum lithium levels because of accidental or deliberate overdose, interactions with drugs that promote raised serum levels (especially diuretics, nonsteroidal antiinflammatory drugs, calcium channel blockers), severe dehydration because of vomiting, diarrhoea, heatstroke, or accumulation because of reduced renal excretion. Prophylactic serum levels are between 0.6 and 1.2 mmol/L. Toxicity typically appears at levels of ≥1.5 mmol/L with headache, nausea and other gastrointestinal upset progressing to tremor, blurred vision, ataxia, impaired consciousness, seizures, cardiac arrhythmias, coma as levels increase. It represents an acute medical emergency.

Lithium use is also associated with a variety of possible adverse effects

1. Hypothyroidism
2. Impaired renal function (typically after sustained use over many years) and that is usually reversible (irreversible in approx. 1% of users)
3. Weight gain and oedema because of fluid retention
4. Polyuria and polydipsia
5. Gastrointestinal upset
6. Sedation and/or lethargy
7. Tremor
8. Benign leucocytosis

9. Cardiac conduction problems (usually benign T-wave changes and prolonged QRS)
10. Teratogenesis.

Lithium monitoring guidelines (Maudsley guidelines)

It is recommended that lithium levels be monitored weekly until stable serum levels are achieved to minimize the potential for side-effects. Thereafter, for most patients (i.e. those without specific issues):

- Lithium levels should be measured every three months.
- Thyroid function, U&E, FBC and LFT should be checked every six months.
- Creatinine clearance and an electrocardiogram should be measured annually.

Lithium levels are measured 12 hours after the last dose, which is usually in the early to mid-morning, as lithium is usually taken before going to bed because of its mild sedative effects. It is important to clarify when the last dose was taken as lithium has a short half-life such that for patients who usually take lithium in the morning, this can artificially elevate levels. Conversely, some patients may erroneously discontinue lithium for a period prior to testing of serum levels.

The glomerular filtration rate (GFR) is a key indicator of renal function. The estimated GFR provides a useful measure of renal function that is relevant to lithium-related change. The eGFR is a mathematically derived entity based on a patient's serum creatinine level, age, sex and race. A normal level is 90 mL/min. Five levels of impaired renal function are noted and can be classified according to eGFR. Levels between 60 and 90 mL/min reflect stage 1 and 2 chronic kidney disease (CKD), which can be consistent with normal ageing. Below 60 mL/min is more concerning (stage 3–5 CKD), but importantly, the longitudinal trend of eGFR is crucial to make decisions over lithium use such that a stable value below this can be acceptable. In contrast, a declining value requires careful consideration of the need to explore lithium discontinuation.

---

3. Caroline also reports weight gain, fatigue, hypersomnia, thinning of her hair and that she has been feeling cold all the time. Investigation reveals that her lithium levels are 0.7 mmol/L and that her thyroid-stimulating hormone levels are significantly elevated with reduced T4 levels. After discussion, she agrees to continue lithium and commence L-Thyroxine along with escitalopram (a serotonin specific reuptake inhibitor; 10 mg per day). However, over the coming weeks, her low mood worsens despite increasing her escitalopram dose to 20 mg per day. After eight weeks, she commences venlafaxine (a serotonin and noradrenaline reuptake inhibitor; 225 mg), which improves her mood.

6. What is the therapeutic range for lithium levels?
7. How does the treatment of bipolar depression differ from that occurring in unipolar illness?
8. What features of a depressive episode suggest that it is more likely to be part of a bipolar than unipolar illness?

The therapeutic range for lithium is widely accepted to be between 0.4 mmol/L and 1.2 mmol/L. Some evidence suggests that patients who are maintained above 0.6 mmol/L have a lower rate of relapse than those who are maintained between 0.4 and 0.6 mmol/L. Moreover, most psychiatrists aim for levels between 0.6 and 1.0 mmol/L.

The distinction between unipolar and bipolar affective disorder is important for many reasons. These include managing the likelihood of the so-called 'switching', whereby antidepressant interventions can precipitate hypomanic or manic episodes, and in identifying optimal treatment for depressive episodes. Depressive episodes occurring in patients with bipolar affective disorder are often more challenging to manage as they are less likely to respond to conventional antidepressants [e.g. serotonin specific reuptake inhibitors (SSRIs)]. In contrast, treatment with more potent antidepressants (e.g. tricyclic agents or SNRIs) is associated with a risk of precipitating (hypo)mania and in extreme cases destabilizing the underlying illness, with the emergence of rapid cycling illness (see below). Furthermore, in patients with suspected bipolar illness, the approach to managing depressive episodes includes optimizing mood stabilizer therapy, being aware that usual antidepressant interventions may be less efficacious and having an open mind about the value of using alternative strategies, such as other antidepressant classes, another mood stabilizer or antipsychotic augmentation strategies. Many clinicians believe that unopposed antidepressant therapy (i.e. without a concomitant mood stabilizer or antipsychotic) should be avoided.

The National Institute for Health and Care Excellence guidelines recommend that bipolar depression is initially treated with an SSRI as first-line therapy and that second-line approaches include either: (i) switching to mirtazapine or venlafaxine or (ii) augmentation with mirtazapine, quetiapine, olanzapine or lithium.

The diagnosis of bipolar illness is often delayed, particularly in patients who present with depressive episodes without evidence of periods of elation. Of note, in many cases, there are episodes of elation. However, these can be overlooked unless specifically explored for (enquire about the following: sustained periods of unusually high levels of energy, reduced sleep requirement, elevated confidence and/or disinhibition with spending, hypersexuality or other risk-taking behaviours). In addition, there are clues in the presentation of depression that suggest a higher likelihood that the actual diagnosis is a bipolar illness. These include a positive family history of bipolar illness; early age of onset; severe episodes, including any with psychosis; relative treatment resistance (e.g. to SSRIs); and presence of atypical features, such as hypersomnia, increased appetite or mixed features. In such cases, it can be useful to manage patients with the likelihood of bipolarity in mind and, therefore, emphasize mood-stabilizing interventions in treatment.

---

4. Ten days later, Caroline is referred for an urgent review. Her mother reports that she has not been sleeping well, is overtalkative and has been purchasing large amounts of expensive lingerie online. Her workmates have expressed concern that she has been inappropriate and overfamiliar with customers, offering substantial price reductions for goods. She reports feeling 'fundamentally liberated' but also upon discussion accepts that she may perhaps be 'a little high'. She does not report any ideas that might be delusional in intensity and denies other psychotic phenomena. She is not keen to be admitted to hospital and her mother volunteers to 'keep an eye on her for a few days'.

    9.   What is your diagnosis and immediate management plan?

These disturbances suggest that Caroline is experiencing an episode of hypomania rather than full mania as she has been able to continue her usual day-to-day routine and does not have evidence of any psychotic symptoms. Her relative insight into the probable nature of her recent behaviour also suggests hypomania, especially given her willingness to take appropriate treatment along with the availability of continuous and well-informed support. It appears reasonable to proceed with community-based treatment, albeit with regular review of her progress in case her circumstances deteriorate.

It is important with bipolar illness to recognize the longer-term picture and to develop a collaborative relationship as this means that help-seeking is likely to be earlier, which can prevent full-blown episodes. Moreover, a key principle of mental health legislation is that treatment should always be provided in the least restrictive environment that is possible, available and rational in terms of perceived risks. Equally, it is important to try to prevent unnecessary loss of social capital. The statistics regarding a substantially elevated risk in patients with bipolar disorder in terms of experiences relating to the loss of employment, financial difficulties and experience of marital failure emphasize the need to minimize exposure to socially damaging situations. This is a balance that requires careful consideration in collaboration with the patient and is frequently enhanced by having good collateral sources of information about the extent of any behavioural changes that are evident. It can be useful to explore preferences for how a 'high' should be managed with the patient when they are stable and normothymic.

5. You agree to manage Caroline's symptoms as an outpatient, and she agrees to commence risperidone (3 mg nocte). Her mental state settles over the following week. At the review, it emerges that she decided not to take the serotonin and noradrenaline reuptake inhibitor as prescribed. There are no other obvious explanations for the deterioration in mental state. She is worried that the 'lithium may have stopped working' and wishes to discuss the pros and cons of alternative approaches to the prevention of episodes. Moreover, she is interested in exploring the implications of lithium for pregnancy as she has been in a stable relationship for three years and has been thinking about settling down and starting a family.

   10.   What are the alternatives to lithium for maintenance treatment of bipolar affective disorder?

   11.   What are the implications of lithium for pregnancy and childbirth?

   12.   What are the implications of discontinuing lithium treatment?

Lithium is the prototype for a class of agents frequently referred to as mood stabilizers. In essence, these are medications that can treat both mania and depression, although the evidence that many of these agents treat both poles of bipolar illness is quite limited and the definition is often extended to include agents that treat either depression or mania and rarely cause the other pole to become worse in the process. Lithium is generally considered the most effective mood-stabilizing agent and, in reality, most mood stabilizers are primarily antimanic agents that also impact upon, mood cycling and shifting, but are not effective at treating acute depression. Lithium, quetiapine and lamotrigine are the principal exceptions with evidence that they are effective in treating both manic and depressive symptoms. A recent detailed systematic review of randomized controlled trials of bipolar maintenance treatment (Severus et al., 2014) highlighted that lithium is more effective than a placebo in preventing overall mood episodes, manic episodes and depressive episodes. Lithium was superior to anticonvulsants in the prevention of manic episodes.

FURTHER READING

For a review of maintenance management of bipolar affective disorder, see: Severus E, Taylor MJ, Sauer C, et al. (2014) Lithium for prevention of mood episodes in bipolar disorders: systematic review and meta-analysis. International Journal of Bipolar Disorders 2(1):15. doi:10.1186/s40345-014-0015-8

Valproate is the agent that is typically used as an alternative to lithium. Interestingly, despite the evidence to favour lithium as a first-line treatment, in the United States and Australia, valproate is the preferred agent perhaps because of concerns about the adverse effects of lithium and/or the need for relatively less intense monitoring. Furthermore, valproate is considered to be more effective in treating 'mixed state' symptoms and rapid cycling. Alternatively, valproate is often used as a second-choice mood stabilizer. In support of its use, a recent study by Geddes and colleagues (2010) found that lithium or the combination of lithium and valproate was superior to valproate alone in preventing relapse in patients with bipolar I disorder.

FURTHER READING

For details of a recent study on relapse prevention in bipolar I disorder, see: Geddes JR, Goodwin GM, Rendell J, et al. (2010) Lithium plus valproate combination therapy versus monotherapy for relapse prevention in bipolar I disorder (BALANCE): a randomised open-label trial. The Lancet 375(9712):385–395. doi:10.1016/S0140-6736(09)61828-6

In addition, a variety of other anticonvulsants are used in the maintenance treatment of bipolar illness with variable effect. However, there is limited evidence for their efficacy. Carbamazepine is frequently used in those who do not respond to lithium and/or valproate in the management of acute mania and mixed affective episodes. Lamotrigine is typically used for bipolar depression while there is minimal evidence for oxcarbazepine, gabapentin and topiramate. In recent years there has been a movement to formally recognize antipsychotic agents as potential mood-stabilizing agents because of evidence that quetiapine, olanzapine, risperidone and aripiprazole are effective for managing mania but may also improve bipolar depression. This practice is an extension of the longstanding empirical use of antipsychotics beyond the acute phase at low dose in bipolar patients, including sometimes by intramuscular depot formulations.

FURTHER READING

For a discussion on issues relating to lithium use in pregnancy and cardiac malformations, see: Patorno E, Huybrechts KF, Bateman BT, et al. (2017) Lithium use in pregnancy and the risk of cardiac malformations. New England Journal of Medicine 376(23):2245−2254. doi:10.1056/NEJMoa1612222

Lithium has well-established teratogenic potential and use in women of childbearing age requires careful consideration of the relative risk−benefit ratio. Lithium exposure during the first trimester of pregnancy is associated with a congenital heart defect called Ebstein's anomaly (a tricuspid valve abnormality) in approximately 1/600−1/1000 cases. However, there are considerable risks associated with discontinuing lithium with relapse rates in lithium responders estimated to be as high as 30% within a month of rapid discontinuation. Even with gradual discontinuation, there is an estimated three-fold greater risk of relapse within a year. Moreover, targeted discontinuation and reinstatement after the first trimester are unrealistic, and for many patients, the continuation of lithium is preferable to discontinuation.

Similarly, valproate is associated with a variety of major and minor malformations. These include a 20-fold increase in neural tube defects, cleft lip and palate, cardiovascular abnormalities, genitourinary defects, developmental delay, endocrinological disorders, limb defects and autism. Additionally, it should be avoided in women who are at risk of becoming pregnant. Carbamazepine is also linked with an elevated risk of neural tube defects, but this is thought to be less than that associated with valproate.

---

6. Over the following six months, Caroline experiences an unstable period alternating between periods of low mood, including an admission with mania. Her mother asks to see you to discuss what is happening. She is concerned about a reference to 'rapid cycling' that she came across on the internet. She also informs you that she suspects that Caroline has not been taking her medication regularly and has discovered a store of unused lithium.
   13. What is 'rapid cycling' and what implication does it have for treatment?
   14. What can be done to address problems with poor adherence?
   15. What are your thoughts about the store of unused lithium?

FURTHER READING

For a review of rapid cycling in bipolar affective disorder, see: Carvalho AF, Dimellis D, Gonda X, et al. (2014) Rapid cycling in bipolar disorder: a systematic review. Journal of Clinical Psychiatry 75(6):e578−586. doi:10.4088/JCP.13r08905

Rapid cycling is a pattern of frequent, distinct episodes in bipolar affective disorder. In rapid cycling, a person with the disorder experiences four or more episodes of mania or depression in one year. Rapid cycling is not a diagnosis or a distinct subtype of the illness but rather a 'course specifier' or descriptor of a more aggressive phasic course of illness. It can occur at any point in the course of bipolar affective disorder and runs a variable and transient course.

Rapid cycling is estimated to occur at some point in around 10% of patients with bipolar illness and is more common in women, those with early-onset illness and with comorbid substance misuse. A few people with rapid cycling alternate between periods of hypomania and major depressive disorder. However, it is far more common to have repeated and distinct episodes of depression dominate the picture such that persistent treatment-resistant depression is an important differential diagnosis. Antidepressant agents have poor efficacy in treating depression that occurs in rapid cycling illness and is thought to be a potential precipitant and/or maintaining factor. Therefore, many experts advise against the use of antidepressants in bipolar patients at risk of rapid cycling. Mood-stabilizing agents are the core of treatment for rapid cycling illness, often in combinations and sometimes with antipsychotic agents.

Adherence has been defined as 'the extent to which a person's behaviour, taking medication, following a diet, and/or executing lifestyle changes, corresponds with agreed recommendations from a health care provider'. It is also sometimes referred to as compliance or concordance. About half of the patients diagnosed with bipolar affective disorder become nonadherent during long-term treatment, a rate largely similar to other chronic illnesses. Nonadherence in bipolar affective disorder is a complex phenomenon determined by a multitude of factors. Four mutually interacting domains can be used to understand nonadherence: (i) patient (e.g. demographic characteristics such as younger age, comorbid substance use, lower socioeconomic group/social disadvantage and personal beliefs and attitudes around illness and treatment, which include insight levels); (ii) illness (e.g. greater severity of symptoms and/or frequency of episodes, earlier phase of illness); (iii) the effect of medications (e.g. side-effects); and (iv) characteristics of the clinicians (e.g. extent to which there is a truly collaborative relationship with patients).

FURTHER READING

For a comprehensive review of the role of psychotherapy in bipolar affective disorder, see: Lauder SD, Berk M, Castle DJ, et al. (2010) The role of psychotherapy in bipolar disorder. Medical Journal of Australia 193(S4):S31. doi:10.5694/j.1326-5377.2010.tb03895.x

Interventions that include psychoeducation, cognitive behavioural therapy, social rhythm therapy and family therapy have all been shown to impact positively upon adherence and relapse rates in bipolar illness. Interpersonal and social rhythm therapy is designed to help people with bipolar affective disorder improve their mood by understanding and stabilizing biological and social rhythms. It aims to create and sustain consistent daily routines (including habits and routines relative to medication), managing sleep/wake cycles and enhancing skills around managing, and where possible, avoiding socially based stressors.

Storing up medication is a major concern, especially if it is deliberate. Lithium is one of the few psychotropic agents (along with clozapine) whereby receiving a prescription for it is associated with a reduced long-term risk of suicide. Beyond the stabilizing effect on illness course that many lithium users experience, the mechanism of action for this effect is not well understood. Lithium is a highly dangerous drug if taken in overdose, and it should be noted that 15% of patients with bipolar affective disorder die through suicide.

7. It emerges that Caroline had been reducing her lithium dose and missing doses because of an increasing preoccupation about her weight. This began after her boyfriend suggested that she might consider starting a diet. She purchased some slimming pills but thought that she ought to check with her psychiatrist to clarify if they would be safe because a friend had told her that they could affect people with mental health problems.
   16. How would you respond to these issues?
   17. How are issues of weight control addressed in patients receiving psychotropic medications?

Weight gain is one of the main reasons that people diagnosed with depression and other mood disorders stop taking their medication. Many of the so-called slimming pills that are available have psychostimulant properties and, therefore, are best avoided in patients with bipolar affective disorder. These include products that contain diethylpropion, benzphetamine, methamphetamine, phentermine, phendimetrazine or topiramate.

Moreover, there are more effective ways to achieve a sustained reduction in weight that involve careful consideration of prescribed medication. Often weight gain is dose-related or can be avoided by switching to agents within the same class. Overall, the largest body of research exists to support an association between weight gain and antipsychotic treatment (olanzapine and clozapine are especially implicated) and for antidepressants (e.g. mirtazapine). In addition, many services provide specific lifestyle programmes that focus upon helping patients to manage their diet better and engage with realistic exercise programmes that assist in weight management.

Weight gain is greatest during acute treatment phases and in the first 3−6 months of treatment. The underlying mechanism behind weight gain in response to psychotropic treatment is unclear. For antipsychotics, an affinity for histamine H1 receptors, serotonin 5-HT2 and dopamine D2 receptor affinity have been identified.

Weight gain with psychotropics is linked to a variety of factors: metabolic effects (e.g. hypertriglyceridemia, impaired glucose/insulin homeostasis, effects on leptin signalling), increased appetite and carbohydrate cravings and through decreased energy expenditure that can happen with reduced activity. Lithium may cause weight gain by an insulin-like effect on carbohydrate metabolism, altered fat cell metabolism and depressed thyroid function.

FURTHER READING

For a comprehensive review of the epidemiology and management of metabolic issues in psychiatric patients, see: Penninx BWJH, Lange SMM. (2018) Metabolic syndrome in psychiatric patients: overview, mechanisms, and implications. Dialogues in Clinical Neuroscience 20(1): 63−73.

Patients with mental illnesses such as schizophrenia and bipolar affective disorder have an increased prevalence of metabolic syndrome (approximately doubled) with a marked increase in the risk of cardiovascular disease and type 2 diabetes. This is an important factor in the marked gap in life expectancy of more than a decade between those with major functional psychiatric disorders, such as bipolar illness and schizophrenia, and the general population. The increased risk of metabolic issues is linked to a combination of lifestyle and medication effects. Moreover, regular monitoring of weight, abdominal girth and glucose and lipid parameters in collaboration with the patient's general practitioner are warranted.

CHAPTER 16

Declan

Mental Illness in Autistic Spectrum Disorders

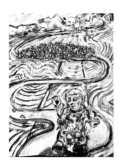

1. Outline the clinical features and course of autistic spectrum disorder (ASD).
2. Outline the epidemiology, including the gender distribution of ASD.
3. Understand the management of ASD.
4. Be familiar with the terminology used in describing ASD.
5. Be able to adapt the history taking and mental state examination techniques in the assessment of those with ASD.
6. Appreciate the role of structured assessments and formal tools in this population.
7. List the disciplines involved in the care of persons with an intellectual disability.

1. When Declan was three years old, he was referred to the local disability service early intervention team for assessment, as his mother was concerned that 'he was not like other boys his age'. The early intervention team assessed Declan. They also spoke at length to his parents who reported that 'Declan seems to have no interest in cuddles or contact; he would rather organize his toy car collection by colour and size than play with his cousins'. His mother also reported that he frequently would flap his hands for no apparent reason.
    1. What is the likely diagnosis given the information thus far and what are the characteristics of this disorder?
    2. How is a diagnosis made?

The most likely explanation is that Declan is on the autistic spectrum, which was created to account for persons with such issues. Specifically, autistic spectrum disorder (ASD) can be associated with a wide range of symptoms, which are grouped into three broad categories: (1) reciprocating social interactions; (2) language and communication issues; and (3) unusual or repetitive behaviours (see Box 16.1).

BOX 16.1 ■ The diagnosis of autistic spectrum disorder is based upon the combination of the following:

Difficulties with reciprocal social interaction can include the following:
Often seeming distant or detached
Having little or no interest in other people and prefer to spend time alone
Finding it difficult to make friends
Not seeking affection in the usual way
Resisting physical contact
Finding it difficult to make eye contact with other people
Wanting to have social contact but have difficulty knowing how to initiate it
Not understanding other people's emotions and struggling with managing their own emotions

Impaired language and communication skills can include the following:
Delayed language development (some remain nonverbal throughout their lives)
Problems initiating or engaging with conversations
Use of odd or made up phrases or words
Using more words than are necessary to explain simple things
Difficulty with understanding or using nonverbal cues, gestures, facial expressions or tones of voice
Difficulty understanding the nuances of language
Concrete or literal interpretation of language

Unusual or repetitive behaviours can include the following:
Limited imaginative play
Playing the same games over and over or playing games designed for children younger than themselves
Becoming upset if their daily routines are interrupted/altered in any way
Showing repetitive/stereotyped behaviours, such as hand flapping or spinning
Developing 'obsessions' with specific objects, lists, timetables or routines

---

The characteristic features of ASD are present from an early age, with differences and delay in social-communicative development associated with a restricted pattern of interest or behaviour. Most people with ASD experience sensory difficulties and may be oversensitive to specific things like touch, certain textures, light intensity or sound. Sensory difficulties can also lead to problems with movement and social interaction. A person with ASD may appear clumsy or have an unusual way of walking.

Asperger's syndrome is a form of ASD. People with Asperger's syndrome will generally not have a learning disability and often have average or above-average intelligence. They will usually have fewer problems with language development. In DSM-5, the diagnosis of Asperger's syndrome has been absorbed into the diagnosis of ASD. There is also a new diagnosis called 'social (pragmatic) communication disorder'. This is categorized as a communication disorder and may serve as an alternative diagnosis for individuals with some Asperger's-like symptoms. This is characterized by prominent difficulties with pragmatics and the social use of language and communication.

FURTHER READING

For a discussion on the diagnosis and concept of autistic spectrum disorder, see: Lord C, Elsabbagh M, Baird G, Veenstra-Vanderweele J. (2018) Autism spectrum disorder. The Lancet 392(10146):508–520. doi:10.1016/S0140-6736(18)31129-2

A child who is ultimately diagnosed with ASD often receives clinical attention initially because of developmental delays highlighted by parents. When ASD is suspected, careful consideration should be given to a range of physical or psychological diagnoses. Sensory difficulties, such as hearing or visual problems, must be ruled out. Prior to giving a diagnosis of ASD careful consideration should be given to taking a detailed medical, developmental and family history. A full physical examination including inspection for dysmorphic features, observation for the presence of atypical behaviours or stereotypies and a detailed neurological examination is essential. The child's social interaction, response to name, joint attention, play skills and use of language should be noted. Formal developmental/psychometric testing as well as the use of standardized tools such as the Autism Observation Diagnostic Schedule, Second Edition (ADOS-2) and Autism Diagnostic Interview-Revised (ADI-R) facilitate diagnosis. Genetic testing may be indicated depending on the clinical picture.

Intelligence testing is vital as the overall intelligence quotient is likely to have a significant impact on the phenotypic presentation and functionality of individuals with ASD.

---

2. Declan receives a diagnosis of autistic spectrum disorder with a mild learning disability. He and his family receive ongoing support from the early intervention team and the local branch of the Autism Society. With the help of a special needs assistant, he then enters mainstream school at the age of six. He does well, and while he struggles academically and with social interaction, he makes good progress.

Declan is now seven years old. Recently, he has been displaying challenging behaviour at school, which the school management has brought to his parents' attention. They note that Declan is refusing to put away the art supplies after art class, a job he seemed to enjoy previously. Declan also has less interest in going out to the playground and is noted to be generally quieter and more irritable. He shouted at other children and pulled one of the girls' hair when she teased him about being 'slow'. He has banged doors at home and hit out at his 9-year-old twin sisters. You are asked to assess the situation, and in the referral letter, it also states that Declan deliberately started to bite his hand, causing minor tissue damage.

3. What are the possible causes of Declan's behaviour based on the information available?
4. What do you understand by the term 'self-injurious behaviour?'
5. What other information would be useful to have at this point?

There are multiple possible causes of Declan's behaviour based on the information above. Possibilities at this point include psychiatric illness (such as depression or attention deficit hyperactivity disorder); environmental changes/changes to routine; substance misuse; interpersonal difficulties; a physical cause, especially, pain, gastric reflux or constipation; or seizure activity.

Self-injurious behaviour is the deliberate alteration or destruction of body tissue without conscious suicidal intent. Self-injurious behaviour, for example, biting, squeezing, head-banging or scratching can occur in the context of mental illness or independent of a diagnosable mental health condition, often as a maladaptive stress-relieving mechanism.

It is important to establish if Declan has any previous history of mental or physical ill-health, if he is taking any regular medications, has had any recent trauma, adverse life events or circumstance changes. The results of any investigations or formal assessments should be obtained.

---

3. Declan does not have a known history of mental illness or any chronic medical conditions. He is not taking any regular medication but has been prescribed oral antibiotics twice within the last six months for respiratory infections. During the meeting with Declan's mother, she informs you that Declan's primary special needs assistant recently went on maternity leave and she wonders if this might be a factor. She also questions you as to whether there is a risk that her twin daughters may develop the condition, although neither has a history of developmental delay.

6. What is the prevalence and cause of autism?
7. What is our current understanding of the brains of children with autistic spectrum disorder compared to controls?

The prevalence of ASD is 5–10 per 10,000 population. The ratio of males to females is approximately 4:1, with the onset of symptoms typically before three years of age. The reason for this gender difference remains unclear but may be partially because of an under-diagnosis in females. Prevalence does not vary significantly with socioeconomic status. Traditionally, it has been considered that most people with ASD (approximately 70%) have an intellectual disability. However, this concept is changing, with the spectrum expanding to include an increasing number of people with some autistic traits but without intellectual or other issues. The overlap with concepts such as schizoid and schizotypal personality is considerable.

Research into the possible genetic basis for ASD has focused on searching for irregular segments of genetic code and investigating the possibility that under certain conditions, a cluster of unstable genes may interfere with brain development. Research is ongoing to better understand the effect of problems during pregnancy, delivery or postpartum and environmental factors, such as viral infections, metabolic imbalances and exposure to chemicals on ASD presentation. Presently, there are no clear, consistent findings and the cause of ASD is still not fully understood.

ASD is a strongly heritable condition, and the concordance for autism in monozygotic twin pairs is typically at least double of that in dizygotic twin pairs. Twin studies estimate the heritability of autism to be high (estimated between 56% and 95%), but also with some environmental contribution (estimated at 30%).

FURTHER READING

For an interesting insight into the difference in brain structure and function in autistic spectrum disorder, see: Ha S, Sohn IJ, Kim N, et al. (2015) Characteristics of brains in autism spectrum disorder: Structure, function and connectivity across the lifespan. Experimental Neurobiology 24(4): 273–284. doi:10.5607/en.2015.24.4.273

Functional imaging of children with ASD and controls found differences in the shape, size and structure of their brains. The most consistent finding is an accelerated total brain volume growth in the early childhood in ASD at around 2–4 years of age. The pathological mechanism that represents an ongoing enlargement of the brain is unclear.

Specific core regions have been suggested to mediate the clinical phenotypes of ASD, such as the frontotemporal lobe, frontoparietal cortex, amygdala, hippocampus, basal ganglia and anterior cingulate cortex. For example, abnormalities in (1) the inferior frontal gyrus, superior temporal sulcus and Wernicke's area might be related to defects in social language processing and social attention; abnormalities in (2) the frontal lobe, superior temporal cortex, parietal cortex and amygdala might mediate impairments of social behaviour; and abnormalities in (3) the orbitofrontal cortex and caudate nucleus have been associated with the restricted and repetitive patterns of behaviour in ASD.

---

4. You then interview Declan. He is superficially cooperative but appears uninterested in talking to you. He repeatedly asks you if you have any model toy cars that you can give him. Your assessment of Declan has included a history, mental state examination and collateral information. Declan does not report any subjective complaints. When asked about his mood, he replies that he does not understand what this means. You then explain this to Declan in terms of sadness or happiness most of the time. Declan responds that he is happy most of the time but that he feels sad because Sarah, his previous special needs assistant, has not been at school recently. He does not endorse any anxiety symptoms or psychomotor abnormalities on the mental state examination. He does not describe any delusions, paranoia or formal thought disorder. As part of a thorough examination, you ask Declan if he ever hears voices when there does not seem to anybody around; he states that he does. Other than this finding on the mental state examination, you do not find any indications of affective illness, and Declan's account, though limited, is consistent with the collateral information given by his carer.

8. How might you explore whether Declan is experiencing auditory hallucinations?

FURTHER READING

For an outline of mental health assessment in individuals with autistic spectrum disorder, see: The United Kingdom's National Autism Society. (2008) Basic guidelines for interviewing a person with an autism spectrum disorder. Available at: https://www.choiceforum.org/docs/iv.pdf.

The following approach is useful when assessing for the presence of auditory hallucinations:

- Observe Declan for a period of time to ascertain if he appears to be experiencing an auditory perception in the absence of an external stimulus (this may manifest itself as talking back to a perceived voice, distress, lability of mood, inappropriate affect).
- Obtain collateral information from staff in the school to establish if Declan appears to be responding to auditory stimuli that do not appear to have a source in the external environment.
- Ask Declan if he can hear a voice when no one else is in the vicinity (external sensory sources).
- Ask Declan if he hears a voice in internal space (his head) or external space (through his ears).
- Ask Declan does he recognize the voice or indeed if it is his voice.
- Ask Declan to describe the content.
- Enquire how often this occurs, whether regularly or infrequently and whether it is associated with going to sleep or while waking up.

---

5. On further discussion with Declan, you establish that he perceives this voice as located inside his head and that he recognizes it as his own voice. He reports that the voice is telling him that he must have done something wrong for Sarah to leave. He reports that he often hears it when he is sitting on his own in his room. Recently, it has been occurring on average a couple of times per day, but previously, it was more frequent in the immediate period after Sarah left. He gets a little upset when he hears this voice, but it does not stop him from carrying on with his activities. You observe Declan tidying his room for 15 minutes. During this time, he appears to talk to himself a lot, asking where to put the objects that he is tidying and answering affirmatively. Collateral information from his parents and teacher confirms that Declan engages in a lot of self-talk, the content of which appears to be of reassuring himself or asking questions about model toy cars for which he supplies answers himself.

9. Is Declan experiencing 'true' or 'pseudo' auditory hallucinations?

Declan is unlikely to be experiencing true auditory hallucinations. True hallucinations are perceived in external space and are not perceived as one's own thoughts. Pseudo-hallucinations are not necessarily psychopathological but they can be a subtle expression of emerging psychosis. In Declan's case, the 'voices' may be explained in the context of the relatively egocentric perspective that occurs in autism.

---

6. You discuss Declan's change in behaviour with him. At first, he is reluctant to discuss this and becomes irritable and expresses that he 'will be good' and not engage in biting his hand or refuse to help tidy away the art supplies from now on. When you clarify that your intention is not to criticize or 'give out to him', but to try and help, he becomes more cooperative. He tells you that he misses Sarah and that this makes him feel sad and that when he feels sad, he bites his hand or stays in his room crying. Declan states that he does not understand why Sarah has left and wanted her to return straight away.

10. What is the significance of Declan's disclosure?
11. What comorbidities are reported with autistic spectrum disorder in general?

Disturbed or self-injurious behaviour is relatively common in people with ASD who have a comorbid intellectual disability. Self-injurious behaviour can be a method to communicate distress for those who lack the skills to communicate their distress verbally. This may be due to the lack of the physical ability to speak, not having the necessary language or not having the ability to link internal distress to spoken words. Self-injurious behaviour may also be caused by sensory difficulties, which are especially common in those with ASD. Those with ASD often have altered senses, either having an increased ability or decreased ability to hear, see, feel, taste and smell. The most reported of these is increased sensitivity to sound and light. A less well-known but very common sensory issue for those with ASD is touch. Those with ASD often find light touch (e.g. stroking the skin) uncomfortable but find deep touch (e.g. deep tissue massage) soothing. Therefore, self-injurious behaviour in those with ASD may be an attempt to experience deep touch and, thus, find a method to self-soothe. Therefore, self-injurious behaviours are largely functional in that they achieve an important immediate outcome for the individual.

People with ASD commonly suffer from other psychiatric disorders, most commonly Attention Deficit Hyperactivity Disorder and Obsessive Compulsive Disorder. Specific phobias are very common. Depression, social phobia and oppositional defiant disorder frequently occur.

---

7. You obtain collateral information from Declan's mother and father who describe that Declan's sleep and appetite are good. They report that Declan is not expressing any lowering of mood and continues to enjoy his model toy collection. Declan has repeatedly been asking about when Sarah is returning to school. When Declan's parents explained that she was taking time off to have a baby, he was visibly upset, feeling he was her baby and explained to you that Sarah would often refer to him affectionately as 'her baby'.

Declan's case is discussed in detail at the weekly multidisciplinary team meeting. Contributions are made by several members of the team. You provide feedback that from your assessment, you think Declan is experiencing an adjustment reaction. You explain that this is a form of adjustment disorder in response to a recent stressful life event. You do not believe that Declan is currently suffering from an affective disorder. On discussion, it is decided that a psychological assessment is warranted as Declan's normal activities are affected. An occupational therapist will also visit Declan at his home and school.

12. What other disciplines do you think will be represented at the multidisciplinary team meeting?
13. What are the diagnostic criteria for adjustment disorder?
14. How might the symptoms of adjustment disorder differ in a person with an intellectual disability than someone without an intellectual impairment?
15. How might have Declan's presentation differed if he was experiencing a moderate depressive episode?

Multidisciplinary team (MDT) members may include social workers, psychologists, occupational therapists, intellectual disability nurses, psychiatrists, social care workers, service managers (day/transport/residential) and general practitioners. The MDT may also include other specialists such as dieticians, physiotherapists, dentists and neurologists.

Adjustment disorder involves a state of subjective distress and emotional disturbance, usually interfering with social functioning and performance, and arising in a period of adaptation to a significant life change or the consequences of a stressful event. The stressor may involve the individual or his/her group or community. Individual predisposition or vulnerability plays a role in the risk of developing adjustment disorder (Box 16.2). Characteristics include depressed mood, anxiety, worry, feelings of inability to cope and some degree of disruption of daily routine.

BOX 16.2 ■ The diagnosis of adjustment disorder is applied where:

1. Functionally significant emotional and/or behavioural symptoms occur soon (within months) after a stressful or upsetting experience
2. Symptoms that do not meet criteria for another mental health disorder (e.g. depressive episode, anxiety disorder), and that are
3. Expected to resolve with physical and temporal removal from the precipitating experience (e.g. within six months)

In people with an intellectual disability, changes in behaviour and signs of regression back to an earlier developmental stage (clingy behaviour with his mother, reduced independence, tantrums) may be prominent features. The onset is usually within one month of the occurrence of the stressful event or life change, and the duration of the symptoms does not usually exceed six months.

If Declan was experiencing a moderate depressive episode, he would be likely to display symptoms such as pervasive anhedonia (which is not evident as he continues to enjoy his toys), persistent depressed mood or, in the absence of this, sustained irritability, changes in appetite and weight, sleep disturbance, anergia, persistent withdrawn behaviour, feelings of excessive and inappropriate guilt, suicidal thoughts and major disruption to social or work life.

---

8. A behavioural support plan involving positive behaviour support was drawn up, including strategies such as modelling, behaviour shaping and self-management of behaviour using video technology. Declan's rate and intensity of self-injurious behaviour and other problem behaviours reduce. He now engages well with his new special-needs assistant. You conduct a follow-up assessment 10 weeks after the first multidisciplinary team meeting. From your assessment, you conclude that he does not display features of adjustment disorder or other mental illness. You plan to continue to follow-up Declan's case every two months for the time being and to continue to liaise with other multidisciplinary team members and with Declan's parents.

CHAPTER 17

Francine

Borderline Personality Disorder

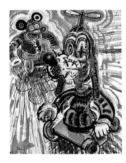

1. Describe the key clinical diagnostic features of personality disorders in general, and specifically, borderline personality disorder (BPD), including differential diagnoses and common comorbid mental and physical disorders.
2. Compare and contrast the main clinical features of the different clusters of personality disorders.
3. Briefly describe the epidemiology of BPD, including the prevalence and gender differences.
4. Describe the key potential aetiological factors in BPD and classify these in terms of medical/biological, social and psychological factors.
5. Beginning with a detailed history, mental state examination and collateral history, list the main investigations involved in the assessment, diagnosis and ongoing treatment of BPD. Moreover, consider these investigations as medical/biological, social and psychological.
6. Describe the main treatments for BPD and consider these in terms of medical/biological, social and psychological approaches.
7. Briefly describe the key prognostic factors for BPD and compare to the prognosis of other major mental disorders.

1. Francine is a 19-year-old, single, music and drama student who is referred by her general practitioner for assessment of 'depression and low self-esteem'. At interview, she describes feeling low recently because of relationship problems with her boyfriend. She describes having repeated arguments because of her accusations that he is 'looking at other women and not properly committed to the relationship'. She states that he thinks she is overpossessive and needs to 'calm down a bit'. She explains that she attended her general practitioner after one such argument but feels fine now as they have resolved these problems. She mentions that she attended child psychiatry services because of an eating disorder when she was younger.

Continued on following page

(Continued)

She reports a recurring pattern of problems in interpersonal relationships whereby she tends to get overinvolved and is easily upset by rejection. She says that her romantic relationships have always tended to end 'messily'.

1. What are the key diagnostic issues in this presentation?
2. What is your preferred immediate management plan?

This presentation indicates a pattern of experiencing adjustment problems and situational crises in the context of ongoing difficulties in interpersonal interactions and vulnerable personality traits that include low self-esteem and fears of rejection. These problems seem to be ongoing as she relates them as a consistent and recurring pattern in relationships. The nature of difficulties around the attendances at Child and Adolescent Mental Health Services (CAMHS) should be clarified, but again suggest longstanding difficulties in personality, self image and in managing relationships.

The transient nature of symptoms and close relationship to situational stressors does not support the presence of sustained major mental illnesses such as depression. Furthermore, although pharmacological intervention is not warranted, it needs to be considered how Francine can be best helped to deal with situational stress, including exploring her self-esteem issues, which seems the most appropriate intervention. The severity of her reported problems suggests that the intervention could be readily provided through community-based primary care services rather than requiring the input of a specialized mental health service.

2. After discussion, you agree to a management plan that includes engaging with a counsellor to explore coping strategies and self-esteem. However, at the inpatient ward round the following Monday, you are informed that Francine has been admitted over the weekend after an overdose and with 'severe depression' and placed on a high observation regimen because of concerns about possible, repeated self-harm. At review, the staff report that Francine has appeared well over the weekend, sleeping at night and engaging with the staff and other patients. At interview, Francine reports that she took 12 ibuprofen tablets after a night out that ended in an argument with her boyfriend when she accused him of being unfaithful. She reports feeling 'very low' with thoughts that she cannot cope with life and wanting to 'end it all'.

3. What is the significance of the disparity between Francine's observed behaviour and reported subjective mental state?
4. What can additional sources of information assist in clarifying the diagnosis and treatment plan?

Hospital admission can serve several important functions: providing a place of safety during an acute crisis, allowing close observation during a period of stabilization of mental state, including monitoring of response to treatment and facilitating the monitoring of mental state and behaviour to clarify if reported symptoms are evidenced in an observed environment.

Although it can be argued that some patients put on a brave face in public, the reality is that for more severe illness, the impact upon expressed mood, affect, motivation, behaviour and biological functioning are usually visibly obvious. A patient with 'severe depression' is unlikely to be capable of appearing 'well' and actively engaging in social interactions. There is often a gap between the subjective quality of sleep, and that observed when specifically monitored (e.g. as an inpatient). The disparity evident in Francine's case suggests that her dysphoria does not reflect a sustained and pervasive disturbance of mood and functioning consistent with a major depressive illness, but rather relates to more transient or situational factors.

Nevertheless, it would be important to assess carefully for other indicators of depressive illness (anhedonia, cognitive distortions) and/or more subtle presentations of mood disorder (e.g. atypical depression, mixed affective states). The pattern of mood disturbances (intensity, duration, precipitants), relationship to life circumstances and lifestyle factors and previous personal and family history of mental ill-health can all assist in an accurate diagnosis. If situational factors are relevant, it will be important to assess their interaction with baseline personality, including coping style under pressure. Collateral history from somebody who knows the person well is a vital source of information along with input from her general practitioner (GP). As Francine attended CAMHS in the past, they should also be contacted for a collateral account and for a copy of previous reports and clinical notes.

---

3. You agree to continue with inpatient care to allow for a period of further observation and to obtain previous case notes and a collateral history. Francine permits you to contact her mother, who explains that Francine attended Child and Adolescent Mental Health Services in the context of problems with low self-esteem, chaotic eating habits, disciplinary problems at school and considerable disharmony at home. After six months of attendance, things 'settled down' until eight months ago when she commenced attending college. At that point, she moved to live independently, and contacts with her family have been intermittent ever since. Her mother describes her as 'highly strung' and 'hypersensitive', especially, in relationships with boyfriends, which have usually 'ended badly'.

The clinical case notes from Child and Adolescent Mental Health Services describe problems with chronic dysthymia without a pattern of sustained clinical depression, intermittent self-harm (superficial wrist cutting) and a bulimic eating pattern. At one appointment, she reported an episode of alleged sexual abuse at age 13 years by a visiting uncle, but this was subsequently denied and withdrawn. Otherwise, her engagement with psychological support was inconsistent with multiple missed appointments. The discharge summary suggests a 'prominent axis II' pathological condition as the principal cause of her difficulties.

5. What are the psychological difficulties accounted for by an 'axis II' classification?
6. What are the diagnostic criteria for personality disorder? What are the main categories and their characteristics? Specifically, describe borderline personality disorder.
7. What are the implications of this information for her immediate management?

Prior to the introduction of the Diagnostic and Statistical Manual of Mental Disorders-5 in 2013, the American Psychiatric Association classification and the diagnostic system was multiaxial, allowing for the recognition of multiple active and significant problems in any one patient. In this system, axis I included major psychiatric disorders, e.g. major depressive disorder, schizophrenia, autistic spectrum disorder; and axis II included intellectual disability and disorders of personality. This distinction has gradually led to patients with prominent personality-driven elements in their presentations as being sometimes referred to as 'axis-two-y'. Axis III was reserved for medical or physical conditions that may affect or be affected by mental health issues. Axis IV allowed for the inclusion of contributing environmental or psychosocial factors, and axis V referred to the global assessment of functioning.

Personality disorder refers to a diagnostic concept that captures psychological and adaptive dysfunction that reflects an enduring abnormality of personality or character (Fig. 17.1). This abnormality is deeply ingrained and enduring in nature such that it typically impacts interpersonal

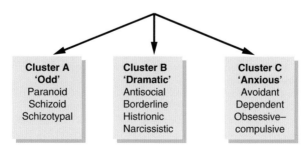

Fig 17.1   DSM-5 categories of personality disorder.

and adaptive functioning across the domains of life (work, home, hobbies). Problems are not provoked by a single situational factor but rather reflect a recurring pattern of dysfunctional engagement. The disturbance is such that it significantly impacts the ability to function and/or causes significant distress to the person or others (Table 17.1 and Box 17.1).

TABLE 17.1 ▪ Details of the Categories of Personality Disorder

Cluster A (odd or eccentric)		
Paranoid	**Schizoid**	**Schizotypal**
Irrational suspicions Mistrust of others	Lack of interest in social relationships Seeing little point in sharing time with others Introspection	Odd behaviour or thinking

Cluster B (dramatic, emotional or erratic disorders)			
Antisocial	**Borderline**	**Histrionic**	**Narcissistic**
Lack of empathy for the perspective of others Pervasive disregard for the law and the rights of others	Relationship instability Poor self-image Self-harm Fear of rejection Impulsivity	Attention-seeking behaviour Seductiveness Shallow or exaggerated emotions	Grandiosity Need for admiration Lack of empathy

Cluster C (anxious or fearful disorders)		
Avoidant	**Dependent**	**Obsessive– Compulsive**
Social inhibition Feelings of inadequacy Extreme sensitivity to negative evaluation Avoidance of social interaction	Psychological dependence on others Fears of abandonment	Rigid conformity to rules, moral codes Excessive orderliness

---

BOX 17.1 ▪ The diagnosis of borderline personality disorder is based upon the following:

1. A deeply ingrained and pervasive pattern of behaviour that impacts upon the socio-adaptive function of a person and or others.
2. The core characteristic involves the following: (a) an unstable sense of personal identity with low self-esteem and chronic feelings of emptiness and (b) fear of rejection.
3. A pattern of unstable and intense interpersonal relationships that typically relates to difficulties in tolerating emotional ambiguity.
4. Affective instability because of a marked reactivity of mood and difficulties in anger management.
5. Impulsivity with a pattern of self-damaging behaviours (e.g. spending, sexual behaviour, substance abuse, binge eating).
6. Recurrent suicidal behaviour, gestures, threats or self-mutilating behaviour.
7. Transient, stress-related paranoid ideation or dissociative symptoms.
8. These behaviours are consistently identifiable over time and across different domains of interpersonal, social and occupational activities and do not occur exclusively during episodes of other mental disorders (e.g. mania, psychosis).

Borderline personality disorder (BPD) has three characteristic domains: (1) hypersensitivity to interpersonal problems (and especially perceived rejection); (2) affective instability with a proneness to emotional dysregulation; and (3) impulsivity. Note how this differs from histrionic personality disorder where the theme of needing attention prevails rather than preventing abandonment. The diagnosis is based upon a relatively enduring pattern of behaviours that are stable in their instability. Recurrent issues with self-harm when accompanied by fears of abandonment are highly suggestive. The pattern should be evident across functional life domains such that it impacts upon social, familial and work-related interactions, and therefore, is not highly situational specific. These features should also significantly impact the ability to function in these domains and/or cause significant distress.

FURTHER READING

For a detailed review of borderline personality disorder, see: Gunderson JG. (2011) Clinical practice. Borderline personality disorder. New England Journal of Medicine 364:2037−2042. doi:10.1056/NEJMcp1007358

This information has important implications for management, whereby it will be important to agree on a clear management plan. There is little evidence to indicate that the hospitalization of people with BPD is particularly effective except where the occurrence of comorbid conditions warrants inpatient care. Moreover, a careful assessment for clinically significant depression can guide ongoing care, including the appropriateness of inpatient or outpatient care.

4. The following evening, Francine leaves the inpatient unit against medical advice after a disagreement with another female patient.
    8. Under what circumstances can a voluntary patient be prevented from leaving an inpatient unit?
    9. What arrangements would you make for follow-up treatment?
    10. What is the relationship between personality disorders and other psychiatric illness?

A voluntary patient can be prevented from leaving a psychiatric unit if they are deemed to meet criteria for detention, i.e. suffering from a significant mental illness that poses a risk (to self or others) or necessary treatment can only be provided as an inpatient, and voluntary means are not possible. Francine's presentation has not indicated that urgent or immediate treatment against her will is required.

Follow-up treatment can be made by direct contact with Francine and her GP. The period immediately after hospital discharge is a key time of increased risk for service dropout and self-harm. Therefore, active and early follow-up is indicated.

FURTHER READING

For a review of comorbidities with borderline personality disorder and other psychiatric conditions, see: Dell' Osso B, Berlin H, Serati M, Altamura AC. (2010) Neuropsychobiological aspects, comorbidity patterns and dimensional models in borderline personality disorder. Neuropsychobiology 61:169−179. doi:10.1159/000297734

Comorbidity is the norm in patients with BPD. Mood disorders (unipolar and bipolar), post-traumatic stress disorder (PTSD), anxiety and substance misuse disorders commonly complicate the clinical picture. The frequency of PTSD (39%) and a mood disorder (approximately 50%) is so high that BPD has been postulated as a complex form of each disorder. Of note, there is an elevated rate of affective disorder in first-degree relatives of patients with BPD, while traumatic experience in childhood is a well-recognized risk factor for both BPD and PTSD.

5. Some weeks later, Francine's general practitioner informs you that she has moved to a neighbouring catchment area and is linking in with services there for follow-up. Some months later, you receive a referral indicating that she has moved back to your locality and is requesting a follow-up appointment. In the interim, she has had three admissions to their service, each in the context of situational stress and including one with 'quasipsychotic' symptoms. The primary diagnosis is of borderline personality disorder. Her ongoing management is discussed at the weekly multidisciplinary team meeting where two team members are resistant to accepting the referral as they are concerned that Francine's problems do not reflect 'proper illness' and 'personality cannot be treated'.

11. What is the significance of the so-called 'quasipsychosis?'
12. How would you respond to the concerns as to Francine's treatability?
13. What evidence is there that psychological treatments are effective in the treatment of borderline personality disorder?

'Quasipsychosis' is a term used to refer to the expression of symptoms that do not have the characteristics of psychosis occurring in functional psychotic disorders. For example, this includes the phenomenon of pseudo-hallucinations whereby the character of experiences differ from true hallucinations by not being perceived in external space or as truly real (e.g. voices inside one's head rather than voices heard through one's ears and perceived as real sensory phenomena). Such quasipsychotic symptoms are indicative of states that occur in people who have personality disorders or other vulnerabilities.

The treatability of personality disorder has long been a source of controversy for both psychiatry and society in general. In its most basic form, the 'mad versus bad' distinction suggests a dichotomy that is vastly over-simplistic since all people with mental illness have personality-based aspects of their profile, while people with abnormal personality profiles have a heightened vulnerability to other mental health problems. This occurs either as part of their illness constellation, a consequence of the same aetiological factors (e.g. adverse or abusive experiences in childhood) or difficulties and adverse life events that relate to personality-driven adversity (substance abuse, interpersonal difficulties, loss events).

It is also important to note that many major mental disorders initially present with a prodromal phase that includes problems that could easily be attributed to personality disorder and the emergence of overt major mental illness often results in one's personality and temperament being expressed in exaggerated terms. Therefore, the person can become a caricature of their usual self.

In simple terms, the lifestyle of people with more severe personality disorders is stressful and can provoke other mental health problems. In addition, people with personality disorders tend to mostly engage with services at times of active depressive illness, for instance. Ultimately, the presence of patients with personality disorder in mental health services mandates that the challenges of trying to manage many of their problems reside within mental health services.

The prevalence of personality disorder in the general population is 10%, increasing to 25% of primary care attenders and 40% of patients attending psychiatric services. The poor outcomes (it is estimated that 10% of patients with BPD end their lives by suicide) emphasize the need for specialist psychiatric input.

The issue of treatability remains contentious with some suggesting that personality disordered patients absorb valuable therapeutic resources disproportionate to the level of benefit experienced. Undoubtedly, patients with more severe personality disorders are high utilizers of mental health services. However, this phenomenon suggests that mental health services need to manage this engagement in a more organized and effective manner. Therefore, understanding the needs of personality disordered patients is key. Gathering evidence that various pharmacological and psychological interventions can improve outcomes in people with a personality disorder is increasingly tilting the balance towards proactively engaging such patients with treatment.

FURTHER READING

For a review of pharmacological approaches in borderline personality disorder, see: Lieb K, Voellm B, Ruecker G, et al. (2010) Pharmacotherapy for borderline personality disorder: Cochrane systematic review of randomised trials. British Journal of Psychiatry 196:4−12. doi:10.1192/bjp.bp.108.062984

Pharmacological treatment is highly symptom-oriented, and as such, there is evidence for the use of antidepressants and mood stabilizers in patients with prominent mood and impulse dyscontrol, with other evidence suggesting that the use of antipsychotic agents can assist in patients with prominent impulsivity.

FURTHER READING

For a review of psychological approaches in borderline personality disorder, see: Paris J. (2010) Effectiveness of different psychotherapy approaches in the treatment of borderline personality disorder. Current Psychiatry Reports 12:56−60. doi:10.1007/s11920-009-0083-0

Psychological approaches form the mainstay of the treatment of BPD. Conversely, pharmacotherapy is targeted towards specific problem areas or comorbidities. Numerous (over 20) randomized controlled trials support the effectiveness of psychotherapeutic interventions, which typically involve prolonged therapy (e.g. one year) with regular and intense contact. Common elements include clarification of the diagnosis and acknowledgement of the associated distress and dysfunction that it causes. This is followed by agreed targets that focus on stress reduction, developing strategies to improve impulse control and developing social outlets and capital.

Specific therapies include dialectical behavioural therapy (DBT) and cognitive approaches that emphasize mentalization, that is, examining and labelling emotional responses to situations. In DBT, the therapist and client work with acceptance and change-oriented strategies. The emphasis is on developing strategies to improve coping with challenging situations, emotional and impulse regulation (including mindfulness). In DBT, the therapist acts as an ally rather than an adversary in the management of difficulties and aims to accept and validate the client's feelings but also identify how some feelings and behaviours are maladaptive and can be substituted by alternatives. The therapist acts as a coach and is available to provide support, for example, by telephone for extensive periods. Positive outcomes include improved emotional and impulse regulation and reduced rates of deliberate self-harm, but there is less convincing evidence that responders no longer meet criteria for BPD.

---

6. Francine re-attends consultation and is linked in with the clinical psychologist. Some weeks later, you are contacted by a student nurse from the team who has been socializing with Francine and is concerned that Francine is not 'connecting' with the psychologist. Francine has confided to her that she has a stockpile of paracetamol that she plans to take if things do not improve. Moreover, you receive correspondence from a solicitor seeking a report in relation to an episode of shoplifting where they have asked that you comment on Francine's illness as a mitigating factor.
  14. What are your thoughts about this information, including its content and how it has been received?
  15. What are your thoughts about the extent to which her legal problems can be explained by a mental disorder?

Psychological engagement with BPD patients is notoriously challenging because of their propensity to challenge therapeutic boundaries, test the therapist's ability to maintain a therapeutic relationship, idealize the therapeutic relationship, and engage in 'splitting' (whereby different information and attitudes are adopted for different staff members). Patients with BPD are prone to re-enacting previous significant relationships during therapeutic encounters. Threats of self-harm or other dysfunctional behaviours can be used in a manipulative manner, often to prevent perceived abandonment or rejection. This information is presented through a messenger with whom the patient has established a relationship that is outside usual therapeutic boundaries and includes information that has a compelling theme of possible self-harm and pressurizing the relationship with the psychologist.

Patients with behavioural problems that occur in the context of having the capacity to understand that they are 'wrong' and are likely to have adverse outcomes should be held accountable for their actions, as to remove responsibility can serve to reinforce aberrant, socially unacceptable or irresponsible behaviour. The presence of a personality disorder can assist in understanding how or why a patient has engaged in such activity but does not absolve them of responsibility.

---

7. Francine attends for review where she reports sustained low mood, loss of interest, low energy, early awakening, loss of appetite with a 4–5 kg weight loss and feelings of futility saying, 'I will never be good enough for other people to like me'. She admits to drinking heavily on most days 'to try and lift my mood'. She relates to the onset of these difficulties in exploring the episode of childhood sexual abuse in therapy. She feels that she may never get better.
    16. What is the significance of these difficulties?
    17. What is the longer-term prognosis of people with borderline personality disorder?

This presentation suggests the emergence of a comorbid depressive illness and a problematic pattern of drinking in the context of dealing with the emotional impact of addressing a previous trauma. Patients with BPD have an increased vulnerability to a range of disorders, especially mood disorders, substance misuse problems, PTSD and eating disorders. A key challenge in managing patients with BPD is to remain vigilant to the possibility of these comorbidities and to diagnose and treat them promptly. It is not unusual for such problems to be misdiagnosed or missed completely, particularly where patients have a history of challenging or otherwise compelling behaviour that can distract clinicians. Specific attention to the character of symptoms and their consistency over time can allow for more accurate detection.

In addition to the problems of timely detection, the prognosis of patients with BPD in relation to response to comorbidities is also impacted upon by the tendency for less consistent engagement with treatment, erratic compliance, need to avoid potentially dangerous therapies, the tendency for less supportive social networks and socio-adaptive capital, and elevated rates of substance misuse.

Traditionally, it has been thought that personality (and by extension personality disorder) reflects an enduring phenomenon that is resistant to intervention. However, follow-up studies indicate that only one-third of patients diagnosed with BPD meet the criteria at 10–20-year follow-up, with up to one-half of the patients no longer meeting any personality disorder criteria. In part, this may reflect that our expression of self is softened with advancing age but also highlights the potential for change. Less encouragingly, only 25% of the patients with BPD have full-time employment at 10 years, and the lifetime suicide rates are estimated at 10%. Poor prognostic indicators include the presence of concomitant antisocial traits and severe and repetitive self-harm.

CHAPTER 18

Trevor

Antisocial Personality Disorder

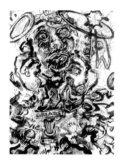

1. Understand the principles of maintaining personal safety during patient interviews.
2. Be able to advise on good sleep hygiene.
3. Recognize the core elements that underpin the concept of personality disorder.
4. Understand the diagnostic criteria for antisocial personality disorder (ASPD).
5. Describe what we know about the cause of ASPD.
6. What are the treatment options for ASPD?
7. Recognize the overlap between personality disorder and other mental health disorders.
8. What is the prognosis of ASPD?

1. You are a nonconsultant hospital doctor in the general adult psychiatry service. You have received a referral from a general practitioner requesting an opinion on a 23-year-old man, Trevor, who presented requesting 'relaxers' as he was subjectively anxious and finding it difficult to sleep following a road traffic accident three months previously.

You arrange to meet Trevor. Trevor lives a 30-min drive away from the clinic. His mother has driven him to the appointment as Trevor is currently off the road for driving under the influence. She takes a seat in the waiting area. Trevor shakes your hand warmly and takes a seat; stating 'I'm delighted to meet you, cos I could really do with a little help'. He explains he is having difficulty sleeping and feels anxious all the time. He is experiencing dizziness and headaches and feels this is because of anxiety. He mentions that he was on tablets before for this and feels he needs them again. You explain to Trevor that you need to ask him some more detailed questions before deciding on the right course of action. He becomes somewhat irritable insisting that 'Xanax' (alprazolam, a benzodiazepine) is the only thing that would help but regains control quickly and you proceed with the assessment.

    1. What are the principles of maintaining personal safety in clinical settings?

FURTHER READING

For excellent advice on safety in the various psychiatric settings, see: Royal College of Psychiatrists. (2005) Safety for Psychiatrists. Available at: https://www.rcpsych.ac.uk

The possibility of being assaulted while at work is very real for mental health-care professionals, with the vast majority experiencing at least one assault during their careers. As such, it is good to plan for 'when, not if' such an incident might occur. Several practical steps could be taken to minimize this risk, including the following:

- Ensure the interview room is set-up safely before you start. This includes making sure that the room is clutter-free. Position the chairs so that they are a safe distance apart and that you have easy, unblocked access to the door. You should always be closer to the door.
- Personal alarms should always be used, and you should seat yourself so that you have easy access to the wall alarm button or are carrying a mobile alarm device. Personal and wall-mounted alarms should be tested regularly to ensure they are operating properly.
- If you feel uneasy during an interview, end the interview politely (if necessary, excuse yourself to go to the bathroom) and ask for help or leave the room.
- Ensure you are not alone in a remote part of the building with a patient.
- If you notice the patient becoming agitated or upset by a line of questioning, it may be advisable to drop that line of enquiry.
- Report any incident compromising your safety, however trivial you think it is. It needs to be documented in an incident form.
- Avoid wearing items that could be used as a ligature, such as ties, long scarves or jewellery around your neck. Avoid high heel shoes as these too could be used as a weapon.
- If possible, gather collateral information about the patient before you see them. If you do not feel comfortable seeing a patient alone, ask another member of the team to sit-in with you.

---

2. You ask Trevor about the accident. He was a front-seat passenger. His friend was driving 'because he was less bombed than me'. The car went out of control and through a stone wall into a field. Trevor lost consciousness for 2–3 minutes. Both men were taken to hospital by ambulance; while Trevor was admitted overnight for observation, his friend Rory sustained serious injuries and was admitted to the intensive care unit before being transferred to the National Rehabilitation Centre. You enquire about Rory's recovery; Trevor responds by saying, 'I don't know how he is; he's a clown; I don't care. What's it to you, anyway? Aren't we here to talk about me and get me something to relax?'

On Mental State Examination, Trevor was not depressed, not overtly anxious and denied symptoms of posttraumatic stress disorder. He did not display psychotic symptoms.

He admitted to smoking cannabis 'to relax' and was spending €80 per week on the drug. He denied current use of alcohol or any other drugs. He had moved back in with his mother after his girlfriend 'broke up with him' 8 weeks previously.

You advise Trevor of the dangers of cannabis use and go on to suggest ways for Trevor to improve his sleep hygiene and suggest anxiety management techniques. Trevor becomes very annoyed and hits the desk between you and him hard. He curses that this was a waste of time and tells you that if you do not give him something to relax, he will end up killing himself and 'it would be your fault'. He stands up from his chair, knocking it over. You activate your alarm and staff from the day hospital come to your aid. Trevor storms out of the door brushing staff aside as he does so and leaves the building.

    2. What are your initial thoughts on Trevor's presentation?
    3. What is the differential diagnosis?
    4. What are the principles of good sleep hygiene?

Trevor does not show due regard for boundaries and seems indifferent to the feelings of others. From what we know to date, Trevor appears manipulative and seems to treat others with callous indifference. He does not seem remorseful or guilty that his 'friend' is badly injured. There is also a significant drug and alcohol element.

The differential diagnosis is quite broad given the information thus far and includes posttraumatic stress disorder (PTSD), or another anxiety disorder, substance use disorder, personality disorder (any of antisocial, narcissistic, borderline or histrionic personality disorder) or no psychiatric illness.

Sleep hygiene includes a variety of different practices that promote good nighttime sleep quality and full daytime alertness. The following are recommendations from the national sleep foundation:

- Limiting daytime naps to 30 minutes. A short nap of 20–30 minutes can help to improve mood, alertness and performance.
- Avoiding stimulants such as caffeine and nicotine close to bedtime. While alcohol is well-known to help you fall asleep faster, too much close to bedtime can disrupt sleep in the second half of the night as the body begins to process the alcohol.
- Exercising to promote good quality sleep. As little as 10 minutes of aerobic exercise, such as walking or cycling, can drastically improve nighttime sleep quality.
- Avoid strenuous workouts close to bedtime.
- Steering clear of food that can be disruptive right before sleep. Heavy or rich foods, fatty or fried meals, spicy dishes, citrus fruits and carbonated drinks can trigger indigestion for some people. When this occurs close to bedtime, it can lead to painful heartburn that disrupts sleep.
- Ensuring adequate exposure to natural light. This is particularly important for individuals who may not venture outside frequently. Exposure to sunlight during the day and darkness at night helps to maintain a healthy sleep–wake cycle.
- Establishing a regular relaxing bedtime routine. A regular nightly routine helps the body recognize that it is bedtime. This could include taking a warm shower or bath, reading a book, or light stretches.
- Try to avoid emotionally demanding or upsetting conversations and activities before attempting to sleep.
- Making sure that the sleep environment is pleasant. Mattress and pillows should be comfortable. The bedroom should be cool. The bright light from lamps, mobile phones and television screens can make it difficult to fall asleep.
- Consider using blackout curtains, eyeshades, earplugs, 'white noise' machines, humidifiers, fans and other devices that can make the bedroom more relaxing.

---

3. Trevor's mother, Ellen, stands at the clinic door and shouts after her son to come back. She starts to cry. You are aware that other patients are looking on and you invite Trevor's mother into your office. She asks what happened, and you explain that you cannot discuss her son without his consent. She blurts out that she does not know what to do with her son. 'Trevor has always been a handful'. You notice bruising on Ellen's wrists; she catches you looking at them. Self-consciously, she pulls down her sleeves but then says 'he didn't do that...it was his father...he loses it sometimes'.

Ellen tells you that 'Trevor can be so charming and thoughtful sometimes and brings me chocolates', but is afraid Trevor will end up in prison again as he was arrested after a pub brawl where he knocked out his cousins front tooth and threw a chair across the bar, breaking several glass bottles.

Ellen tells you that Trevor was a difficult child and hated school. He had many acquaintances but no real friends. He would stay out late and be picked up by the police on several occasions in his teens for the destruction of property, theft and antisocial behaviour. He was convicted of the violent assault of a shop owner and was sentenced to 18 months in prison 'but was inside for three years because he did something else'. Ellen's distress heightens and you suggest leaving it there for now, but she responds by saying 'I have to let this out; I cannot take it anymore' and continues to talk about Trevor.

    5. What is 'personality disorder?'
    6. Do we know the cause of antisocial personality disorder?
    7. What are the features of antisocial personality disorder?
    8. What other terminology is used to describe antisocial personality disorder?

A personality disorder is a type of mental disorder in which the difficulties reflect characterological issues rather than a phasic illness. The person has a deeply ingrained pattern of maladaptive behaviours that impact upon their socioadaptive functioning in terms of relationships, social activities, work and school. Typically, the difficulties are evident from early adulthood (or earlier) and occur across the person's life (i.e. they are not just caused by a specific situation such as an unpleasant job or a bad relationship).

Personality disorder is, thus, defined by longstanding patterns of behaviour and is grouped into three clusters based on similar characteristics and symptoms. These are the following:

- Cluster A is characterized by odd or eccentric behaviour and includes paranoid personality disorder, schizoid personality disorder and schizotypal personality disorder.
- Cluster B is characterized by dramatic, overly emotional, unpredictable thinking or behaviour and includes ASPD, borderline personality disorder, histrionic personality disorder and narcissistic personality disorder.
- Cluster C is characterized by anxious, fearful thinking or behaviour. They include avoidant personality disorder, dependent personality disorder and obsessive–compulsive personality disorder.

Many people with one personality disorder also have signs and symptoms of at least one additional personality disorder.

Cause of ASPD

The causes of ASPD are not well understood. A combination of genetics, temperament, early life experiences and an early lack of empathy are all linked to the development of the disorder.

FURTHER READING

For a study on gene-to-gene interactions in ASPD, see: Arias JMC, Acosta CA, Valencia JG, et al. (2011) Exploring epistasis in candidate genes for antisocial personality disorder. Psychiatric Genetics 21(3):115–112. doi:10.1097/YPG.0b013e3283437175

In a meta-analysis of twin and adoption studies, Mason and Frick (1994, see below) discovered that 50% of the variance found in measures of antisocial behaviour could be attributed to genetic effects. Viding et al. (2007) identified callous and unemotional personality traits, which appeared to be genetically based. Neocortical vulnerability possibly arising from genetic, *in utero* exposure to substances or subtle frontal lobe injury coupled with early chronic stress may result in a chronically hypoaroused state and lack of emotional response; such children may learn to down-regulate their feelings.

FURTHER READING

For study results on genetic effect, see: Mason DA, Frick PJ. (1994) The heritability of antisocial behavior: A meta-analysis of twin and adoption studies. Journal of Psychopathology and Behavioral Assessment 16(4):301–323. doi.org/10.1007/BF02239409
and
Viding E, Frick PJ, Plomin R. (2007) Aetiology of the relationship between callous-unemotional traits and conduct problems in childhood. British Journal of Psychiatry 49: s33–38. doi: 10.1192/bjp.190.5.s33

A study by Arias et al. (2011, see above) suggests that epistatic gene interactions between genetic variants of the catechol-O-methyltransferase (COMT), 5-HTR2a and tryptophan hydroxylase genes could be associated with ASPD and influence the dopamine reward pathways and modulate serotonin levels in ASPD. Their study supports an important role of polymorphism in serotonin receptors and low enzyme activity of COMT for susceptibility to ASPD.

Violence and neglect within the family are two of the most consistent factors predicting later antisocial behaviour. Early life experiences, including inconsistent supervision, harsh punishment, being from a large family (four or more), early institutional living, parental rejection, inconsistent parental figures (e.g. shifting from parents to grandparents to friends) and the presence of an alcoholic father, may all be contributory. Parental ASPD, parental conflict, domestic violence, single parenthood, maternal depression and socioeconomic status may also be contributory as could parental substance misuse.

Prenatal factors may also influence the development of ASPD. Exposure to alcohol and other drugs *in utero*, low birth weight, premature birth and childhood exposure to toxins are also potentially contributory.

Impulse control dysfunction and the presence of hyperactivity and inattention are the most highly related predisposing factors for the presentation of antisocial behaviour. Children with attention deficit hyperactivity disorder and a comorbid conduct disorder are more likely to develop ASPD. Negative emotionality (anxiety, irritability and anger) has been found to be related to the commission of crime. In addition, impulsivity was most strongly correlated with the manifestation of antisocial behaviour between the ages of 9–15 years.

The low arousal theory posits that people with ASPD seek self-stimulation by excessive activity to counteract an abnormally low baseline level of arousal. Moreover, the provocative behaviours of ASPD are thought to be aimed at addressing a chronic state of so-called 'stimulus-hunger'. In support, people diagnosed with ASPD typically score low on fear conditioning and have been shown to have less physiological arousal to pictures of people crying than non-ASPD subjects.

Below average intelligence quotient and poor language skills during the preschool years are associated with future delinquency. Conduct disorder (CD), such as disruptiveness and truancy, may then contribute to further worsening of academic achievement and ultimately the persistence of CD behaviours into adulthood, which then fall under the remit of ASPD.

Features of ASPD

ASPD is a condition wherein the individual has a longstanding pattern of failure to conform to social norms, often bringing the individual in contact with law enforcement agencies. There is typically a marked lack of empathy and history of impulsivity, with a low threshold for the discharge of aggression. There is often a reckless disregard for the safety of self or others and problems with accepting personal responsibility for one's actions. An inability to show guilt or remorse for their actions may be evident. Substance abuse is frequently a comorbid feature.

Of note, people with ASPD can also be quite charming, but this is typically goal-directed and not sustained once they have achieved their goal. The personal history of people with ASPD often includes multiple relationships and employment periods that typically end badly. Diagnosis should be based upon longstanding and repetitive patterns of behaviour, and often this may require collateral history and careful attention to personal history as the person may not accurately report events (Box 18.1).

Terminology

Both 'psychopath' and 'sociopath' are other terms or ways to describe people with the profile of ASPD. ASPD is the term used in the Diagnostic and Statistical Manual of Mental Disorders–5. Dissocial personality disorder is the term used in the International Classification of Diseases–10. These different labels are essentially interchangeable.

BOX 18.1 ■ The diagnosis of antisocial personality disorder is based upon the following:

1. A deeply ingrained and pervasive pattern of behaviour that impacts upon the socioadaptive function of the person and or others.
2. Typical behaviours indicate a disregard for societal norms and/or the wellbeing of others. They can include criminal behaviour, impulsivity, aggression, dishonesty, taking advantage of others for personal profit or pleasure, reckless or irresponsible behaviour often as a means of self-stimulation or gratification, difficulties in maintaining interpersonal relationships or employment.
3. The core characteristic involves a lack of empathy or remorse with respect to the perspective of others that can include a callous disregard.
4. The diagnosis is restricted to adults, but there is frequently a pattern of conduct disorder during childhood/adolescence.
5. Antisocial behaviours are consistently identifiable over time and across different domains of interpersonal, social and occupational activities and not occur exclusively during episodes of other mental disorders (e.g. mania, psychosis).

---

4. Before Ellen leaves, she remarks, 'He's not a bad boy, I think it might be drugs, and he gets down'. She did not know when he started using drugs but thinks he was about 14 years old. She reports how 'sometimes he came home and was as high as a kite' and other times he would be very 'relaxed and eat us out of house and home'. He has a good relationship with his father overall, but they can get into arguments, and this has ended in physical fights on occasion. He has a younger sister whom he is not close to.

As you need to continue with the morning clinic, you ask the crisis nurse on the team to take Ellen to the relaxation room and stay with her until she is ready to leave.

9. What are the common comorbidities seen with antisocial personality disorder?

FURTHER READING

For a paper which aims to highlight ASPD and psychopathy as related but distinct disorders, see: Werner KB, FEW LR, Bucholz KK. (2015) Epidemiology, comorbidity, and behavioural genetics of antisocial personality disorder and psychopathy. Psychiatric Annals 45(4):195–199. doi:10.3928/00485713-20150401-08

Individuals with ASPD are four times more likely to experience a mood disorder, 13 times more likely to experience a substance use disorder and 7 and 9 times more likely to experience suicidal ideations and attempt suicide, respectively. There is significant overlap with other personality disorders. In general, longitudinal studies indicate that the concept of personality disorder is stable over time, often becoming less prominent with older age as the person 'softens'.

---

5. You are concerned about Trevor's threat of suicide and ask the team crisis nurse to make telephone contact with him in the afternoon. The crisis nurse contacts Trevor after the meeting. His speech is slurred and he curses at the nurse saying, 'tell that so-called doctor to shove her anxiety management'. The nurse offers Trevor a further appointment, which he refuses. She enquires about suicidal ideation and thoughts of harming others. Trevor curses 'No, what's it to you anyway, don't call me again' and hangs up.

Along with the crisis nurse, you discuss the case with a consultant after the phone call. You explain that you suspect antisocial personality disorder but point out that you only had a limited time with Trevor. You are advised to complete an incident report and telephone the general practitioner to advise her of the consultation and that you are discharging Trevor back to her care.

Two months later, you receive a letter from consultant forensic psychiatrist, Dr Bell. Trevor is on remand on violent assault charges, and the court is requesting a psychiatric assessment. Enclosed with the letter is a consent form signed by Trevor, allowing you to discuss the case. You call Dr Bell and explain your limited interaction with Trevor and his mother and agree to send on a detailed letter.

    10. How might the forensic psychiatrist proceed from here?

    11. What is the prevalence of antisocial personality disorder?

Assessment

When assessing a person with a possible ASPD, each of the following areas warrants attention:

- Clear elucidation of antisocial behaviours.
- Personality functioning, coping strategies, strengths and vulnerabilities.
- Assessment for comorbid mental disorders (including depression and anxiety, drug or alcohol misuse, PTSD and other personality disorders).
- The need for psychological treatment (and whether the individual is suitable for this), social support and occupational rehabilitation or development.
- Establish if domestic violence may be an issue.
- Establish if there are any child protection issues.

It is inadvisable to attempt to diagnose a personality disorder based on a single interview. The use of structured assessment methods is advised to increase the validity of the assessment. In forensic services, structured personality inventories, such as the Minnesota multiphasic personality inventory, may be used to aid diagnoses and structured judgement tools, such as the psychopathy checklist (PCL)-R or PCL-SV, to assess whether there is significant 'psychopathy'. The latter is a psychological construct, not a clinical diagnosis, that can be used to inform risk and treatability decisions.

The prevalence of ASPD in the general population is 3% in males and 1% in females. The prevalence in prisons is far higher and is approximately 50% of male and 25% of female prisoners.

6. Several months later, you learn through your crisis nurse (who met Ellen in the supermarket) that Trevor has been convicted of aggravated assault and sentenced to 5 years in prison. According to his mother, he is receiving 'some kind of counselling, so I hope it helps when he gets out'.

    12. What are the treatment options for antisocial personality disorder?

    13. What is the prognosis?

Treatment

ASPD is difficult to treat. People with this condition usually do not seek treatment on their own and may only engage with therapy when required to do so by the court, and even then, can be difficult to engage. Most treatment approaches are psychological and seek to promote pro-social behaviours and attitudes. They are often delivered by the criminal justice system on a group therapy basis. Behavioural treatments, such as those that reward appropriate behaviour and have negative consequences for inappropriate behaviour, can be effective in some individuals.

FURTHER READING

For guidance on ASPD, see: National Institute for Health and Care Excellence (NICE). (2009) Antisocial personality disorder: treatment, management and prevention, CG77, Available at: https://www.nice.org.uk/guidance/cg77.

There is only modest evidence for the effectiveness of group-based cognitive behavioural skill interventions, delivered in the community and institutional settings, in reducing offending for adults in the criminal justice system.

Group-based cognitive behavioural skill interventions for offending behaviour have a small but positive effect on the rate of re-offending for adult male offenders. There is also some evidence for structured residential therapeutic programmes. Moreover, this works on the prosocial principle, and residents can expect timely behavioural feedback from other residents and staff when rules are broken.

There is little evidence to support the use of pharmacotherapy in ASPD, and no drugs are licenced for this indication. Comorbid mood or psychotic disorders are common and should be treated. Borderline personality traits are common in those with ASPD, as is substance misuse. All these need to be considered when formulating a management plan.

In general, the focus is on management, rather than treatment, of ASPD and should, as a core principle, avoid antitherapeutic practices such as overprescribing medication, especially any with addictive potential. In the future, the role of interventions such as dialectical behaviour therapy may alter this perspective of ASPD.

Prognosis

The difficulties of ASPD tend to peak during the late teenage years and early 20s. They sometimes improve on their own by the time a person is in their 40s. Comorbidity with mental illness or substance misuse confers a poorer prognosis. Positive prognostic predictors are a recognition of the problem by the individual, a genuine desire to change and sustained engagement with a therapeutic programme.

Frank

Gender Dysphoria

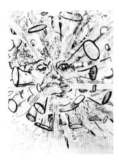

1. Appreciate the differences between sex, gender identity and sexual orientation.
2. Understand what is meant by dual role and fetishistic transvestism.
3. Appreciate the complexity of the concept of transgender behaviour, including transsexualism.
4. Recognize how to assess gender dysphoria (GD).
5. Appreciate the known epidemiology of gender variance.
6. Recognize how GD is managed, including the different stages of transition.
7. Describe the outcome of gender realignment interventions.

1. You receive a phone call from the consultant endocrinologist at your hospital. A 24-year-old male patient, Frank, was admitted under his care yesterday evening after an overdose of oestrogen. He is reassured that this was not a suicide attempt. However, the patient has a previous psychiatric history and the consultant would like your opinion.

You retrieve Frank's old chart and note a history of a single episode of elation two years previously. During this episode, Frank had beliefs that he was especially in tune with the thoughts and feelings of female patients in the ward. He had requested a bed in the female ward, and most of his contact on the ward was with female patients, with whom he would have, what he referred to, as 'girl talk'. His discharge letter noted that the episode was very mild, and he was not maintained on psychotropic medication.

You meet with the house officer on the endocrine team, and he feels that Frank is very depressed with unusual thought processes concerning his 'sexuality'.

   1. What are your immediate thoughts about this presentation?

This initial presentation raises several possibilities. In simple terms, this is a liaison referral for a young man with a psychiatric history who has taken an overdose. The chart review suggests a possible bipolar illness with an episode of elation accompanied by prominent ideas of identification with female patients. However Frank was not maintained on psychotropic medication, which suggests that this first presentation was not thought to represent a psychotic episode. Even though the team feels that Frank is significantly depressed, they do not feel that the overdose was a suicide attempt and oestrogen would not be a common agent used in overdose. It again appears that his mood disturbance is accompanied by unusual thought content regarding his sexual identity.

Of note, 'sex' is the term we use to refer to a person's sexual anatomy, including sex chromosomes, sex organs and hormonal make-up. 'Gender' is the term we use to refer to how a person feels about themself as a boy/man or girl/woman. 'Gender identity' is the term for how a person self-identifies in terms of being a boy/man or girl/woman. 'Gender role' refers to social roles that are assigned by society according to gender. 'Gender assignment' is the social process by which children are labelled as boys or girls at birth. 'Sexual orientation' is the term we use to refer to a person's sexual (erotic) feelings and preferences. Therefore, when we talk about a person being homosexual, heterosexual, or bisexual, we are referring to that person's sexual orientation.

---

2. When you arrive in the ward, Frank has been taken down to the radiology department for a liver ultrasound as he has pronounced gynaecomastia and testicular atrophy along with abnormal liver function tests. His girlfriend is in the ward and you take the opportunity to take a collateral history. She says that Frank has been very distant for the last few months and appears to her to be depressed with intermittent periods when he seems very activated and energized. She is also visibly upset and confides that on one occasion, she returned home early from work and found Frank wearing one of her dresses. When she confronted him about this, he told her that he had done this on several occasions and attempted to reassure her by saying that there was no sexual motivation for wearing the clothes.

   2. What are the possible causes for this presentation?

   3. What do you understand about the terms transvestite and transsexual?

   4. What do you understand about gender dysphoria and how common is it?

The team are investigating for possible organic underpinnings to Frank's presentation. Gynaecomastia and testicular atrophy may be stigmata of chronic liver disease or may suggest chromosomal abnormalities, such as Klinefelter's syndrome. It is important to keep in mind Frank's past psychiatric history and that he is showing signs of affective disturbance. Nonetheless, there is also a prominent theme around gender identity (see Table 19.1).

In short, sex is about your body, gender is about whom you feel yourself to be, and sexual orientation is about to whom you are attracted sexually.

Gender, gender role, gender identity and gender expression may have complex and often independent relationships. Increasingly, some individuals may not label their gender in binary terms, and those who express their gender in this way come under the umbrella term 'nonbinary'. This is not necessarily a modern construct, with different cultures recognizing 'third genders'. These include (but are not limited to) the 'Fa'afafine' in Samoan society (anatomically male, dress and behaviour typically feminine) and the 'Hijras' in South Asia (majority are anatomically male, with occupations of singing, dancing and running households).

TABLE 19.1 ■ Gender Issues

Gender identity	Female/Male/Other
Gender expression	Feminine/Masculine/Other
Sex assigned at birth	Male/Female/Intersex
Physically attracted to:	Women/Men/Other genders
Emotionally attracted to:	Women/Men/Other genders

'Gender fluid' individuals may express the wish to remain flexible in their gender identity. 'Bigender' individuals shift between masculinity and femininity and 'trigenders' move between these and a third gender.

Others do not identify as having any gender or gender identity and may be referred to as 'agender' individuals.

Transvestism

> **BOX 19.1** ■ **Transvestism (International Classification of Diseases-10; F.64.1)**
>
> The individual wears clothes of the opposite sex to experience temporary membership in the opposite sex.
> There is no sexual motivation for the cross-dressing.
> The individual has no desire for a permanent change to the opposite sex.

Transvestism (Box 19.1) is the practice of dressing and acting in a style or manner traditionally associated with the opposite sex. Transvestism can be divided into two principal patterns: 'dual role' and 'fetishistic' transvestism. In dual role transvestism, the person wears clothes of the opposite sex to experience being the opposite sex temporarily but does not have a sexual motive. In fetishistic transvestism, the individual gains sexual excitement from wearing clothes of the opposite sex. In many cases, the term has been replaced by the phrase 'cross-dresser' as this makes no presumptions around motives and might be less stigmatizing. Interestingly, the term is rarely applied to females who dress in typically male clothes.

Gender dysphoria

Gender dysphoria (GD) is a condition where a person experiences discomfort or distress because they perceive a mismatch between their biological sex and gender identity. It is sometimes known as gender incongruence. It can be described as pervasive, profound unhappiness or unease that one's body does not match one's psychological state. It is underpinned by personal dissatisfaction with sexual identity (not sexuality), sex-/gender-specific body characteristics and gender roles (behaviour). It is a rare variant of human nature, is unremarkable in some cultures and may coexist with mental illness.

GD is represented in a continuum; from those experiencing discomfort with their gender role/presentation, through to those 'transgendered' individuals who wish to present and be accepted as a member of the opposite sex to those who wish to modify their body to appear in line with their desired gender. The latter group are referred to as transsexuals (Box 19.2).

A survey of 10,000 people, undertaken in 2012 by the Equality and Human Rights Commission in the United Kingdom (UK) found that 1% of the population surveyed was gender variant, to some extent. While this suggests that GD is uncommon, the number of people seeking help with the condition is increasing because of growing public awareness.

FURTHER READING

For a review of the historical development of the concept of GD, see: Beek TF, Cohen-Kettenis PT, Kreukels BPC. (2016) Gender incongruence/gender dysphoria and its classification history. International Review of Psychiatry 28(1):5–12. doi:10.3109/09540261.2015.1091293

BOX 19.2 ■ Transsexualism (International Classification of Diseases-10; F.64.0)

Three criteria:
1. The desire to live and be accepted as a member of the opposite sex, usually accompanied by the wish to make the body as congruent as possible with the preferred sex through surgery and hormone treatment.
2. The transsexual identity has been present persistently for at least two years.
3. The disorder is not a symptom of another mental disorder or chromosomal abnormality.

As psychiatrists have traditionally been responsible for managing the care of transgender patients, GD currently remains classified as a mental disorder along with other disorders of gender identity. Whether GD should remain classified as such is a controversial area, representing an area of discomfort to both GD individuals and mental health practitioners. From the professional position, the classification may influence the general approach to patient management, whereas GD individuals may have concerns about the impact the classification has on their interface with medicine and society. This issue resonates with the previous inclusion of homosexuality as a psychiatric disorder until the 1970s, with many psychiatry services before then offering 'treatment' to address what were considered pathological homosexual ideas and behaviours.

The incidence of transsexualism in the UK is estimated to be approximately 1:10,000 (i.e. there are between five and six thousand transsexuals currently living in the UK). However, because of the considerable interest in the idea of less rigid approaches to gender identification and considerable destigmatization (even reverse stigmatization), these estimates are increasing.

European studies would suggest that 70% of transsexuals are male to female (MTF) and 30% female to male (FTM). Data from the London Gender clinic provide a 7:1 ratio for MTF: FTM.

The mechanisms underpinning GD are unknown and are likely to reflect a complex range of interlinking factors. Historically, GD was thought to arise from psychopathology. In simplistic terms, the 'patient' has an unconsciously motivated delusion that they are in the 'wrong' physical gender. Psychosocial factors hypothesized to influence the development of this psychopathology include parental factors, such as an emotionally distant father, parents with an unfulfilled desire for a child of the opposite sex and parental encouragement of the child participating in the opposite gender role. Childhood abuse has also been implicated in the development of GD.

However, there is growing evidence that the condition has neurobiological underpinnings. These include hormonal causes, such as increased exposure to prenatal androgens, and genetic and neurobiological studies of people with gender identity issues. It is thought that the extent to which men and women exhibit masculine or feminine behaviour is dependent on the organization of the brain into male or female patterns. A recent study examined sex differences in brain activation patterns of young transgender people. Adolescent boys and girls with GD were examined using magnetic resonance imaging scans to assess brain activation patterns in response to a pheromone known to produce gender-specific activity. The pattern of brain activation in both transgender adolescent boys and girls more closely resembled that of non transgender boys and girls of their desired gender. In addition, GD adolescent girls showed a male-typical brain activation pattern during a visual/spatial memory exercise.

Other studies support a significant genetic basis for the development of GD. In one recent study comparing concordance between monozygotic and dizygotic twin pairs, of 23 monozygotic female and male twins, nine (39.1%) were concordant for GD, while in contrast, none of the 21 same-sex dizygotic female and male twins were concordant for GD.

FURTHER READING

For a detailed review of gender dysphoria, including its neurobiology, see: Zucker KJ, Lawrence AA, Kreukels BPC. (2016) Gender dysphoria in adults. Annual Review of Clinical Psychology 12:217–247. doi:10.1146/annurev-clinpsy-021815-093034

Differential diagnoses

3. Frank returns to the ward and agrees (enthusiastically) to an interview with you. His mood is labile but not overtly depressed. He tells you that he has a profound sense of 'being a woman in a man's body' and that he experiences intense feelings of disgust at his genitalia.

He is happy to be in the hospital because he would like to see a surgeon to discuss the possibility of gender realignment surgery. He is hoping that this can be performed during his current admission as he has private health insurance. He has a letter from a surgeon who mentions a 'capacity assessment'.

5. What is the likely diagnosis and how would you proceed?
6. Would a history of bipolar disorder have ramifications in terms of diagnosis or capacity to request treatment?

Transgender beliefs were originally attributed to psychosis and, indeed, several psychiatric illnesses can (rarely) present with symptoms of cross-gender identification, including schizophrenia and other delusional disorders, bipolar disorder, dissociative and personality disorders. Studies have demonstrated that a significant percentage of patients requesting gender reassignment had a psychiatric diagnosis other than GD that accounted for their desire for a transition to the opposite sex, with the most frequent diagnosis being one of personality disorder. Furthermore, despite the Diagnostic and Statistical Manual of Mental Disorders, assertion that 'delusions of belonging to the other sex' are rarely seen in schizophrenia, there are occasional cases.

It appears that the diagnosis is GD, as Frank describes a longstanding desire to exist as a member of the opposite sex, and also wants to make his body as congruent as possible with his preferred (female) sex. Nevertheless, it remains important to take a careful developmental history exploring aspects of the individual's life that pertain to their gender feelings and experiences (Box 19.3).

BOX 19.3 ■ **Key issues to be covered in the assessment of a person with gender dysphoria include the following:**

1. The type of play as a child (conforming to gender role or nonconforming)
2. Preferred dress as a child
3. Gender identity as a child, adolescent and adult
4. The reactions of others regarding the patient's gender and behaviour
5. Experiences of puberty
6. Any history of cross-dressing, and whether this was associated with sexual arousal
7. Later life cross-gender experiences such as going shopping or socializing in public as a member of the opposite sex
8. Any progress towards adopting the opposite gender role, such as changing name or hair removal, should be clarified
9. Contact with other transgender people
10. Aspects of self that are perceived to be masculine and those perceived to be feminine
11. Clarify what the patient's goals and expectations are regarding making the transition to the opposite gender

As noted above, transsexualism may coexist with mental illness but whether this is coincidental or a primary or secondary factor in GD requires careful consideration. For example, mental illness may occur in individuals with GD because of the inherent stress caused by their gender conflict and the reactions of those around them. Where mental illness occurs alongside (or secondary to) GD, the issues most frequently seen include depression, anxiety, substance misuse and self-harming behaviours.

Patients may be reluctant to reveal symptoms of mental illness, for fear that this may jeopardize treatment of the gender disorder. Where psychiatric illness is diagnosed, gender reassignment surgery/hormonal therapy is not contraindicated, although those with comorbid illness may experience more difficulties during the gender reassignment progression. The psychiatric disorder should be stabilized for an extended period before the medical treatment of gender disorder is commenced.

FURTHER READING

For a review of psychiatric comorbidity with gender dysphoria, see: Dhejne C, Van Vlerken R, Heylens G, Arcelus J. (2016) Mental health and gender dysphoria: A review of the literature. International Review of Psychiatry 28(1):44–57. doi:10.3109/09540261.2015.1115753

Depression

Depression appears to be particularly common among those with GD. The incidence of clinical depression has been variously reported to be between 21% and 44%. As with the 'normal' population, depression may be related to genetic liability. However, the condition may be overrepresented in those with GD concerning (for example) suppression of transgender feelings and behaviours, social isolation and hopelessness.

Suicide attempts

It has been reported that very high numbers (in the region of one-third) of GD individuals have attempted suicide at least once in adulthood which is significantly higher than the 'normal' population. The experience of gender-based victimization is independently linked with suicide. There is some evidence that initiation of GD related treatment lowers self-injurious behaviour.

Substance misuse

Substance misuse and alcohol misuse also appear to be common, with studies reporting drug or alcohol misuse in around 50% of those with GD. The vast majority attribute such misuse to trying to cope with their gender issues.

Definition of capacity

A diagnosis of severe mental illness does not preclude capacity. A person is deemed to lack capacity to decide if he or she is unable to do any of the following:
1. Understand the information relevant to the decision
2. Retain that information long enough to enable making a decision
3. Use or weigh that information as part of the process of making the decision
4. Communicate the decision by any means.

> **BOX 19.4 ▪ Triadic therapy**
>
> 1. Sustained experience of living in an identity-congruent gender role.
> 2. Administration of hormones of the desired gender.
> 3. Surgery to change the genitalia and other sexual characteristics.

4. After a lengthy interview, you cannot elicit any signs of psychiatric illness. Frank has admitted that he was taking oestrogen prior to his psychiatric admission two years ago and tells you that it led to a very labile mood. He does not give any convincing history of bipolar illness.

Frank gives a lengthy history of gender dysphoria and is convinced that he should proceed towards gender reassignment surgery.

7. What should you advise?

Individuals with GD may take their treatment to several different levels. Some remain transgender despite dysphoria. Others continue cross-gendered living full-time/part-time, with or without hormones, with or without chest surgery and with or without genital surgery.

The advised approach for those seeking surgical gender reassignment involves making a social, hormonal and physical transition. This is typically progressed using 'triadic therapy' (see Box 19.4).

While the above treatment pathway should be suggested, individuals will probably have already initiated hormone treatment themselves. Nonetheless, patients should be guided through the benefits and limitations of treatments, have their readiness to progress assessed and be linked in with psychotherapeutic services.

Living in an identity-congruent gender role

The World Professional Association for Transgender Health (2011) emphasizes the importance of sustained experience living in the desired gender when preparing for gender reassignment to experience the issues involved in belonging to their preferred gender and make an informed decision about their capacity to function in it. Much of this phase concerns the provision of appropriate information, for example, on how one's legal name and gender can be changed and how to cope with appearing as the opposite gender in the workplace.

Hormone therapy

This should involve the services of an endocrinologist, who will monitor for any potential iatrogenic haematological, biochemical or physical consequences. Patients may also be referred to other specialists such as dieticians, drama/speech therapists and for minor cosmetic advice, such as hair removal.

Psychotherapy

Psychotherapy is aimed at facilitating comfort in one's reassigned gender identity, allowing for more realistic chances to succeed in relationships, education and work. Therapy should focus on coping strategies, support and providing the patient with information about their treatment options.

Of note, many studies link psychotherapy with more favourable outcomes after surgery. There is also evidence for including partners and parents in therapy.

5. Frank attends a psychologist for a few sessions along with a speech therapist. He attends an endocrinologist. Although their relationship has ended, his ex-girlfriend has remained supportive. A date has been booked for surgery and she is worried about the incidence of regret after the operation.
    8. What would you advise in terms of prognosis?

Follow-up studies suggest that most patients who undergo gender reassignment surgery are generally satisfied with the outcome. A recent longitudinal study of over 1000 persons who underwent sex reassignment surgery found that most reported beneficial effects in terms of emotional well-being, sexuality and general quality of life. Nonetheless, it appears that around 10% of patients may experience a worsening of their psychosocial functioning after surgery. Postsurgical regret has been associated with an incorrect diagnosis, prior mental health problems, surgical complications, inadequate family support, weak social networks and unrealistic expectations of surgery.

CHAPTER 20

Eric

Dementia

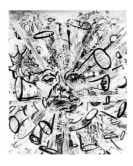

1. Give a general clinical definition and list the diagnostic criteria for dementia.
2. Give a clinical definition and list the diagnostic criteria for the common subtypes of dementia (Alzheimer's, vascular, mixed, dementia with Lewy bodies, frontotemporal dementia).
3. Describe the common presenting cognitive and psychiatric problems seen in individuals with dementia.
4. Define mild cognitive impairment, its subtypes and prognostic significance.
5. Describe the epidemiology of dementia.
6. Outline the societal and economic costs of dementia.
7. Describe bedside cognitive tests that are used in everyday clinical practice, relating them to the main higher cognitive functions.
8. Describe the common aetiological factors and neuropathological condition involved in dementia.
9. List the main investigations involved in dementia workup.
10. Describe general health measures in the management and prevention of dementia, using a biopsychosocial approach.
11. Describe the pharmacology of the dementia-specific medical treatments currently available for the treatment of dementia.
12. Outline the course and prognosis of the common dementias, including factors that prompt long-term care.
13. Describe a biopsychosocial approach to the management of behavioural and psychological symptoms in dementia.

1. Eric is a 71-year-old retired health, safety and environment administrator who has been a widower since his wife died 18 months ago. His daughter contacts you, his general practitioner, to arrange a consultation because she is concerned that in the last 6–12 months, he has 'not quite been himself', and in particular, has seemed forgetful at times, mixing up his grandchildren's names.
    1. What are your initial thoughts regarding the possible explanations for this presentation?
    2. What additional information might you seek?
    3. How can you assess his current level of cognitive functioning?

Memory and other cognitive problems in older people are often minimized and attributed to 'old age', by both the individual and their family. Furthermore, the individual may be seemingly unaware of the cognitive problems, and family members may be the ones who initiate presentation for assessment. The loss of a spouse or close supporting relative may expose the cognitive problems in an individual, in that a spouse may have been supporting and compensating for memory and other cognitive problems in the affected individual.

Key elements of the initial assessment include a history of the nature, duration and progression of the cognitive difficulties, baseline cognitive function and comorbid medical and psychiatric disorders. As with other areas of psychiatric assessment, obtaining a comprehensive collateral history from family is vital, focussing on the key cognitive domains, along with an assessment of any functional loss.

Several brief cognitive screening measures are outlined in Box 20.1. These assessments can be easily conducted by a general practitioner (GP) or at a psychiatric clinic. Abnormalities on these initial assessments may lead to a specialist referral to old age psychiatry, neurology, geriatric medicine or a memory/cognitive assessment clinic for further more detailed neuropsychological testing that may need to be repeated over a one to two year period to check for any evidence of change or progression in the cognitive deficits.

2. With further questioning, Eric's daughter tells you that he has started to become flustered when out driving ever since new traffic lights were installed at the end of his road, that he has stopped attending mass each morning, which had been his usual routine, and that he recently switched from the cryptic to the simple crossword in the *Irish Times* newspaper. Eric himself seems unworried and explains that his daughter 'has always been a bit of a fusspot'. On formal testing, his mini-mental state examination score is 25/30.
    4. What is the normal range for the mini-mental state examination? What are the main differences between the mini-mental state examination and the Montreal cognitive assessment?
    5. What additional brief cognitive tests might be useful to assess his attention, executive function, recent memory and visuospatial function?
    6. What is mild cognitive impairment and how is it defined?

BOX 20.1 ■ How do we assess cognition at the bedside/in clinic?

- Both the mini-mental state examination and Montreal cognitive assessment test allow for testing of a variety of cognitive domains and have cut-off scores that are linked to significant cognitive impairment. Note that both tools are subject to restrictions regarding their use in terms of cost and training, respectively.
- The clock drawing test is also sometimes used as a general test of cognition as it tests executive function, planning, memory and visuospatial awareness.
- Otherwise, single tests can be used for specific cognitive domains, such as the months backward test for attention, remembering named items over 3–5 minutes (short-term memory) and listing words that begin with 'F' or types of animals (executive function). (See Chapter 6 on Delirium for more detail about bedside cognitive tests.)

FURTHER READING

For a review of cognitive assessments, see: Young J, Meagher D, MacLullich A. (2011) Cognitive assessment of older people. The British Medical Journal 343:d5042. doi:10.1136/bmj.d5042

Mild cognitive impairment (MCI), which is also referred to as 'mild cognitive disorder' in the International Classification of Diseases-10 and 'minor neurocognitive disorder' in the Diagnostic and Statistical Manual of Mental Disorders (DSM)-5 involves (despite the name) significant cognitive impairment on one or more domains that occur in the absence of significant functional impairment. It is the absence of functional impairment that distinguishes MCI from dementia.

A detailed assessment of everyday routines and activities is needed to identify functional impairment. In previously high functioning individuals, declining function may be subtle (e.g. moving to a simpler crossword type). With the progression of dementia, there will be increasing evidence of deficits in physical self-maintenance (e.g. self-hygiene, dressing), in addition to the (generally earlier) decline in everyday activities (e.g. driving, cooking, engagement with social activities).

Individuals with MCI have a 10-fold increased risk of progression to dementia in the subsequent year. The pattern of deficits on testing in MCI may also suggest future dementia subtype; for example, amnestic deficits suggesting a relatively higher risk of Alzheimer's dementia (Box 20.2).

3. Eric's daughter wonders if he should have a 'brain scan' and tells you that he was a heavy smoker until his late 50s when he developed angina, and that he was also commenced on a statin for high cholesterol. He had an operation to remove a nodule from his thyroid gland 30 years ago.
   7. What physical conditions might relate to his presentation and what are the causes of the so-called 'reversible dementia?'
   8. What investigations would you perform?

Eric's vascular risk factors (history of heavy smoking, angina and dyslipidaemia) are risk factors for vascular dementia, Alzheimer's dementia and dementia of mixed vascular/Alzheimer's aetiology. The identification and tight control of vascular risk factors are important at a primary and secondary prevention level in the treatment of MCI and dementia. Thyroid dysfunction (perhaps relevant in this case) may also present with cognitive deficits (e.g. cognitive slowing and memory problems in hypothyroidism).

BOX 20.2 ■ Diagnosis of neurocognitive disorder (dementia and mild cognitive impairment)

- Evidence of significant decline from a previous level of performance in one or more of the following cognitive domains: learning and memory, language, executive function or social cognition. These deficits are evident with formal testing.
- In major neurocognitive disorder, the cognitive deficits are of a severity that they impact upon independence in everyday functioning, for example, self-care and managing personal affairs. In minor neurocognitive disorder, everyday functioning is relatively preserved and does not require assistance from others.
- The cognitive deficits are sustained and typically progressive over time.
- Cognitive deficits are not better explained by another mental disorder (e.g. delirium, depressive illness).

Other routine blood screen measures include a full blood count, renal function, liver function, vitamin B12, folate, erythrocyte sedimentation rate, C-reactive protein and fasting glucose. Identification and treatment of abnormalities in these measures may not necessarily reverse dementia, but appropriate treatment may nevertheless lead to improvements in general health and subsequent cognitive health.

Along with the blood screen measures outlined above, additional health screening measures (and potential contributors to cognitive impairment) should be taken, including syphilis serology, human immunodeficiency virus testing, calcium screen, chest X-ray and electrocardiogram (ECG).

In addition, neuroimaging is an essential component of the screening and workup process. Computed tomography or (preferably) brain magnetic resonance imaging can reveal potentially treatable causes of cognitive impairment (e.g. tumour or normal pressure hydrocephalus). It can also indicate the level of cardiovascular disease and any significant morphological changes, such as cortical atrophy and ventricular enlargement.

The dementia screening and workup process can thus be seen to have three primary functions. First, potentially reversible and treatable causes of cognitive impairment can be identified and managed. Second, managing comorbid health problems in an individual with dementia or MCI may lead to improvements in their general and cognitive health and potentially delay cognitive deterioration. Third, baseline cognitive and physical testing is important in tracking the progress of dementia and in monitoring treatment response.

---

4. His daughter is also concerned that Eric has seemed less energetic and withdrawn in recent times. Having stopped going to mass this year, he has not accompanied his friends on their usual weekend fishing trips. She says that he is easily upset and seems less confident in himself. She wonders if he might be depressed.

    9. How can you clarify if he has clinical depression?

    10. What is the relationship between mood disorder and cognitive difficulties in the elderly?

Depression is common in established dementia and may occur in up to half of the cases. Depression in earlier or mid-life may also be a risk factor for cognitive impairment and depression later in life. The diagnosis of depression in dementia may be more complicated than in non-dementia populations because of the overlap between certain depressive and dementia-related features (e.g. apathy, withdrawal and functional impairment). The key to diagnosis is a detailed history, collateral history and mental state examination, focussing on biological symptoms of depression and subjective reports from the patient and family of emotional and behavioural changes. When diagnosed, depression should be treated as it would be in non dementia populations, with serotonin specific reuptake inhibitors or serotonin and noradrenaline reuptake inhibitors. Tricyclic antidepressants should be avoided because of their anticholinergic side-effects and potential to worsen cognitive function.

---

5. Upon questioning, it is apparent that Eric does not have evidence to indicate any sustained lowering of mood or change to his usual energy, sleeping patterns or appetite. He still enjoys things but is worried that he might get mixed up doing things or become lost when he goes out, as this has happened once or twice. In addition to his vascular risk factors, he tells you that he has an older brother who has been in a local nursing home for the past four years 'with Alzheimer's'.

    11. What are the different types of dementia and how are they relevant to treatment and prognosis?

    12. How can they be distinguished in clinical practice?

Alzheimer's dementia (AD) accounts for half to two-thirds of the cases of dementia, with vascular dementia accounting for at least one-quarter. Improved neuroimaging in recent years has led to increased diagnoses of mixed Alzheimer's and vascular dementia. Less common types (e.g.

dementia with Lewy bodies [DLB], frontotemporal dementia [FTD] and Creutzfeldt–Jakob disease) account for 5%–15% of dementia cases overall.

Key aspects of the history (nature and progression of cognitive deficits) and cognitive profile may help elucidate the dementia subtype with blood tests and neuroimaging providing further clarification.

The cognitive deficits seen in AD tend to be predominantly related to short-term memory in the early stages and progress slowly over time. Traditionally, cognitive deficits in vascular dementia are described as having a stepwise progression, with abrupt drops in cognitive function followed by plateau phases. In clinical practice, this distinction is not always clear, especially in cases of mixed aetiology.

DLB may have one or more of a characteristic triad of fluctuating cognitive profiles, Parkinsonism and visual hallucinations, thus making a distinction from delirium difficult at times. FTD often presents with changes in personality and behaviour. There may be a 'disinhibited' presentation with elements of disinhibition and coarsening of personality and behaviour and/or an apathetic presentation with social withdrawal. Generally, in FTD, there is a notable lack of insight/awareness in the patient and relatively preserved performance on standard cognitive testing (e.g. mini-mental state examination [MMSE]) at least in the early stages.

While acetylcholinesterase inhibitors (donepezil, rivastigmine and galantamine) are not disease-modifying, they are indicated early during dementia and may have a symptomatic role in AD, vascular, mixed AD/vascular dementia and DLB. The mode of action of these drugs is to increase acetylcholine levels through inhibition of acetylcholinesterase.

All three agents are available in an oral formulation, and rivastigmine has an additional transdermal patch formulation. No agent is clearly superior in terms of efficacy or side-effect profile. Given the absence of a cholinergic deficit, these drugs are not indicated in FTD.

Donepezil has the longest half-life (70 hours) and, therefore, can be used on a once-daily basis. Modest short-term improvements in cognition and clinician ratings have been demonstrated, with additional benefits at the 10 mg dosage than the starting 5 mg dosage. The most common side-effects are related to peripheral cholinergic activity and include nausea, vomiting, diarrhoea and anorexia. Pulse (and an ECG) should be checked before starting acetylcholinesterase inhibitors as they can cause syncope because of cardiac effects, particularly, in those with supraventricular conduction abnormalities.

Rivastigmine has effects on both acetylcholinesterase and butyrylcholinesterase, although the latter is clinically insignificant. Its side-effect profile is similar to donepezil and galantamine. Rivastigmine tends to be the agent of choice in Parkinson's disease dementia and DLB.

Galantamine has a half-life intermediate between that of donepezil and rivastigmine. Its side-effects and efficacy profile are similar to those of the other two agents.

Memantine (an N-methyl-D-aspartate receptor antagonist) has a potentially symptomatic role in moderate to severe dementia of Alzheimer's and vascular aetiology. The effect is mediated through its anti glutamatergic and, thus, potentially, neuroprotective action. In practice, acetylcholinesterase inhibitors and memantine are frequently used together from the early stages and throughout the clinical course of dementia.

---

6. A month later, Eric re-attends with his daughter to review his test results. The blood tests are essentially normal, but the magnetic resonance imaging scan shows 'generalized mild atrophy with sulcal widening and with evidence of white matter hyperintensity'.
   13. Does Eric fulfil the criteria for dementia?
   14. Should he commence a cognitive enhancing agent?
   15. What are the current treatment considerations in terms of his practical everyday life, while ensuring his safety and legal issues?

Eric fulfils the diagnostic criteria for dementia in that he has sustained significant cognitive impairment with associated functional loss that is not better accounted for by acute or reversible conditions (see Box 20.2 for the DSM-5 criteria of major neurocognitive disorder). The neuroimaging findings are consistent with the atrophic changes seen in AD and coexistent vascular changes, and there is no evidence of an acute or reversible pathological condition. His initial relatively high score on MMSE (25/30) may be related to his high premorbid levels of intellect, education and functioning.

FURTHER READING

For a review of the pharmacological strategies for dementia, see: Rodda J, Carter J. (2012) Cholinesterase inhibitors and memantine for symptomatic treatment of dementia. The British Medical Journal 344:e2986. doi:10.1136/bmj.e2986

Acetylcholinesterase inhibitors are indicated as first-line treatment in mild to moderate dementia of Alzheimer's, vascular and mixed Alzheimer's/vascular aetiology. While memantine is indicated in moderate—severe Alzheimer's, vascular and mixed Alzheimer's, it is commonly used earlier in the course of dementia as an adjunctive treatment with acetylcholinesterase inhibitors.

At this relatively early stage in his dementia, Eric should be referred to relevant agencies, such as public health, to assess his general health and functional needs. While his GP will coordinate his medical care, referral to old age psychiatry may be helpful in further clarifying the diagnosis (exact nature and severity of dementia), performing a functional assessment (through occupational therapy) and in managing behavioural and psychological symptoms of dementia (BPSD) if and when they arise (see below).

A balance should be struck between facilitating Eric's ability to live and function independently while also being mindful of his increasing and likely progressive disability and frailty. Specifically, detailed discussions should be had with Eric and his family regarding his driving; his ability to care for himself, manage his house and live independently and his plans regarding his finances, future care and legal issues such as his will and inheritance. These complex issues should be addressed as part of a sequential process. Generally, Eric should be facilitated to maintain as much of his independence, for as long as possible.

---

7. Eric's family are keen to meet with you to discuss his diagnosis and treatment plan. They are divided as to whether he should be present as they do not want to upset him. They are wondering about how best to plan for his future in terms of managing his personal and financial affairs.
  16. Should Eric be present at the meeting? What are the main principles to be considered in dealing with his family?
  17. What is an enduring power of attorney?

Giving a dementia diagnosis should be done as part of a careful process that involves Eric and his family as much as possible. While his family may have the well-meaning intention to 'protect' Eric from being given a diagnosis, he has the right to have all his questions and concerns addressed by the treating medical team. The language of such meetings can involve euphemisms such as 'memory problems' and 'thinking problems'. Technical terms, medical jargon and overly definitive statements on prognosis and life expectancy should be avoided. As a general guide, any questions of Eric's should be addressed openly and clearly, and he should not be overloaded with unsolicited information on his diagnosis, treatment and prognosis. Moreover, there may be a process involved in gradually imparting information to Eric and his family on the nature and prognosis of his dementia.

Eric and his family should also be advised that he should now arrange an enduring power of attorney (EPOA). Essentially, this involves Eric liaising with a solicitor and assigning key individuals (generally family members) to manage his financial and legal affairs if he loses the capacity to do so in future. An EPOA should be arranged as a priority once the dementia diagnosis has been clarified before his capacity is significantly diminished. If an individual with dementia loses capacity and has not already made arrangements for an EPOA, it may be required that they are made a Ward of Court, and this is a costly and cumbersome process. The Ward of Courts system is to be replaced by legislation around capacity that it is hoped will allow for the more timely and proactive care of people with cognitive issues.

---

8. Nine months later, you are called at night to come and see Eric urgently. He returned home from the local hospital a week previously after a 5-day admission with a respiratory tract infection. His neighbours are concerned that he has been in the back garden in his underpants shouting for his dog 'Hugo' who has been dead for more than 10 years. When you arrive, the neighbours also tell you that he has been stopping passing traffic to enquire whether they have 'submitted an up-to-date logbook to go with their HSE mileage claims'.

    18. What is the differential diagnosis at this point?

The immediate presentation is highly suggestive of delirium superimposed on background dementia. (See Chapter 6 for further details.)

The longer-term history of abnormal behaviour (stopping passing traffic) is more suggestive of BPSD. BPSD are common complications of all types of dementia, and most patients will develop one or more BPSD at some point. BPSD symptoms vary in nature and severity and include depression, agitation, wandering, aggression and psychotic symptoms.

FURTHER READING

For a review of the best practice in managing behavioural and psychological symptoms of dementia, see: Tible OP, Riese F, Savaskan E, von Gunten A. (2017) Best practice in the management of behavioural and psychological symptoms of dementia. Therapeutic Advances in Neurological Disorders 10(8):297–309. doi:10.1177/1756285617712979

A general approach to managing BPSD includes a clear definition of target symptoms (based on history, collateral history and mental state examination) and the ruling out of physical or modifiable factors such as delirium, pain, dehydration or constipation. Thereafter, psychiatric diagnoses should be considered, such as depression or psychosis.

Antidepressants or antipsychotic agents can be considered, along with environmental strategies (e.g. addressing routines, habits and re-orientation techniques). The use of antipsychotics is best avoided as evidence of their beneficial effects is lacking, and they are associated with an increased risk of cerebrovascular incidents when used in people with dementia. Moreover, antipsychotic agents are poorly tolerated in patients with Parkinson's disease or DLB.

Linda

Opiate Misuse and Pregnancy

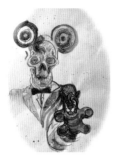

1. Recognize the signs of opioid intoxication.
2. Describe the epidemiology (incidence and prevalence) of opioid use.
3. Recognize the signs of an opioid overdose.
4. Outline the criteria used to define opioid dependence.
5. Describe the principles that underpin the treatment of opioid addiction, including methadone substitution and other interventions.
6. Describe how to manage opioid addiction in pregnancy.
7. Recognize the features of neonatal abstinence syndrome.
8. Understand the factors that impact prognosis in opioid use.

1. Linda is a 22-year-old female who was referred by her general practitioner to a drug treatment clinic for homeless services. When she presents at the treatment centre, she is sleepy, relaxed, euthymic and has pupillary constriction. On examination, she is bradycardic and hypotensive. She has been homeless for six years following a period of 10 years in foster care. Her longest stable period in foster care was 18 months. She is no longer in contact with any of the foster care families.

Linda commenced drinking alcohol at 11 years of age. She was introduced to cannabis by the teenage son of her foster care family at the age of 12 and she smoked cannabis daily from the age of 12 to 14. She has smoked heroin since the age of 15 and was introduced to intravenous heroin by her birth mother at the age of 17 while on a visit organized by the social work department. Her mother is currently in prison for manslaughter. She does not know who her biological father is and she is unaware if she has any siblings.

    1. What are the signs of opioid intoxication?
    2. How do opioids exert their effects?

Continued on following page

(Continued)

3. What are your initial thoughts regarding the management of this case and what further information should be obtained?
4. What are the criteria for substance 'dependency?'

Linda is demonstrating signs of opiate intoxication (Box 21.1). The term 'opioid' refers to natural and synthetic substances with morphine-like actions that activate the mu-opioid receptors in the central nervous system and gastrointestinal tract. 'Opiate' refers to a subclass of opioids consisting of alkaloid compounds derived from opium that include morphine, codeine, and semisynthetic derivatives, such as heroin, methadone, fentanyl, hydromorphone and buprenorphine.

Heroin (diamorphine) is the most widely abused opiate with its substantial euphoric and analgesic properties. Although commonly smoked, it may also be used orally, snorted or parenterally (intravenous 'mainlining', intramuscular use or subcutaneous 'skin popping'). Many users begin by smoking but progress to intravenous use because of the increased bioavailability from this mode of administration. When used intravenously, it is 3−5 times more potent than its parent compound.

Heroin was first synthesized in 1874 and was initially marketed as a safer, nonaddictive version of morphine. By 1914, it was prohibited to be used without a prescription and by 1920 it was prohibited under the dangerous drugs act in the United States. In Ireland, there are about 20,000 users of heroin, 15,000 of whom reside in Dublin. The cost of heroin is usually in the region of €25−35 for a 0.25 g 'bag'.

Opiates exert their effect by binding to receptors, particularly in the limbic system, hypothalamus, sensory system and gastrointestinal tract. There are three main opiate receptor subtypes (mu, delta and kappa) of which the mu and kappa receptors have an established role in dependence. Stimulation of the mu receptors accounts for most of the analgesic and euphoric properties.

Individuals with opiate addiction issues are generally managed in specialist services because of the complex challenges that they frequently pose in terms of obtaining good outcomes and effectively monitoring care. Management in this initial phase should include an assessment of the extent of the problem and suitability for available treatment pathways. This includes taking a full history of substance misuse, which would detail the class of drugs taken, age of first use of each drug, the quantities of each drug taken and how regularly. All patients should be alerted to the numerous physical complications that may arise from intravenous drug use. These include abscesses at injection sites (particularly, underarm, and in the groin area), venous thrombosis, blood-borne infections (including those caused by human immunodeficiency virus [HIV] and hepatitis virus) and soft tissue infections such as cellulitis.

Patient education should include general education/information on the substances being misused, alongside specific information on the medical consequences and comorbid risks of consuming drugs.

BOX 21.1 ■ Signs of opiate intoxication

- Pupillary constriction
- Hypotension
- Bradycardia
- Slurred speech
- Impaired coordination
- Mood change—intense pleasure/euphoria
- Cough reflex suppression
- Nausea and vomiting
- Emotional numbing
- Analgesia/increased pain tolerance

Many centres will also advise on 'safe' methods of intravenous use of drugs, including how to prepare heroin. Clean needles are often supplied and safe disposal of used needles may be facilitated. Patients should be advised of all available facilities in their area. A urine toxicology screen is routinely obtained when the patient visits an outpatient clinic and the results of these should be discussed with the patient.

A multidisciplinary approach may provide support for patients in the community as many individuals present with a complex constellation of problems and benefit from the inputs of a social worker and community mental health nurse. Problems associated with drug use, homelessness, social isolation and forensic issues should be elicited and often would be discussed by a multidisciplinary team to construct a suitable care plan.

---

2. A few days later, Linda is brought into the Accident and Emergency department by ambulance after being found unconscious on the street. She has a weak pulse, shallow respirations, bradycardia, hypotension and pupillary constriction. Track marks are visible on her arms.

When she regains consciousness, Linda is informed that she has been admitted to the hospital and advised to remain hospitalized for further medical care. Linda requests information on commencing a programme of stabilization on methadone. She has taken street methadone before but has never been on a formal stabilization programme. She is commenced on a low dose of methadone in the ward.

Unfortunately, Linda then takes discharge against medical advice, but she does agree to follow-up in a drug treatment clinic to continue her methadone maintenance treatment.

5. What are the signs of an opiate overdose?
6. How would you manage an opiate overdose?
7. What considerations need to be taken when commencing methadone?
8. What are the alternative agents to methadone in opioid substitution treatments?

Tolerance occurs when the reaction to a concentration of a specific drug is progressively reduced such that an increased dose is needed to achieve the desired effect (see Box 21.2 for other features of substance dependance). Tolerance develops quickly with heroin use, and when the drug is stopped, it diminishes (see Box 21.3 for features of opiate withdrawal). This leads to an increase likelihood of overdose following a period of abstinence. Opiate overdose is most common in people who inject heroin, particularly at times when tolerance is likely to be low, for example, after a period in rehabilitation or prison. It is also more common when heroin is used with other central nervous system depressants like benzodiazepines or alcohol.

Following an overdose (Box 21.4), cardiopulmonary resuscitation and supportive care are usually warranted. An opiate antagonist, most commonly intravenous naloxone, may be administered. However, intravenous access may be compromised in drug users and the intramuscular route is often preferable. Of note, naloxone is short-acting and repeated doses may be necessary if the patient reverts into a withdrawal state. There has been recent interest in providing heroin users with 'home kits' of naloxone with evidence that these may reduce the number of heroin-related overdose deaths.

BOX 21.2 ▪ The diagnosis of substance dependence is based upon the following:

1. Substance use for longer periods or in greater amounts than intended
2. Loss of control over use
3. Craving for the substance when abstinent
4. Excessive time spent around substance use, both in terms of consumption and recovery from its effects
5. Interference with social or occupational functioning, with evidence of increasing primacy of alcohol over other activities
6. Continued use despite adverse effects that may be social, psychological or physical
7. Evidence of physical addiction with increasing tolerance to acute effects
8. Evidence of physical addiction with symptoms of withdrawal upon cessation of use

---

BOX 21.3 ■ Features of opioid withdrawal

- Restlessness
- Insomnia
- Intense craving for the drug
- Muscular and joint pain
- Eye and nasal lacrimation
- Diaphoresis (sweating)
- Abdominal cramps
- Vomiting and diarrhoea
- Piloerection
- Dilated pupils
- Tachycardia
- Instability of temperature control

BOX 21.4 ■ Signs of opiate overdose

- Respiratory arrest with a pulse
- Constricted ('pinpoint') pupils that are unreactive to light
- Snoring giving way to shallow respirations [rate <8/min]
- Bradycardia
- Hypotensive
- Reduced consciousness/coma

In the prevention of heroin-associated morbidity, there are two main strategies. One is to reduce use by limiting its availability. Another perhaps more realistic approach is to reduce the harm the substance causes through comorbid conditions (such as HIV, hepatitis B and hepatitis C infection) with strategies such as needle exchange programmes. A further strategy is to provide an alternative to heroin.

Maintenance programmes consist of providing a substitute drug, usually opioid-based, to help to resist heroin-use. This substitution is routinely combined with psychological, social and medical support. It is important to remember that opioid withdrawal, while extremely unpleasant, is not life-threatening, but without careful supervision, overdose of opioid-based heroin substitutes may be fatal.

Patient motivation should be assessed prior to commencing a substitution programme, and the goals of treatment need to be agreed. Methadone is a synthetic derivative of opium and a mu receptor agonist. Methadone substitution programmes involve commencing methadone at a low dose and slowly increasing to a maintenance dose that is based on the quantity of daily heroin intake. Methadone is usually dispensed in a liquid form and taken orally. It takes longer to cross the blood−brain barrier than heroin and therefore does not provide the same levels of euphoria/analgesia, while effectively preventing withdrawal. Nonetheless, methadone is widely abused and carries a high risk of dependency and toxicity. Methadone availability is typically restricted to approved outpatient treatment programmes, where it is dispensed to patients daily. It is generally considered safe to prescribe in pregnancy.

The main alternative to methadone is buprenorphine, which is a partial mu agonist and has lower abuse and dependency potential. Buprenorphine also has a lower risk of toxicity because of a ceiling effect. In practice, buprenorphine is combined with naloxone, which induces withdrawal symptoms if the medication is injected to 'get high'. These symptoms are averted when the drug is prescribed for sublingual administration. It is not safe to prescribe in pregnancy.

It is important to recognize that engaging users in maintenance programmes present an opportunity to link them with psychological and social supports that can be crucial to addressing issues that underpin opiate use.

---

3. On a return appointment to the drug treatment clinic, a routine blood screen, urine toxicology, alcometer and pregnancy tests are obtained. The urine screen is positive for opiates, and Linda is human chorionic gonadotropin-positive. She is human immunodeficiency virus, and Hepatitis B and C virus negative. The general practitioner she occasionally attends had completed a course of Hepatitis B vaccination.
   9. What are the principal considerations when using methadone in pregnancy?

The use of illicit opiates during pregnancy has significant risks for both the mother and baby. These include exposure to blood-borne infections, stillbirth, preterm labour, miscarriage, postpartum haemorrhage, intrauterine growth restriction, preterm labour microcephaly and neonatal withdrawal. Many drug treatment services offer priority treatment to pregnant women and coordinated care between medical teams, nurses, social support and antenatal services.

A methadone programme offers the benefit of reducing heroin use and improves overall health in pregnant heroin-dependent women. However, methadone use can result in babies born with low birth weight and neonatal abstinence syndrome. Nonetheless, it has been demonstrated that switching from heroin to methadone use during pregnancy is associated with improved neonatal outcomes. Infants require a shorter duration of stay in neonatal units, develop less severe neonatal abstinence syndrome and are more likely to be discharged into their mother's care than those whose mothers continue heroin use up to delivery.

Detoxification, if requested, is usually carried out in the second trimester in an attempt to avoid miscarriage in the first trimester or preterm labour, following withdrawal in the third trimester. However, many services prefer to continue with methadone maintenance throughout the pregnancy and discuss detoxification once safe delivery of the baby has been achieved. Maternal metabolism will increase in the third trimester, and an increased dose of methadone is usually necessary. It is recommended that potential problems should be considered for women taking prescribed opioids during pregnancy concerning opioid pain relief during birth. There is no evidence of an increase in congenital defects with methadone. However, the newborn may experience withdrawal syndrome.

Methadone is considered compatible with breastfeeding as the exposure of infants to methadone through their mothers' breast milk is minimal. Breastfeeding should not be discouraged in women using methadone for the treatment of opioid dependence, as the benefits of breastfeeding largely outweigh any minimal theoretical risks.

---

4. At 36 weeks of gestation, Linda goes into labour and delivers a baby boy who weighs 2 kg. He has respiratory distress at birth and is transferred to the neonatal care unit. Linda names the baby Dylan. She is very concerned regarding how the baby is doing.
   10. What is neonatal abstinence syndrome?

Neonatal abstinence syndrome is characterized by excessive crying, a hyperactive reflex, tremors, variation in muscle tone, frequent yawning, sweating, nasal stuffiness, tachypnoea, diarrhoea, vomiting, loose stools and failure to thrive.

These signs typically occur a few days after birth if the mother was using heroin. However, withdrawal is often delayed when the mother is using methadone as it has a longer half-life. Management is initially with the provision of a supportive, soothing environment, and there is evidence for breastfeeding and 'rooming in' in this context. If medical management is necessary, morphine weaning is usually initiated.

---

5. Linda attends the follow-up three months after the birth of her son. She has continued on methadone and is coping with the change in her circumstances. She appears highly motivated with respect to 'moving on' with her life and is requesting complete methadone withdrawal. She is particularly interested in lofexidine as a friend has confided to her that that was key to their finally stopping heroin use. Linda would also like advice about any medications that may help prevent a relapse into heroin use.

    11. What is a typical regime for methadone withdrawal?
    12. What additional pharmacological agents may be considered and what other treatment options are available?
    13. What is the natural history of opiate dependency?

Owing to the risk of overdose, the starting dose of methadone is between 10 mg and 30 mg daily. Given its interactions with other sedative drugs, including benzodiazepines or alcohol, the starting dose may need to be reduced if patients are using these agents. The dose can then be titrated upwards to optimal levels, usually between 60 mg and 120 mg. Methadone should initially be prescribed daily. Methadone use should be supervised for at least the first three months and until the patient has gained stability.

Where methadone withdrawal is attempted, a reduction programme should be commenced with the patient in terms of targets. Although typical reductions are in 5−10 mg increments weekly, these may be highly variable. Flexibility is required according to the individual's physical and psychological needs and their access to social support. It is not uncommon for temporary dose increases to be part of an overall withdrawal plan. In particular, towards the end of the reduction programme, dose reduction may be more gradual.

Symptoms of opiate withdrawal are related to surges in noradrenaline release from the locus coeruleus. Lofexidine, an α2 adrenergic agonist, can counteract this adrenergic hyperactivity and is licensed for withdrawal management, although adjunctive medications may be needed for symptoms, such as diarrhoea, that are not attenuated by its action.

Naltrexone is a cost-effective medical strategy for maintaining abstinence in motivated individuals. Several factors should be considered before it is prescribed. A sufficient period of abstinence from opiates (e.g. 10 days in the case of methadone use) should be documented before it is introduced to avoid precipitating withdrawal syndrome. Individuals should be warned that tolerance for opiates will be considerably reduced and that there is a risk of overdose if heroin is used again. This is of importance as the medication may cause insomnia and dysphoria, which may make individuals more vulnerable to relapse.

FURTHER READING

For additional information on treatments, see: National Institute on Drug Abuse. Available at: https://www.drugabuse.gov/nidamed-medical-health-professionals/treatment/opioid-use-disorder-treatment.

There is clear evidence for psychosocial and behavioural interventions in relapse prevention and any medication advice should be within the context of such support. Effective treatments available for heroin addiction include contingency management and cognitive behavioural therapy (CBT), which have synergistic effects with pharmacological approaches. Contingency management employs a voucher-based system, with individuals earning 'credits' for negative drug tests, which may be exchanged for items that encourage healthy living. CBT focuses on the patient's expectations and behaviours related to drug use and aims to increase coping skills for life stressors.

As was illustrated in Linda's narrative, family and social dysfunction, along with earlier use of alcohol and cannabis, predicts heroin dependency. Early use of opiates is associated with longer use trajectories. At a population level, when cannabis use decreases overtime and cocaine use increases before a decline in the fifth decade, heroin use is more stable. There are significant associations with childhood conduct disorder, antisocial personality disorder and protracted use of opiates.

In the United States, studies indicate that over 5 million (almost 2% of the adult population) have used heroin at some point in their lives, with 0.1% reporting its use in the last month. More than half of those who use heroin develop misuse problems and/or dependency. In addition, over two million adults meet the criteria for prescription opioid dependence. Prescription opioids are most often obtained from a relative or friend rather than directly from a clinician. Studies indicate that between 10% and 20% of the patients who are prescribed opioids for noncancerous pain control develop misuse issues. Approximately two-thirds of the people who primarily use heroin also use prescription opioids.

Among patients prescribed opioid analgesics, risk factors for misuse include a previous history of substance use disorder, younger age, more severe pain and comorbid psychiatric illness.

Individuals who use illicit opioids have up to 15 times the risk of premature mortality than the general population, principally because of the higher rates of overdose and trauma. An opioid epidemic is growing in the United States, as demonstrated by a three-fold increase in opioid overdose deaths (almost 30,000 per annum).

CHAPTER 22

Larry

Mental Illness in Intellectual Disability

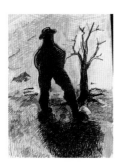

1. Understand the increased risk of having other specific physical and mental disorders in people with Down syndrome.
2. Acknowledge that bouts of episodic mental ill-health will present differently for people with an intellectual disability than that for the general population.
3. Recognize the importance of collateral information in intellectual disability psychiatry.
4. Understand the link between physical conditions (particularly, neurological and endocrine) and episodes of mental ill-health.
5. Acknowledge the complexity of prescribing psychotropic medications for those with an intellectual disability, particularly, if they have co-occurring medical complications.
6. Understand the importance of involving family carers and other professionals in mental health treatment plans for those with an intellectual disability.
7. Recognize the link between Down syndrome and dementia.
8. Describe the deficits in intellectual and adaptive functioning that occur in people with intellectual disability.

1. You have been asked to assess Larry, a 34-year-old man with Down syndrome. He lives with his elderly parents and attends 'An Sli Eile', a local day service for people with intellectual disability. Over the past few weeks, Larry has had daily episodes of irritability, tearfulness and agitation. He is also reported to have disturbed sleep, reduced appetite and episodes of shouting, which is out of character for him. When asked by his parents or care staff what is wrong, Larry repeatedly replies with the word 'sad'.

    1. What are the general principles of assessment when assessing a person with an intellectual disability?
    2. What historical information would be important to establish in this case?

When assessing a person with an intellectual disability, it is always important, as with any clinical assessment, to obtain an accurate and careful clinical history. Many people with an intellectual disability can give a good history, but some cannot. Therefore, these people depend on their family or paid caregivers to give as accurate a collateral history as possible. People with an intellectual disability must be supported at clinical examinations and assessments by family or support staff who know them well. The ability of people with an intellectual disability to give a good history will depend on their verbal skills and their level of intellectual disability.

Many people with an intellectual disability report that family or support staff frequently talk about them at hospital or clinical appointments as though they are not present, or that they talk about upsetting things in front of them. Therefore, always remember to introduce yourself to the patient and ask them if they would like to see you alone or if they would prefer family or support staff present.

It is also important to remember that an assessment of individuals with an intellectual disability and mental health problems takes longer than those who do not have an intellectual disability. Therefore, patience and understanding are important.

Relevant historical information includes the following:

Recent life events: Explore for any significant events (especially losses) in Larry's family and social pool.

Medical history: Has Larry had any cardiac problems, e.g. ventricular septal defect, atrial septal defect? Is there a history of seizures or gastrointestinal problems, e.g. hiatus hernia, gastritis or constipation? Has he had any thyroid problems—hypo or hyperthyroidism?

Surgical history: Has Larry had any past or recent surgery (e.g. cardiac)?

Psychiatric history: Have there been any other behavioural or mental health issues or similar episodes in the past?

Medications: Is Larry taking any regular medications?

Family history: Is there any family history of mental health problems, e.g. mood disorders, schizoaffective disorders, schizophrenia or addiction.

Premorbid personality: Try to ascertain what Larry's personality was like before this. Ask Larry or his family member/caregiver to describe this if possible. What are his interests and hobbies? Who are his friends? What type of work does he do? Have these been affected by the current change in Larry? Has he had any recent difficulties with his memory or any episodes of confusion?

Social history: Ascertain the home circumstances and details of support available to Larry and his parents.

---

2. Collateral information from Larry's parents and his records indicate that he has an intellectual disability in the low–moderate range, and that he has grand mal epilepsy and has been seizure-free for three years. He also has a history of hypothyroidism. He has no significant psychiatric history. Larry had a ventricular septal defect repaired when he was four years old, and he had frequent hospitalizations in his early years, mainly because of his cardiac condition. All major developmental milestones were significantly delayed, and he attended a local school for children with intellectual disabilities from age six until 18 years. He then transitioned to the current day centre. Larry has two older siblings living abroad who visit annually.

Larry's current medications are as follows: sodium valproate (300 mg; twice a day) for seizure prophylaxis and L-Thyroxine (50 μg; daily). He attends the day centre three days per week for six hours and generally enjoys this. In the last few weeks, the staff at the day centre have reported that Larry has been very talkative, restless and fidgety, with poor concentration in the tasks that he previously performed with ease.

3. Why is Larry's medical history of particular relevance?
4. What is your differential diagnosis at this stage?

FURTHER READING

For a review of the prevalence of health conditions in intellectual disability, see: Oeseburg B, Dijkstra GJ, Groothoff JW, et al. (2011) Prevalence of chronic health conditions in children with intellectual disability: A systematic literature review. Intellectual and Developmental Disabilities 49(2):59–85. doi:10.1352/1934-9556-49.2.59

Both hypothyroidism and epilepsy can affect a person's mood and behaviour, along with the medications used to treat these conditions. People with Down syndrome have an increased prevalence of both congenital and acquired hypothyroidism. The lifelong prevalence has been reported as ranging from 13% to 63% (this is approximately 4% in the general population). The prevalence of epilepsy among those with an intellectual disability is higher than that in the general population. Community-based studies of epilepsy in adults with an intellectual disability show a prevalence of 16%–26%. Some studies have shown a higher rate of behavioural and psychological problems in those with epilepsy than those without epilepsy. However, other studies have not shown this trend. There is also an increased rate of psychiatric illness among adults with an intellectual disability, which has been reported to be between 15% and 40%.

The differential diagnoses at this stage include the following:
- Situational or adjustment difficulties with challenging behaviour
- Affective disorder, e.g. depression, mixed affective state, manic episode
- Severe anxiety disorder
- Psychotic disorder
- Organic disorder, including substance use and delirium.

---

3. Larry has been distractible and reluctant to follow advice or requests. He has been tearful on several occasions during the day and is persistently complaining of sadness or distress. Larry has not shown any challenging behaviour (verbal or physical aggression, or any self-injurious behaviour) at home or in the day centre but has required a high level of support and redirection from staff in the centre and his parents at home. He has difficulty getting off to sleep, with recurrent episodes of waking and pacing throughout the night. The behaviours described are markedly different from Larry's usual pattern as he normally engages very well with his daytime routine. He has not expressed any suicidal thoughts or ideas of self-harm. Larry did not have any distressing or similar behaviour or mood change at home or in the day centre prior to this episode.

Larry has no history of substance misuse and has not attended mental health services in the past or been prescribed psychotropic medication. Larry's physical health was described as good at his annual health check, which was undertaken by his general practitioner one month ago. He underwent routine blood tests, the results of which were reported as unremarkable.

5. What are the diagnostic criteria for intellectual disability and how is intellectual disability classified?
6. What is the prevalence of intellectual disability?
7. What are the models of service delivery for those with an intellectual disability?
8. What do you know about the cause of intellectual disability?

The diagnosis of intellectual disability is shown in Box 22.1.

Intellectual disability is classified in several ways that include consideration of the intelligence quotient as well as social and adaptive or functional abilities as outlined in Table 22.1.

Historically, because of social stigma at the time, many people with intellectual disabilities were removed from their families, often at a very young age, and were cared for in residential homes for people with disabilities or in psychiatric hospitals. Intellectual disability services in Ireland were run by religious organizations or state-run institutions. In recent years, the model of service has been changing and is becoming a community or home-based service, which is more person-centred. Employment and vocational training and day centres with the support of specialist multidisciplinary

BOX 22.1 ■ The diagnosis of intellectual disability is applied in cases of the following:

1. Evidence of functional impairment on intellectual functions (comprehension, learning, problem-solving, planning, abstract thinking and judgement) that is evident with formal testing.
2. There is impaired socio-adaptive function secondary to these intellectual impairments.
3. Impairments are evident during development and are typically present from birth/early childhood and are persistent over time and consistent over domains of activity.

TABLE 22.1 ■ Classification and Prevalence of Intellectual Disability

	IQ[a]	Social and Adaptive Abilities	Prevalence
Mild	50–69	Delayed speech Independent Academic difficulties Mental age: 9–12 years	3%
Moderate	35–49	Deficits in language comprehension difficulties Requires supervision Mental age: 6–9 years	0.3%
Severe	20–34	Motor deficits and associated disabilities Limited language that impedes communication Requires help with ADL Mental age: 3–6 years	0.1%
Profound	<20	Very limited language and comprehension Severe neurological and physical disability, immobile, incontinent Mental age <3 years	0.05%

[a]Clinical judgement should be exercised in the interpretation of IQ tests. IQ, intelligence quotient; ADL, activities of daily living

intellectual disability teams are now being developed. Education is based on ability; it needs and includes mainstream or special education schooling options.

There are multiple potential causes of intellectual disability. However, a specific reason is identified in about 25% of cases (see Box 22.2).

---

4. Larry attends an appointment at the local mental health clinic. He is accompanied by his parents and a key worker from his day service. On the mental state examination, Larry is observed to be restless and agitated and does not sit down or stay still for very long during the appointment. He is somewhat amenable to reassurance from the care-worker who accompanies him. He does not engage in conversation very well and repeatedly repeats the word 'sad' during the appointment. Larry repeats this word in response to most questions posed and does not give expansive answers to many of the questions asked. Larry does not appear to be experiencing hallucinations in any modality. He is fully conscious and alert and does not appear disorientated. Psychomotor activity is increased and Larry is tearful and labile in his affect. He does not describe any suicidal thoughts or thoughts of self-harm.
9. What does the psychiatric assessment of a patient with an intellectual disability entail?
10. What further assessments and investigations would be relevant, given the information thus far?
11. What other people involved in Larry's care could be good sources for collateral information?
12. What do you know about the epidemiology of mental illness in patients with an intellectual disability?

BOX 22.2 ■ Potential causes of intellectual disability			
Genetic	Antenatal	Perinatal	Postnatal
Chromosomal (e.g. Down syndrome, Fragile X, Turner's)	Infections (e.g. ToRCH[a])	Birth asphyxia (e.g. cerebral palsy)	Head injury Infection
Autosomal recessive disorders (e.g. phenylketonuria)	Intoxicants (e.g. alcohol)	Severe prematurity	Toxins Deprivation
Deletions or duplications (e.g. Angelman's, DiGeorge syndrome)	Placental dysfunction Preeclampsia CNS malformations		
Autosomal dominant disorders (e.g. tuberous sclerosis, Noonan's syndrome)			
X-linked (e.g. Rett's syndrome)			

[a]Toxoplasmosis, other agents, rubella, cytomegalovirus and herpes simplex

The principles of psychiatric assessment in those with an intellectual disability involve establishing the pattern of symptomology and changes in behaviour. The impact of their intellectual disability on symptoms needs to be established. Close observation of appearance and behaviour, serial assessments and assessment in the patient's natural environment may be important.

A full physical examination should be carried out by the general practitioner (GP) prior to the mental health assessment. The GP may carry out routine bloods as clinically indicated, i.e. in Larry's case, thyroid function test, valproic acid levels (to rule out valproate toxicity), full blood count and urea and electrolytes should be prioritized. Given Larry's preexisting conditions, a computed tomography brain scan, electrocardiogram or echocardiogram may be clinically helpful depending on the findings on physical examination. It may be helpful to refer to any existing psychological, social work, occupational therapy or speech and language assessments.

Other potential sources of collateral information would include day service managers, other day centre staff and support workers, Larry's GP, family members, who although abroad may still have clinically relevant input and also respite staff who may have important information relating to Larry's premorbid state.

All categories of mental illness occur in people with intellectual disabilities, and many disorders are more common. For example, people with an intellectual disability are four times more likely to suffer from depression or anxiety. The prevalence of schizophrenia is three times higher, and bipolar affective disorder is also more common.

5. The physical examination is unremarkable apart from the presence on auscultation of Larry's preexisting cardiac murmur. Larry's valproic acid level is in the subtherapeutic range, and his full blood count, urea and electrolytes and thyroid function tests are normal. The electrocardiogram is normal, and brain computed tomography, electroencephalogram and echocardiogram are requested. Referral to neurology is also requested as Larry has not attended a review appointment for approximately two years.

Continued on following page

(Continued)

Having carefully considered Larry's history, mental state examination results, and collateral information, together with physical examination and investigations, you make a diagnosis of a mixed affective episode. You liaise with the consultant psychiatrist in intellectual disability who concurs with your diagnosis. You draw up a management plan together. Prompt treatment is a priority. After phlebotomy, you increase Larry's sodium valproate up to 500 mg orally twice daily and prescribe a low dose of antipsychotic—olanzapine or quetiapine. You also prescribe an as-needed medication for severe agitation or in the event of symptoms not resolving (lorazepam or an antipsychotic). You plan to follow-up on the investigations requested to rule out a potential organic cause.

13. Can you explain the logic behind the medication changes?

In the treatment of an acute manic episode, the optimization of medication used for mood stabilization is paramount. Sodium valproate is widely used as a mood stabilizer and has shown efficacy in rapid-cycling bipolar affective disorder. It may be possible to titrate up the dose of this medication because Larry is already receiving it for epilepsy, and because it appears effective in preventing seizures. Plasma levels of valproate are less precise in terms of defining its therapeutic range in epilepsy than lithium levels are for a mood-stabilizing effect.

As Larry is presenting with agitated behaviour, in the acute phase, the use of short-term benzodiazepines such as clonazepam may be useful in reducing agitation and improving sleep. Alternative benzodiazepines to clonazepam, such as lorazepam or diazepam, may be considered. Alternative mood-stabilizing medications could also be considered in this situation as first- or second-line treatments. These alternatives include the use of atypical antipsychotics, lithium, carbamazepine, lamotrigine and other antiepileptic medications. When prescribing psychotropic medication, it is extremely important to consider their potential effect on seizure threshold (e.g. this is usually lowered by antipsychotics) and the psychological side-effect profile.

---

6. You arrange a case conference/multidisciplinary team meeting and invite Larry's parents to attend. You have previously explained to Larry's parents that you and the consultant have concluded that Larry is experiencing an episode of mood disturbance and that you have decided to change Larry's medications. You recommend that Larry avail of respite if it is available. You discuss the possible pros and cons of the changes to Larry's medications and your reasoning behind the changes. You also draw up guidelines around when it would be appropriate to administer the as-needed medication. You also explain that further investigations have been requested to rule out other potential causes. The social worker attached to Larry's day service proposes that he will liaise with Larry and his family regarding the arrangements for respite. The respite manager is also present at the case conference and, given the circumstances, agrees to facilitate acute respite for Larry but outlines that respite resources are very limited within the service, and that only short-term respite will be possible.

14. What chromosomal abnormalities can occur in Down syndrome and how does prevalence increase with maternal age?
15. What are the clinical features of Down syndrome?

Down syndrome is the most common genetic cause of intellectual disability. Furthermore, 95% of Down syndrome cases are associated with the nondisjunction of chromosome 21 (trisomy 21), with 75%—85% of nondisjunction's being maternal in origin. Approximately 5% of Down syndrome cases are as a result of a Robertsonian translocation, and 1%—3% is associated with mosaicism. The risk of Down syndrome increases with maternal age; in the <30 years age group, its prevalence is 0.7 per 1000, rising to 35 per 1000 in those over 45 years.

Clinical features of Down syndrome include: short stature; small head, ears and mouth; a protruding tongue, broad neck, epicanthal folds, congenital heart defects, hearing deficits, strabismus, oesophageal atresia, Hirschsprung's disease, obesity, hypothyroidism and epilepsy.

7. Unfortunately, Larry cannot be facilitated in his usual respite house and is admitted to one nearby instead. The plan is for daily assessment by the consultant psychiatrist or nonconsultant hospital doctor. For the first two days, Larry's symptoms remain largely unchanged with the persistence of insomnia and agitation. This presents significant management difficulties for staff, particularly at night, and some residents who are staying for planned respite are distressed by Larry's behaviour. You titrate Larry's sodium valproate up to 800 mg orally twice daily to stabilize Larry's mood. A repeat plasma valproic acid tests is ordered as this increase is in the mid-therapeutic range. Larry's sleep improves on the fourth day of respite and his degree of agitation reduces. He requires frequent lorazepam during his first five days of respite. Larry's lability of affect dissipates at day five, and he becomes less restless and does not have repetitive speech anymore. He continues to express that he 'feels sad'.

After one week in respite, the respite manager contacts you and asks if Larry's care could be continued with management in the community. You agree to a trial of community management under close supervision. The social worker agrees to liaise with Larry's family regarding these arrangements and support from the community mental health nursing service is also arranged.

Larry's father enquires about the possibility of residential placement for Larry and cites his own and his wife's ages as the reasoning behind this. He says that even prior to this episode, they were having significant difficulties in assisting Larry in his activities of daily living because of their physical limitations. You state that you will present a report to the residential admissions committee citing Larry's parents' concerns together with your clinical opinion. You will also ask the occupational therapist to visit the home and reassess Larry's activities of daily living needs.

Larry's symptoms settle over the next four weeks and he returns to his baseline state. The results of awaited physical investigations are normal. Larry returns to his day centre placement. There are no indications of functional change or cognitive decline from his premorbid state. However, you still feel it is prudent to arrange a cognitive assessment for Larry. You also request regular periods of respite for Larry. You advise the team that Larry is likely to require more home resources as time advances. Given Larry's age, he is at a high risk of developing Alzheimer's-type dementia in the future. You arrange for Larry to have regular follow-up psychiatry appointments in the future.

16.   What would a cognitive assessment involve?

17.   What are the general principles of management in patients with an intellectual disability?

Cognitive testing can be achieved using a specific scale for people with Down syndrome called the Down syndrome dementia scale along with other formal tools and a baseline assessment of functional abilities, mobility and language skills. Establishing a history of changes in cognitive ability is important. It is important to exclude psychiatric disorders, e.g. depression and organic disorders, e.g. hypothyroidism or delirium, as these can present with cognitive problems.

FURTHER READING

For a review of cognitive testing and dementia in Down Syndrome, see: Hithersay R, Hamburg S, Knight B, Strydom A. (2017) Cognitive decline and dementia in Down syndrome. Current Opinions in Psychiatry 30(2):102–107. doi:10.1097/YCO.0000000000000307

Estimates suggest that $\geq 50\%$ individuals with Down syndrome will develop Alzheimer's dementia as they age. This is linked to the activity of chromosome 21, which carries the amyloid precursor protein (APP) gene, which codes for the APP protein, and can lead to beta-amyloid plaque formation in the brain. Symptoms often occur earlier than in the general population, typically beginning in the 50s or 60s. The risk of someone with Down syndrome developing dementia increases from 20% at the age of 50 years to 80% by the age of 65 years.

Management principles in dealing with individuals with an intellectual disability include the following:

- The use of multidisciplinary teams
- Community inclusion as an important aspect of management to allow individuals with an intellectual disability to feel they have a valued social role with dignity and respect
- Psychological interventions, including behavioural therapies, cognitive behavioural therapy, family education, therapy or psychodynamic therapies, e.g. relaxation therapy, art, drama, and music therapy, are frequently available and therapeutic
- Treatment of underlying mental illness
- When prescribing, it is important to use a 'start low go slow' approach and give due consideration to the following:
  - Increased or reduced sensitivity to therapeutic effects
  - A higher rate of adverse effects
  - Increased sensitivity to side-effects of medications.

Luke

A Case of Suicide

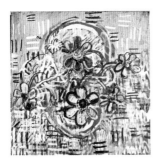

1. Define suicide and self-harm.
2. Distinguish passive death wish, thoughts of self-harm and suicidal intent.
3. Understand how to assess suicide risk.
4. Discuss the epidemiology of self-harm and suicidal behaviour.
5. Discuss risk factors associated with completed suicide.
6. Describe the statutory requirements for reporting a death by suicide.

1. You are working as a general practitioner in a busy city. Your sixth patient that morning is Luke. Luke is a 48-year-old man who has presented to you with a minor upper respiratory tract infection. While talking to Luke, you note that he has a flattened affect and appears lethargic. He has no known psychiatric or medical history of note. On further questioning, Luke admits that life has been quite difficult recently. He has missed out on a promotion at work and feels down about this. He separated from his wife three years ago and has had little contact with his two children since. He drinks about eight units of alcohol a week, usually in the form of beer. In recent months, he has not been going out socially, stopped watching football, which he previously enjoyed as an avid supporter of 'The Hammers' (West Ham United Football Club), and has stopped drinking alcohol completely. He admits to sometimes feeling that life is not worth living and wonders 'what's the point?'

   1. What is known about the epidemiology of deliberate self-harm and suicide?
   2. What is the relationship between mental illness and suicide?

Suicide constitutes about 1% of deaths from all causes annually. However, official suicide statistics likely underestimate the number of actual suicides, in part, because of the stigma that continues to surround suicide. According to the World Health Organization (WHO), an estimated 800,000 people die by suicide every year, with one person dying from suicide every 40 seconds. Suicide is the second leading cause of death among 15–29-year-old individuals around the world. The most common method of suicide is drug overdose (two-thirds of females and one-third of males). Other methods include hanging, shooting and drowning.

Approximately 450 people die in Ireland each year because of suicide. The suicide rate among males is substantially higher (3–4 ×) than in females. Given the significant rate, suicide is a serious global public health problem. The magnitude of the problem is even more significant when the number of attempted but uncompleted suicides, which is 20 times more common, is included.

FURTHER READING

For a review of the many challenges associated with suicide prevention approaches, see: Hawton K, van Heeringen K. (2009) Suicide. The Lancet 373(9672):P1372–1381. doi:10.1016/S0140-6736(09)60372-X

Suicide is considered rare in people under the age of 14 years, but the rates have been increasing. Moreover, there is likely to be gross underreporting of suicides among this demographic. Requirements for recording a death as a suicide vary between countries. For example, in research published by Hawton et al. (2009), it was found that some countries require evidence of intent like a suicide note, e.g. Luxembourg. They also suggested a nine-fold underreporting of suicide in rural areas of India, where suicide is illegal.

Compared with the general population, people with severe depression are 20 times more likely to commit suicide. The risk is especially high for those with comorbid anxiety disorders and agitation. Those with bipolar disorder are 15 times more likely to die from suicide than members of the general population. Among those with schizophrenia, the lifetime risk of suicide is reported as 10%, with the greatest risk usually near the illness onset and immediately following discharge from hospital. Anorexia nervosa shows a strong association with suicide, at 40 times greater than the general population.

Personality disorders, particularly borderline, antisocial and narcissistic subtypes, are associated with increased suicide risk especially in those with comorbid drug addiction, comorbid major mood disorders, a history of childhood sexual abuse, impulsive and antisocial personality traits and recent reduction of psychiatric care, such as recent discharge from hospital. A history of alcohol abuse is common among people who commit suicide, and moreover, alcohol intoxication at the time of a suicide attempt is common.

At the time of suicide, 50% of people have a current known mental illness, one-third have a history of suicidal thoughts or plans, and one-third have significant substance or alcohol misuse issues.

---

2. On further questioning, Luke reveals that he has been having thoughts of suicide. He describes feeling lonely at home since the breakdown of his marriage and has feelings of hopelessness regarding the future. Two weeks ago, he took some tablets he had at home and consumed a litre of vodka in an 'impulsive' suicide attempt. He stated that he took 10 paracetamol and 20 diazepam tablets. He fell asleep at home following this and describes feeling disappointed when he woke up. He has had one previous episode of self-harm where he tried to cut his wrists with a knife during a row with his wife. Currently, Luke reports that he is 'having thoughts of ending it all' at a frequency of 2–3 occasions per week and has occasional suicidal ideation. These consist of thoughts of either overdosing on medication or hanging himself. He denies any plans or intent.

Luke refuses to allow you to contact a family member to obtain a collateral history or to discuss the situation with them. He consents to be referred for an outpatient assessment with a psychiatrist. He does not feel that he needs to attend your local hospital for emergency assessment and in your opinion, he does not require detention under the Mental Health Act as the history does not indicate that he poses an immediate risk to himself and has a good awareness of his difficulties and how they can be addressed.

You decide to commence Luke on escitalopram. You explain how this works and the possible adverse effects. You also advise Luke that if he feels worse on the medication or if his suicidal ideation becomes worse, that he should come back into the clinic or attend the emergency department.

3. What is parasuicide?
4. How would you assess this patient for suicide risk?
5. What are the risk factors for deliberate self-harm and suicide?
6. How might you assess suicidal intent following an act of deliberate self-harm?
7. How would you manage this patient?

The WHO defines suicide as the deliberate act of killing oneself. Parasuicide is an act with a non-fatal outcome, in which an individual deliberately engages in behaviour that, without intervention from others, will cause self-harm. Parasuicide is the strongest known predictor for completed suicide. As society has developed a more informed understanding of self-harm behaviours, the distinction between suicidal and parasuicidal behaviour, which is largely based upon intent, has become blurred as it is clear that many people who engage in self-harm have complex and mixed feelings about the likely outcome. Many people engage in risky behaviours as they are ambivalent about life (e.g. an intoxicated young man driving recklessly late at night on his way home after a relationship break up comments, 'I don't really want to die, but if it happens it is not the worst outcome'). Similarly, many people who engage in behaviour with a high likelihood of lethality are primarily seeking relief from mental anguish (sometimes called 'psychache') rather than permanent death. As Voltaire observed 'The man, who in a fit of melancholy, kills himself today, would have wished to live had he waited a week'.

FURTHER READING

For further information on risk assessments, see: Morriss R, Kapur N, Byng R. (2013) Assessing risk of suicide or self harm in adults. The British Medical Journal 347:f4572. doi:10.1136/bmj.f4572

A risk assessment is an important part of a psychiatric evaluation. Studies indicate that two-thirds of patients who complete suicide have attended their general practitioner in the previous month, and one in eight have attended a psychiatrist in the previous week. One in six people leave a suicide note. Moreover, between one-third and half of patients who complete suicide have a history of self-harm defined as any act of self-poisoning or self-injury, irrespective of motivation.

A passive death wish is characterized by a desire to be dead, but without the urge to cause one's own death, i.e. their perspective is passive rather than active. An example of this would be a patient who wishes that they would not wake up in the morning.

In contrast, suicidal ideation is a more active desire where thoughts of taking one's own life are present. An individual may experience thoughts of self-harm, for example, a patient may have thoughts about hanging themselves or taking an overdose, and the intensity and frequency of these thoughts must be explored during the assessment (see Box 23.1). Vague suicidal thoughts may evolve to the commencement of planning for suicide. Often suicidal ideation occurs without obvious intent such that the person is distressed by the thoughts and communicates that they do not want to end their life (e.g. 'I could never do that, I love my children too much').

Suicidal intent occurs when suicidal ideation has progressed into a plan for suicide, usually with action towards completion of the plan having been taken. These so-called 'final acts' include preparing a will, writing a suicide note, acquiring the means of suicide (e.g. tablets, weapon) and identifying an area to complete the suicide. Progression from a passive death wish to suicidal ideation, and the intent is likely to convey the increasing risk of future completed suicide in an individual.

BOX 23.1 ■ Risk factors for deliberate self-harm

1. Female: male, 1.3:1
2. Aged 15–24 years
3. Drug or alcohol abuse
4. A sense of hopelessness
5. Aggressive tendencies
6. Impulsiveness
7. Relationship difficulties
8. Sexual, physical or emotional abuse
9. Loss of a parent at a young age
10. Psychiatric family history
11. Chronic physical illness, e.g. epilepsy
12. Less help-seeking behaviour
13. Drinking alcohol within three hours of the attempt

BOX 23.2 ■ Risk factors for completed suicide

1. Male: Female, 2–4:1
2. Aged 15–24-year-old females, 25–34-year-old males
3. Mental illness: major depressive disorder, 10–15%; schizophrenia, 10%; bipolar disorder, 10–20%; and alcohol dependence, 15%
4. Previous suicide attempt
5. History of deliberate self-harm (DSH) (up to 60% have at least one recorded DSH attempt, 30% will repeat DSH within one year)
6. Social isolation
7. Lack of social support
8. Stressful life events
9. Physical illness (e.g. chronic pain, epilepsy)
10. Family violence
11. Access to means of suicide
12. Unbearable psychological pain, termed 'psychache' by Schneidman in 1993
13. Postpartum
14. Overcrowded inner-city areas, social deprivation and poor economic situation
15. Prisoners
16. Bullying in school children
17. Unresolved grief

FURTHER READING

For further details on factors influencing suicidal thoughts, see: Gunnell D, Harbord R, Singleton N, et al. (2004) Factors influencing the development and amelioration of suicidal thoughts in the general population: a cohort study. The British Journal of Psychiatry 185 (5):385–393.

Other types of risk that should be explored in suicidal individuals include, but are not limited to, risk of self-neglect, risk of neglecting children under their care and risk of causing harm to dependents, such as children, alongside the suicidal act.

Risk factors associated with suicide are varied and are listed in Box 23.2. Despite these associations, most people with these risk factors will not die by suicide, because despite its seriousness, suicide is a statistically rare event. This is true even for people who have suicidal ideation because the proportion of people with suicidal thoughts who go on to complete suicide is less than one in 200 (Gunnell et al. 2004, see above).

The assessment of suicidal risk usually begins with open-ended probes about the person's general sense of well-being and self-perception to more specific questions about how the person views the future, what they are looking forward to and for any sense of hopelessness, worthlessness or that life is not worth living. It is important to probe for any sense of passive death wish ('do you ever think that if you were to die that it might not be a bad thing' or 'do you ever wish that you could go to sleep and not wake up?'). The assessment then progresses to specific questions about actual thoughts of suicide (suicidal ideation), with attention to the person's attitude towards these thoughts (if present), any planning concerning the method and final acts and then asking about actual suicidal intent. It is useful to consider protective factors such as not wanting to leave or hurt loved ones.

General principles in the management of a suicidal patient

- Conduct a risk assessment, including a detailed history, a collateral history (if possible), a mental state examination, a detailed assessment of current suicidal ideation or intent and details of any previous attempts. Details about the patient's social support network and coping strategies would be important along with any current life stressors.
- Consider admission to hospital, and if declined, consider whether involuntary admission would be warranted.
- Continuity of care is critical. Schedule further regular outpatient appointments and consider the need for referral to a specialist centre.
- Treat any underlying psychiatric conditions if present.
- Offer psychological treatment with an experienced therapist if appropriate.
- Rally support from family and friends.
- If dealing with a minor, address any issues of risk, including sexual or physical abuse, neglect or bullying.
- Care in prescribing is warranted. Use of time-limited prescriptions and drugs with less serious overdose consequences are recommended.
- Provide patient with details of the local emergency department or 24-hour suicide support line.
- Provide psychoeducation to allow the patient to understand the illness and the necessity of treatment, compliance with medications and need for support.

FURTHER READING

For a review of the suicide risk assessment tools, see: Roos L, Sareen J, Bolton J. (2013) Suicide risk assessment tools, predictive validity findings and utility today: time for a revamp? Neuropsychiatry 3(5):1–13. doi:10.2217/NPY.13.60

Several structured approaches to the assessment of suicide risk exist. These tools are a useful means of structuring the assessment, but their use as a measure of suicide likelihood is disputed as the considerable complexity of suicide risk assessment requires flexibility in how different factors are weighted. The Beck's suicide intent scale, shown in Table 23.1, is an example of a structured approach to the assessment of suicidal risk. It is important to recognize that the risk assessment has many ethical and legal complexities. Risk assessment tools are biased towards overestimating risk ('playing safe'), but this has important implications in terms of rationing of

TABLE 23.1 ■ Beck's Suicide Intent Scale

1 Isolation	Somebody present	0
	Somebody nearby or in contact (as by phone)	1
	No one nearby or in contact	2
2 Timing	Timed so that intervention is probable	0
	Timed so that intervention is not likely	1
	Timed so that intervention is highly unlikely	2
3 Precautions against discovery and/or intervention	No precautions	0
	Passive precautions, e.g. avoiding others but doing nothing to prevent their intervention (alone in the room, door unlocked)	1
	Active prevention, such as locking doors	2
4 Acting to gain help during or after the attempt	Notified potential helper	0
	Contacted but did not specifically notify potential helper regarding an attempt	1
	Did not contact or notify potential helper	2
5 Final acts in anticipation of death	None	0
	Partial preparation or ideations	1
	Definite plans made (e.g. changes in will, taking out insurance)	2
6 Suicide note	None	0
	Note written but torn up	1
	Present	2

psychiatric resources (e.g. admission, staff time for interventions) and in terms of civil liberty whereby those considered at-risk can be subjected to involuntary inpatient treatment. Some observers have even recommended that the risk assessment is so inaccurate that it should be abandoned.

---

3. Two days later, you receive a call from a psychiatrist to say that Luke has committed suicide in the local psychiatric unit. Luke had been admitted to hospital the day before, following an assessment in the emergency department for increased suicidal ideation. Luke's next of kin have been informed and they are very upset. They also expressed concern regarding Luke having been commenced on antidepressant medication prior to the suicide as they have heard that these medications can increase suicide risk.

    8. What strategies are available for suicide prevention?
    9. What do you know about antidepressant medication and suicide risk?
  10. What statutory obligations are in place for doctors regarding the reporting of a suspected suicide?

No single intervention appears to be effective in reducing the suicide rate according to research. Recommendations focus on targeting at-risk individuals. These focus on behavioural change, coping strategies and improved ego strength. Programmes focusing on skills training and social support for at-risk students in schools are effective in reducing risk factors and enhancing protective factors. In many societies, it is considered taboo to discuss suicide openly, and only a minority of countries have included the prevention of suicide among their priorities. As previously mentioned, there are also questions about the reliability of suicide certification and reporting. Of note, recent evidence in Ireland is that the longstanding trend towards increasing suicide rates, especially in younger persons, is now starting to reverse with a sustained reduction noted over recent years. The extent to which this reflects the increased awareness of mental well-being and ill-health as an important issue, greater availability of psychological supports or other factors remains unclear.

Recognized effective approaches to suicide prevention

FURTHER READING

Recommended reading: Kelly BD. (2017) Are we finally making progress with suicide and self-harm? An overview of the history, epidemiology and evidence for prevention of suicide. Irish Journal of Psychological Medicine 35(2):95–101. doi:10.1017/ipm.2017.51.

1. Reduce access to the means of suicide in at-risk individuals. For example, time-limited prescriptions, single packaging of tablets, reduce access to guns, pesticides.
2. Any underlying psychiatric condition should be treated.
3. Any individual who has had recent parasuicide should be monitored by the appropriate medical service.
4. Primary healthcare workers need to be trained to recognize and offer support to at-risk individuals.
5. Responsible media reporting about suicide to minimize copycat suicides.
6. Provision of an emergency contact card.
7. Psychotherapeutic interventions where appropriate.
8. School-based suicide prevention programmes.

FURTHER READING

For a discussion of the relationship between antidepressant use and increased suicidality, see: Lu CY, Zhang F, Lakoma MD, et al. (2014) Changes in antidepressant use by young people and suicidal behavior after FDA warnings and media coverage: quasi-experimental study. The British Medical Journal 348:g3596. doi: https://doi.org/10.1136/bmj.g3596

It has been reported that a percentage of patients experience worsening suicidal thoughts soon after commencing antidepressant medication. The extent to which this can be attributed to the underlying depressive illness versus a direct medication effect is contentious. In 2004, the Food and Drug Administration issued a black box warning on antidepressant medication stating that: 'antidepressants increased the risk of suicidal thinking and behaviour (suicidality) in short-term studies in children and young people with major depressive disorder and other psychiatric disorders. Anyone considering the use of antidepressant medications in this group is advised to balance this risk with the clinical need'.

Patients who commence antidepressants should be observed closely for clinical worsening, suicidality or unusual changes in behaviour. Lu et al. (2014) reported that safety warnings about antidepressants and the ensuing media reporting have been associated with a reduction in antidepressant use and an increase in suicide attempts in young people. However, completed suicides did not change in any age group.

4. The month following Luke's suicide, his ex-wife attends your clinic.
   The children are currently attending a counsellor after their father's death and appeared to be coping relatively well up to one week previously when her eldest child came home from school very tearful and upset. It transpired that another boy in the school committed suicide, and although her son was not friendly with him, he did know him. The local media had reported a story three weeks previously of a

Continued on following page

(Continued)

16-year-old who killed himself by carbon monoxide poisoning. Apparently, he was a cousin of the boy at her son's school, and his father had also committed suicide.

Luke's ex-wife is now very concerned about her children and whether they would be at-risk of deliberate self-harm, suicide or any psychiatric disorders, following what happened to their father and these further two recent suicides. Moreover, she has heard that there will be an inquest after her ex-husband's death and is looking for further information.

    11. What do we know about the genetic predisposition to suicide?

    12. What is meant by the term 'copycat suicide' or 'cluster suicide' and what interventions can be helpful in young people?

    13. What is the role of the coroner and an inquest after a suspected suicide?

Several studies have focused on whether genetic factors contribute to the complex cause of suicide. The bulk of work has focused on the serotonergic pathway. The two major genes implicated are the tryptophan hydroxylase-one gene and a polymorphism of the serotonin transporter gene. The monoamine oxidase-A gene is linked with impulsive—aggressive personality traits, and while not linked to suicide, it may be associated with violent and repeated suicide attempts. Genetic factors may be related to personality traits such as impulsiveness and aggressiveness, which in turn may lead to suicide attempts.

Suicide clusters are sometimes referred to as 'contagion' or 'copycat' suicides, denoting imitative behaviour. Suicide clusters are most commonly seen in people under the age of 25 years. Others at increased risk include psychiatric inpatients, members of minority groups, prison inmates and soldiers deployed on extended missions overseas.

FURTHER READING

For a review of school-based interventions aimed at suicide prevention, see: Robinson J, Cox G, Malone A, et al. (2013) A systematic review of school-based interventions aimed at preventing, treating, and responding to suicide-related behavior in young people. Crisis 34 (3):164—182. doi:10.1027/0227-5910/a000168

From a review in Australia of 155 research studies that explored how additional deaths could be prevented, the following six recommendations were made:

1. Developing a community plan using 'response teams' to develop a coordinated plan to deal with suicide clusters.

2. Young people affected by suicide can be referred for educational/psychological debriefing (either individually or groups) to help them deal with grief and suicidal thoughts. Debriefing sessions involve providing information on suicide prevention, stress and grief coping strategies and whom to contact if further help is needed.

3. Young people asking for extra help can receive psychological counselling. Group and individual counselling for young people affected by suicide can include addressing guilt and responsibility, recognizing grief reactions, learning that suicide cannot always be prevented, and how to deal with personal suicidal thoughts.

4. Teachers, parents and counsellors can often recognize high-risk cases that seem particularly in need of help. Having a strategy in place for referring high-risk cases for further screening by mental health professionals is especially important.

5. Ensuring responsible media reporting of suicide clusters through collaborative agreements about reporting practices.

6. Recognizing that the problem can continue despite the suicide cluster being contained. Anniversaries, irresponsible media stories, and failure to address the issues that triggered the suicide cluster to begin with need to be identified.

The Irish Association of Suicidology Media Guidelines for Reporting Suicide is now widely adopted to ensure responsible reporting of suicide in Ireland, with similar guidelines in many countries. Several interventions aimed at young people are being delivered in schools and community groups. 'Storm' is one such evidence-based suicide prevention-training programme developed at the University of Liverpool (see: stormskillstraining.com).

'Connecting for life', an Irish suicide prevention strategy, aims to help teachers identify risk factors for suicide among vulnerable students, while also seeking to promote problem-solving among students themselves rather than using alcohol or drugs to relieve stress. Independent experts rather than teachers deliver the programme, as research indicates students often respond better to outside facilitators. All secondary school students are eligible to receive training on how to cope with stress and improve resilience as part of a new five-year Government strategy to reduce the number of people taking their own lives.

Reporting of suicides

A doctor must report any unexpected death to the Gardaí, and an inquest will follow. The Gardaí will ask a relative or a family member to identify the body and take formal statements from those individuals. The coroner will be informed of the death by the Gardaí, as is the case in all deaths from unnatural causes and will subsequently investigate the cause of death. The coroner will request a postmortem, and an inquest into the deceased's death will follow.

An inquest is an official, public enquiry, presided over by the coroner. If the death cannot be explained, an inquest may be held to establish the facts of death, such as where and how the death occurred. Witnesses may be required to attend the inquest to give testimony under oath regarding the circumstances and cause of the death. When a jury is present at an inquest, it is the jury, rather than the coroner, who delivers the verdict. Nobody is found guilty or innocent at an inquest, and no criminal or civil liability is determined. The family of the deceased are entitled to attend the inquest, but they are not legally obliged to be there. If the family attend the inquest, they do not require legal representation on their behalf. However, if legal action is being taken as a result of the death, the family may engage a solicitor to attend the inquest.

When the proceedings have been completed, a verdict is returned regarding the identity of the deceased, and how, when and where the death occurred. The range of verdicts open to the coroner or jury includes accidental death, misadventure, suicide, open verdict, natural causes and unlawful killing. A general recommendation designed to prevent similar deaths occurring may be made by the coroner or jury. When the inquest is completed, the coroner issues a certificate so that the death can be properly registered.

CHAPTER 24

Pious, Bernadette, Dervla, Emmett and Karim

Adverse Effects of Medication

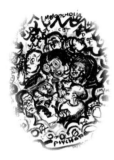

1. Define the terms akathisia and dyskinesia in terms of their core clinical features and distinguish between acute and tardive presentations along with important differential diagnoses.
2. List the main risk factors for the conditions listed above.
3. Outline the immediate and longer-term management strategies for the conditions listed above.
4. Describe the main clinical features of an acute dystonic reaction, including differential diagnoses and risk factors.
5. Describe the immediate and longer-term medical management of an acute dystonic reaction.
6. Describe the core clinical features of neuroleptic malignant syndrome (NMS), including differential diagnoses and risk factors.
7. Describe the immediate and longer-term medical management of NMS, including prognosis.
8. Describe the core clinical features of serotonin syndrome (SS), including differential diagnoses and risk factors.
9. Describe the immediate and longer-term medical management of SS, including prognosis.
10. Construct a table summarising the main medical emergencies encountered in psychiatry care, i.e. NMS, SS and acute dystonic reactions. For each condition, list the key discriminating clinical features, risk factors and immediate treatment approaches.

1. Pious

You are working as a basic specialist trainee in psychiatry and are taking the day to do several joint assessments with the local community mental health nurse, Josephine. Your first call is to Pious, a 20-year-old man who has recently been discharged from the inpatient psychiatric unit after his first presentation with a psychotic illness. Pious had been admitted for six weeks with florid spiritual delusions and hallucinations. However, he improved relatively quickly after receiving high dose atypical antipsychotic treatment (risperidone; 6 mg daily). The psychiatric social worker had been involved with his family, and he is benefitting from cognitive behavioural therapy with Josephine.

Pious initially appears to be cooperative and engaged with your assessment. However, he crosses and uncrosses his legs on numerous occasions and frequently stands up throughout the consultation despite his mother's increasingly vocal encouragement to remain seated. He eventually apologizes and walks out. From the window, you observe him pacing around the yard, smoking a cigarette. His mother tells you 'he can't sit down for a second, I think he's having a relapse, he keeps telling me he can't control his legs, I'm shouting at him to sit down all day'. She does concede that he has been very helpful with work around the small farm and that he has 'been talking sense' since returning home.

With Josephine's encouragement, you continue your assessment with Pious, walking around with him outside, where he can converse more easily. He describes an 'inner restlessness', which has been present since his risperidone dose was increased in the last two weeks of his hospitalization.

1. What are your thoughts regarding this presentation?
2. What treatment options would be available to Pious?

FURTHER READING

For rating of severity, see the Barnes Akathisia Rating Scale: Barnes TR. (1989) A rating scale for drug-induced akathisia. British Journal of Psychiatry 154:672–676.

Pious is experiencing agitation and restlessness after a recent episode of psychosis. There is a relatively wide range of conditions to consider, including several 'functional' psychiatric conditions. As the symptoms of inner and motor restlessness have occurred without evidence of active or worsening psychosis and in tandem with a recent increase in antipsychotic dosage, the likely diagnosis is of 'acute akathisia'. Akathisia is a movement disorder characterized by a feeling of inner restlessness and a compelling need to be in constant motion, often accompanied by a sense of dysphoria. Akathisia has a spectrum of intensity, varying from a mild sense of unease to extreme discomfort, often focused on the legs. The discomfort, which can last all day, might be somewhat relieved by pacing and individuals may walk for hours until they are extremely fatigued. Occasionally affected individuals describe symptoms similar to neuropathic pain or fibromyalgia.

Some patients may not exhibit outer restlessness but instead develop an inner sense of discomfort, which may present as intense dysphoria, anxiety and a sense of despair. Notably, Pious' mother is concerned that he is experiencing a psychotic relapse and it is not unusual for the symptoms of akathisia to be misinterpreted as agitation associated with anxiety or affective/psychotic experiences. Therefore individuals may inadvertently be prescribed increased dosages of the causative medications, further exacerbating their condition. Others may be prescribed anxiolytic medication which may be ineffective.

Types of Akathisia

Acute Akathisia

Most akathisia develops after starting or increasing antipsychotic medication and has a duration of less than six months. It is classically associated with a sense of restlessness, intense dysphoria and complex, semipurposeful motor fidgetiness.

Chronic Akathisia

Persists for over six months after last dosage increment, with less pronounced degrees of dysphoria and subjective restlessness. It may be accompanied by limb and orofacial dyskinesia.

Tardive Akathisia

Has a delayed onset and is not related to a recent change in medication.

Withdrawal Akathisia

Is associated with switching antipsychotic medications and discontinuation of anticholinergic treatment. It can also occur in withdrawal from dependency associated drugs.

Causes

Akathisia is most commonly associated with the use of potent dopamine receptor antagonists, such as first-generation antipsychotics (FGAs) although as is the case with Pious, second-generation antipsychotics (SGAs) may also be implicated. The pathophysiology of akathisia remains unsubstantiated. There is a clear association with the dopamine system but the response to beta-adrenergic blockers suggests that other transmitter systems are also involved.

Antidepressant treatment may also cause akathisia, which may frequently be misinterpreted as agitation, anxiety or hypomanic switching. This implication of the serotonin system is further substantiated by the observation that serotonin antagonists can also be an effective treatment for the condition.

Drug withdrawal has been associated with akathisia. Cocaine is associated with increased dopamine signalling, and subsequent withdrawal may model dopamine antagonism, precipitating the akathisia symptoms.

Treatment of antipsychotic-induced akathisia

- **Reduce** the dose of antipsychotic.
- Switch to **quetiapine, olanzapine or clozapine** (which are less prone to inducing extrapyramidal symptoms [EPS], including akathisia).
- **Beta-blockers,** particularly propranolol, are considered first-line therapy for drug-induced akathisia. Although multiple small studies and case reports support the use of beta-blockers to treat drug-induced akathisia the quality of evidence of their efficacy is controversial. Consider the risk of hypotension, bradycardia and asthma along with drug interactions.
- **Anticholinergics:** Benztropine, biperiden, and procyclidine are frequently used for the prevention and treatment of EPS. However, a Cochrane review concluded that there was insufficient data to support the use of anticholinergics for akathisia. Although multiple case reports have shown anticholinergics to be effective in treating drug-induced akathisia their association with cognitive side-effects suggests a need for caution.
- **Serotonin antagonists and agonists:** The blockade of 5-HT2 receptors can attenuate akathisia symptoms. Mianserin, ritanserin and most recently low dose mirtazapine have an evidence base.
- **Benzodiazepines:** Through their sedative and anxiolytic properties, benzodiazepines are thought to partially alleviate akathisia symptoms. Dependency on these medications is a clear reason for caution in their use.
- **α-Adrenergic agonists:** Clonidine, a selective alpha-2 adrenergic agonist, may also be used, usually when other treatment methods have failed. Side-effects include sedation and hypotension.
- **D2 agonists:** Akathisia and restless legs syndrome have similar pathophysiology, and patients with akathisia may benefit from D2 agonists such as pramipexole and ropinirole.

However, D2 agonists can precipitate or worsen psychosis thus limiting their usefulness in this instance.

2. Bernadette

Your next home visit is to Bernadette, who has a diagnosis of chronic schizophrenia. Josephine informs you that Bernadette's condition is largely characterized by negative symptoms of social withdrawal and self-neglect, and she has been adequately treated with low dose depot flupenthixol for years. She lives with her twin sister Rita, in an isolated cottage, and there are no acute issues apparent; therefore this is a routine visit.

At the assessment, Bernadette has no concerns. However, Rita (who is seated at the opposite side of the large fireplace from her sister) tells you 'she keeps making faces at me, sticking out her tongue and chewing at her face'.

At the assessment, Bernadette is unconcerned. However, you note that she repeatedly puckers her lips, rolls her tongue and makes grimacing movements with her face while blinking her eyes excessively.

3. What is the likely diagnosis?
4. What treatment options are available to Bernadette?

FURTHER READING

For a review of how to manage common extrapyramidal symptoms of antipsychotic medications, see: Stroup TS, Gray N. (2018) Management of common adverse effects of antipsychotic medications. World Psychiatry 17(3):341–356. doi:10.1002/wps.20567

'Dyskinesia' is a general term that describes any abnormal involuntary movement. Dystonia is a type of dyskinesia that involves sustained muscle contractions, often with repetitive, abnormal twisting movements or postures. Tardive refers to the timing of appearance of symptoms (i.e. late occurring).

Tardive dyskinesia (TD) is characterized by repetitive, involuntary movements typically involving the face, trunk and limbs. Examples include grimacing, tongue movements, lip-smacking, lip-puckering and excessive eye blinking. These facial movements are sometimes classified as classic TD or oro-buccolingual stereotypy. In cases where TD involves the muscles of the trunk and lower limbs, involuntary movements can be hidden from the clinician by the typical office desk.

Facial dyskinesia may be accompanied by rapid, involuntary movements of the limbs and digits (limb stereotypies) or rocking of the torso (trunk stereotypy), along with respiratory symptoms such as grunting and shortness of breath. Other closely related neurological disorders have been recognized as variants of TD. Tardive dystonia is similar to standard dystonia but permanent and the syndrome of tardive akathisia is described above.

The precise mechanism underpinning TD remains unclear. The condition was first described in the 1950s shortly after the introduction of chlorpromazine, and most evidence suggests that TD may be the result of antipsychotic-induced dopamine super-sensitivity in the nigrostriatal pathway. First-generation antipsychotics (FGAs) have a higher occupancy at striatal D2 receptors (60%–80% at therapeutic dosages) and are associated with a higher risk for TD than second-generation antipsychotics (SGAs). This theory is further substantiated by the observation that increasing the dose of dopamine blocking agents may temporarily improve the condition (and acute medication withdrawal may worsen it) but does not explain the occasional persistence of TD for years after the offending drug has been discontinued. Other accepted pathogenic mechanisms include damage to γ-aminobutyric acid (GABA) containing neurones and free radical formation from catecholamine metabolism. The risk of TD for individuals taking FGAs for more than three years is estimated at 14%.

Other theories have been postulated to explain the persistence of the condition, including the possibility that long-term antipsychotic exposure may contribute to neurodegeneration. This is consistent with postmortem studies demonstrating neuronal loss in the basal ganglia of TD patients. Of note extrapyramidal disorders, including TD, have been observed in patients with chronic psychotic illness who have not been exposed to neuroleptic medications indicating that the underlying neurobiology of psychotic illnesses contributes in part to the vulnerability to TD.

Epidemiological studies demonstrate a prevalence of TD between 20% and 50% in those treated with antipsychotic medications. Risk factors include advancing age, female sex, decreased functional reserve or cognitive dysfunction, traumatic brain injuries, cigarette smoking, diabetes mellitus and those with prominent negative symptoms of schizophrenia. Interestingly, TD is also more common in those that experience acute neurological side-effects from antipsychotic drug treatment, such as acute dystonias or akathisia. Racial discrepancies in TD rates also exist, with Africans and African Americans having higher rates of TD after exposure to antipsychotics. Certain genetic risk factors for TD have been identified, including gene polymorphisms involving antipsychotic metabolism and dopamine functioning.

Treatment

Prevention: Prevention of TD is achieved by using the lowest effective dose of an SGA for the shortest time. However, this may not be practical. If TD is diagnosed, the causative drug should be discontinued, but the condition may persist after withdrawal of the drug for months or years with the possibility of permanent symptoms. It is standard practice to withdraw any anticholinergic drugs and to reduce the dose of the offending antipsychotic as the initial step in those with early signs of TD. As with the dopamine super-sensitivity hypothesis noted above, this dose reduction may initially worsen TD. It is often advisable to substitute the antipsychotic prescribed when TD was first observed with another drug that has weak striatal dopamine receptor affinity, particularly clozapine, with quetiapine as an alternative agent.

Additional agents: Tetrabenazine is the only licensed treatment for TD in the United Kingdom. It is a dopamine-depleting agent and has antipsychotic properties but is linked to depression, drowsiness and akathisia.

Benzodiazepines are widely used as GABA-enhancing agents and are considered to be effective. However, there is little empirical data to support its use.

Vitamin E: Numerous studies suggest its use as an antioxidant, but its efficacy remains inconclusively established.

3. Dervla

While driving between visits, Josephine pulls over to take a call on her mobile from a distressed relative of a 20-year-old patient, Dervla, who has recently been assessed for a hypomanic relapse of bipolar affective disorder and received treatment from the out-of-hours general practitioner service very early this morning. The caller tells you that Dervla is 'extremely unwell, lying on her back on the ground, twisting her head and crying'.

Josephine swiftly diverts the car, and you arrive at the house shortly after. On arrival, Dervla is lying on the kitchen floor, crying in pain, with her pet Jack Russell, licking her face. Her head is twisted back to the left-hand side, while her eyes are fixed in an upward stare. Both Dervla and her aunt are agitated, and the emotional state in the house is highly charged. Thankfully, Josephine takes control of the situation, stating that she has seen this presentation numerous times in the past. She calls the local general practitioner and notes that Dervla had received an injection of haloperidol earlier this morning for 'racing thoughts'. She advises you about appropriate treatment and assures everyone that things should settle quickly.

5. What is the likely diagnosis?
6. What treatment options are available?

Dervla has experienced distressing physical symptoms shortly after receiving a high-potency antipsychotic. The most likely diagnosis is that of an acute dystonic reaction. Other conditions should be considered, including stroke, central nervous system (CNS) infection, tetanus, metabolic causes (e.g. hypocalcaemia) and hyperventilation leading to a carpopedal spasm. As many as one in three patients experience at least a mild dystonic reaction in the first few days after starting antipsychotic medication.

Dystonia refers to sustained muscle contractions, frequently causing twisting, repetitive movements or abnormal postures. They may affect any part of the body. As is the case with Dervla, patients experiencing acute dystonic reactions are often frightened and fearful and may be in considerable pain. Although theoretically airway or respiratory compromise may occur (e.g. with laryngeal dystonia), dystonia is rarely life-threatening.

Acute dystonic reactions can present in several different ways:

- Laryngeal dystonia: A rare but potentially life-threatening variant characterized by throat pain, dyspnoea, stridor and dysphonia.
- Oculogyric crisis: Classically presents with a deviated or upturned gaze.
- Blepharospasm and other facial spasms: Spasm of the eyelids or other facial muscles.
- Buccolingual crisis: Protruding or pulling sensation of the tongue.
- Torticollis: Twisting of the neck, or the head forced forwards or backwards.
- Opisthotonic crisis: Spasm of the entire body characterized by back-arching, flexion of the upper limbs and extension of the lower limbs.

Several of these presentations may coexist, as is the case with Dervla, who demonstrates an oculogyric crisis, torticollis and opisthotonos.

The dominant mechanism resulting in acute dystonic reactions is thought to be nigrostriatal D2 receptor blockade, which leads to excess striatal cholinergic output.

As with acute akathisia and TD, high-potency D2 receptor antagonists are most likely to produce acute dystonic reactions. Higher dosages are often linked to acute dystonic reactions, but the relationship is unpredictable, and reactions are generally idiosyncratic.

Acute dystonic reactions usually occur within a few hours of receiving an antipsychotic but onset can be delayed a few days. Left untreated, the condition gradually resolves over a few days.

Several other medications may cause dystonia, including the following:

Antiemetics: e.g. metoclopramide, prochlorperazine

Antidepressants and serotonin-receptor agonists: e.g. serotonin specific reuptake inhibitors (SSRIs), buspirone, sumatriptan

Antibiotics: e.g. erythromycin

Anticonvulsants: e.g. carbamazepine, vigabatrin

H2 receptor antagonists: e.g. ranitidine, cimetidine

Recreational drugs: e.g. cocaine.

Not all patients receiving these medications develop side-effects. Increased susceptibility to dystonia is found in those of male gender, younger age, those who are antipsychotic-naive, those with a previous episodes of acute dystonia and those receiving higher potency D2 receptor antagonists in high doses. A family history of dystonia is also considered a risk factor.

Treatment

Anticholinergics: Benztropine or another anticholinergic agent is considered the first-line treatment of acute dystonic reactions. The response is often dramatic and generally occurs within five minutes of an intravenous injection and 20 minutes of an intramuscular administration. If symptoms persist, a second dose may be given after 30 minutes. If there is an ongoing lack of response, an alternative diagnosis should be considered. The exact mechanism of action of anticholinergic drugs in the relief of dystonic symptoms remains undetermined, although it is believed that their effect is centrally mediated and restores the imbalance between striatal dopamine and acetylcholine. Benztropine, for example, reduces cholinergic activity in the basal ganglia and has also been shown to increase the availability of dopamine by blocking its reuptake and storage in central sites.

Benzodiazepines: They are not recommended as first-line treatment, as early use may lead to diagnostic uncertainty. They are of use as a second-line treatment for those whose symptoms are slow to respond to anticholinergics and may help relieve muscle spasm and anxiety.

Antihistamines: H1 receptor antagonists with anticholinergic activity, such as promethazine, may be used if anticholinergics are not available.

As the half-life of many antipsychotics may exceed that of benztropine, it is prudent to continue the anticholinergic medication for at least two to three days.

Patients requiring ongoing antipsychotic treatment may require long-term anticholinergic treatment to prevent symptoms or an alternative, preferably second-generation antipsychotic agent, may be used.

4. Emmett

After taking a break in a nearby village, Josephine takes a call from a local general practitioner, Dr Egerton-Jones, who is looking for collateral information on a 50-year-old patient, Emmett, whom he is sending into the emergency department. The general practitioner recently re-located from Devon and is finding it difficult to understand Emmett's sister's accent.

Emmett has been brought to the surgery feeling very unwell, sweating excessively and complaining of stiff muscles. Dr Egerton-Jones has observed that Emmett appears confused and disorientated, has a temperature of 40 degrees, tachycardia and is diaphoretic with muscle rigidity. He has called an ambulance, which is 30 minutes away.

Josephine informs the general practitioner that Emmett has a history of schizoaffective disorder and in recent times has been quite unwell, leading to an increase in his antipsychotic (depot haloperidol). He is also maintained on the antidepressant, sertraline.

Given the length of time before the ambulance will arrive, Dr Egerton-Jones is keen to initiate further investigations and management.

7. What diagnoses would you consider?
8. What would you advise Dr Egerton-Jones?

Dr Egerton-Jones is appropriately treating this presentation as a medical emergency. Several physical conditions may lead to a similar presentation, including CNS infection, systemic infection, malignant hyperthermia, catatonia, drug withdrawal and autoimmune conditions. Given the recent increase in the high-potency antipsychotic agent, haloperidol, neuroleptic malignant syndrome (NMS) should be considered. Of note, Emmett has also been prescribed the SSRI, sertraline. Therefore, serotonin syndrome (SS) should also be considered.

Appropriate investigations include a full blood count (FBC; leucocytosis), urea and electrolytes (U&E), blood cultures, live function tests (LFTs; altered), serum creatine kinase (CK; markedly elevated and typically >1000 IU), urine myoglobin and coagulation studies. Once Emmett has reached the hospital, further investigations should include a chest X-ray, electrocardiogram (ECG), computed tomography, brain magnetic resonance imaging and a lumbar puncture.

You follow up with a phone call to the registrar in the emergency department. They have reviewed the initial investigations: Emmett has a very high creatinine phosphokinase level of 2100 IU and metabolic acidosis, along with a leucocytosis and myoglobinuria.

While they are aware of the limitations of your role as a psychiatry trainee, they would like your thoughts on the initial management. They also would like advice about managing Emmett's behaviour as he is significantly restless, and they are considering sedating agents.

9. What is the most likely diagnosis?
10. What management would you suggest?
11. What would you advise regarding the management of Emmett's agitation?

The most likely diagnosis at this point is NMS. NMS is a rare, life-threatening, idiosyncratic reaction to antipsychotic medications or the abrupt withdrawal of dopamine agonists such as levo-dopa. Rarely antidepressants and methylphenidate have precipitated NMS.

There is an increased risk of the condition with rapid antipsychotic dose escalation, use of high-potency agents and depot preparations. Males are twice as likely as females to develop NMS and those with a previous history of NMS, catatonia, alcoholism, or organic brain disease are more susceptible.

There is significant mortality associated with NMS, estimated at between 5% and 20%. Causes of death include respiratory failure, cardiovascular collapse, myoglobinuric renal failure, arrhythmia and disseminated intravascular coagulation.

FURTHER READING

For a review of neuroleptic malignant syndrome, see: Berman BD. (2011) Neuroleptic malignant syndrome: A review for neurohospitals. Neurohospitalist 1:41–47. doi:10.1177/ 1941875210386491

The syndrome is thought to be the result of an intensive reduction of dopaminergic activity within the nigrostriatal, hypothalamic and mesolimbic/cortical pathways. D2 antagonism does not explain all the symptoms of NMS and it is also of note that medications with no dopamine receptor affinity, such as lithium, can sometimes cause the syndrome. This has led to several other postulated mechanisms for the development of NMS, including sympathoadrenal hyperactivity and defective calcium regulatory proteins.

Management

After the investigations outlined above, initial management would be to stop the antipsychotics or restart antiparkinsonian agents, monitor temperature, blood pressure, pulse and consider benzodia-zepines for acute behavioural disturbance.

More specialist medical management includes temperature reduction and correction of volume deple-tion. Furthermore, rhabdomyolysis should be treated with vigorous hydration to prevent renal failure.

Several agents may be considered to alleviate muscle rigidity including dantrolene, bromocrip-tine or amantadine.

If there is major behavioural or psychotic disturbance it is advisable to avoid restarting antipsy-chotic medication for at least five days. If the treatment of psychosis is a priority, electroconvulsive therapy should be considered.

After improvement from NMS any re-introduction of an antipsychotic agent should begin very slowly, with a low dose of a drug with low D2 affinity (clozapine or quetiapine).

5. Karim

Your final visit of the day is to a gentleman that Josephine is eager for you to meet. Karim has a diagnosis of recurrent depressive disorder, which has been resistant to treatment. However, his condition has improved in recent months. He runs a successful vegan restaurant and is pursuing a career as a psy-chotherapist, where he hopes to use his personal experience of illness to help others in similar situations. Over the years, he has been an insightful patient and has been compliant with treatment despite his unease with the potential side-effects of prescribed medications, which he feels are at odds with his ethics.

As Karim greets you at his door, he appears quite anxious and is sweating profusely. When he sits down outside, you notice occasional myoclonic jerks from his arms and his speech is very rapid. He excuses himself to go to his bathroom, mentioning frequent diarrhoea over the last two days. When he returns, Karim tells you that he started to come off his antidepressant paroxetine a few weeks ago and supplemented it with 'a good high dose of St John's Wort'. He has continued the lithium he is prescribed for treatment resistance, as he is happy that it is a naturally-occurring salt. He recently had his serum lithium tested (within normal range) and had not noticed any deterioration in his mood. The uncomfortable physical symptoms have come on over the last 24 hours.

12. What are the principal diagnostic considerations at this point?

Again, several diagnoses should be considered that are in line with the NMS case. Both Emmett and Karim have presented with changes in mental status and hyperthermia. The absence of antipsychotic exposure makes NMS unlikely in this case, although it may be caused by antidepressant use in rare cases. Given the recent reduction of antidepressant, there is a possibility of discontinuation syndrome.

Antidepressants are not addictive, in the sense that tolerance is not observed. However, abrupt discontinuation (particularly of antidepressants with shorter half-lives, such as paroxetine and venlafaxine) may lead to several distressing symptoms, including the following:

- Sensory symptoms: paraesthesia, electric shock sensations, palinopsia
- Disequilibrium symptoms: dizziness, vertigo
- General somatic symptoms: lethargy, sweating
- Gastrointestinal symptoms: nausea, diarrhoea
- Sleep disturbance: insomnia, excessive dreaming
- Affective symptoms: irritability, low mood.

Given the slow reduction and cross-titration he has initiated, discontinuation syndrome is unlikely in Karim's case. Lithium toxicity may present with diarrhoea, but his recent serum levels were within the normal range. Given the combination of lithium and dual antidepressant use, the most likely diagnosis is of serotonin syndrome (SS).

FURTHER READING

For a review of serotonin syndrome, see: Buckley NA, Dawson AH, Isbister GK. (2014) Serotonin syndrome. The British Medical Journal 348:g1626. doi:10.1136/bmj.g1626

A diagnosis of SS requires at least three of the following symptoms to be present: agitation/restlessness, sweating, tremor, fever, shivering, diarrhoea, hyperreflexia, myoclonus, ataxia and mental state changes (confusion, hypomania). Organic causes should be ruled out, and there should be an absence of concurrent antipsychotic dose changes.

In contrast with NMS, mortality is rare in SS, at <1 in 1000. Onset is usually acute, and most cases resolve within 24–36 hours, with supportive measures. This contrasts with NMS where onset typically is slow, i.e. days to weeks.

Any mechanism that increases the quantity or activity of serotonin can lead to the syndrome, such as:

- Increased production (L-tryptophan)
- Decreased metabolism of serotonin (monoamine oxidase inhibitors, selegiline)
- Increased release of serotonin (amphetamines, cocaine, 3,4-methylenedioxymethamphetamine)
- Reuptake inhibition (SSRIs, tricyclic antidepressants, serotonin noradrenaline reuptake inhibitors, noradrenergic and specific serotonergic antidepressants, St John's Wort)
- Direct stimulation of serotonin receptors
- Unknown mechanisms (lithium)

Investigations

FBC, U&E, LFTs, glucose, pH, CK, drug toxicology screen, chest X-ray, ECG.

Treatment

Although most cases are self-limiting, severe symptoms are best managed in an emergency department. Overdose should be managed with gastric lavage/activated charcoal. Further management is similar to that of NMS with volume correction and maintenance of high urinary output. Benzodiazepines may be used to prevent seizures, agitation and muscular rigidity or myoclonus.

CHAPTER 25

Piotr

Schizophrenia

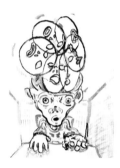

1. Understand the different symptom constellations in schizophrenia.
2. Describe the negative symptoms of schizophrenia.
3. Describe the differential diagnosis of patients with severe and enduring mental illness presenting with reduced emotional expression and motivation.
4. Outline the relationship between schizophrenia and depression.
5. Understand what we know about the management of negative symptoms, both pharmacological and nonpharmacological.
6. Appreciate our understanding of the cause and neurobiology of schizophrenia.
7. Recognize the relative usefulness of different classes of antipsychotics.
8. Appreciate the practicalities of clozapine treatment.
9. Recognize the main extrapyramidal symptoms and their management.
10. Describe the main components of a 'recovery-based' approach to the treatment of schizophrenia.
11. Outline the prognosis of schizophrenia over time.

1. Piotr is a 45-year-old man with a longstanding diagnosis of schizophrenia. His family asks to meet with you as they are concerned that 'although he doesn't have any strange thoughts or experiences, he has seemed chronically depressed for the past few years'. They mention that he is extremely inactive with poor self-care and hygiene, does not seem to enjoy anything and expresses little, if any, emotion. When you meet Piotr, he is dishevelled, wearing both a beanie hat and a cap despite the warm weather, with a long beard and dry skin. He has poverty of thought and speech. He attends his local

Continued on following page

(Continued)

day hospital every six weeks, but his key worker there tells you he does not participate in any of the scheduled activities.
1. What are your initial thoughts regarding this presentation?
2. What is this collection of symptoms called?
3. What is known about the management of such a constellation of symptoms?

Schizophrenia, as a syndrome, includes three constellations of symptoms that are thought to represent distinct neurobiologies:

1. Positive symptoms, which include hallucinations, delusions and disorganized thinking, speech and behaviour.
2. Negative symptoms, which include avolition (reduced drive and activity), affective blunting, alogia (reduced vocabulary), anhedonia (reduced interest and enjoyment) and asociality.
3. Neurocognitive deficits, which include inattention, impaired executive function and reduced skill acquisition.

Piotr exhibits a pattern that is suggestive of negative symptoms of schizophrenia, which include blunting of affect, avolition, lack of drive, apathy, anhedonia and alogia. In practice, it may be difficult to distinguish these symptoms from depression, which may not always present with typical biological symptoms and is common in severe and enduring mental illness (Table 25.1).

In Piotr's case, a thorough assessment should be conducted to rule out a comorbid depressive illness and/or substance abuse. However, the longstanding nature of these symptoms suggests these are negative symptoms of schizophrenia rather than part of a depressive syndrome.

Negative symptoms have been observed in as many as 30% of patients with schizophrenia and in around 15% of those experiencing their first episode. These 'deficit' symptoms are thought to be related to cortical cell loss, as the illness progresses. Accordingly, there is evidence that earlier diagnosis and treatment (e.g. the duration of untreated psychosis; see Chapter 2) may impact functioning and the course of symptoms, including negative symptoms.

In 15%–20% of patients with schizophrenia negative symptoms persist and have been shown to limit recovery and reduce social functioning.

It is important to recognize that, while the positive symptoms of schizophrenia present a compelling therapeutic target, for the majority of patients these symptoms occur during periods of relapse and can usually be well controlled. Conversely, negative symptoms represent a much more challenging long-term therapeutic target that accounts more substantially for adaptive functioning and quality of life over time.

TABLE 25.1 ■ **Some Differences Between Negative Symptoms and Depression**

Negative Symptoms	Depression
Blunted affect	Flat affect
Amotivation	Depressed mood
Anticipatory anhedonia	Anhedonia
Apathy	Guilt
Social withdrawal	Weight loss or gain
Attentional impairment	Decreased concentration
Longitudinally stable	Longitudinally unstable
Medication unresponsive	Medication responsive
Brain structural changes	Structural change less consistent
Cognitive deficits	Cognitive deficits less stable/pronounced

Negative symptoms may be considered primary (inherent to the illness) or secondary to the following: (1) depression; (2) a side-effect of medication, also known as extrapyramidal symptoms (EPS; e.g. bradykinesia); (3) as a result of positive symptoms such as hallucinations/delusions, wherein a patient withdraws socially; (4) institutionalization; or (5) chronic substance misuse. Secondary symptoms should be treated by addressing the relevant cause.

Treatment of negative symptoms

FURTHER READING

For a detailed review of negative symptoms and their management, see: Aleman A, Lincoln TM, Bruggeman R, et al. (2017) Treatment of negative symptoms: Where do we stand, and where do we go? Schizophrenia Research 186:55–62. doi:10.1016/j.schres.2016.05.015

The pharmacological management of negative symptoms requires careful consideration of the extent to which current treatments are causing secondary negative symptoms and the extent to which changes in treatment might impact upon primary negative symptoms in schizophrenia. The latter is a controversial issue with limited evidence that any pharmacological intervention impacts reliably upon primary negative features. A detailed meta-analysis of placebo-controlled studies demonstrated small (but not clinically significant) benefits with second-generation antipsychotics, antidepressants, combinations of pharmacological agents, glutamatergic medications and psychological interventions.

As outlined below, all antipsychotics act as D_2 receptor antagonists. In addition, 5-HT2A antagonism and/or 5-HT1A agonism may contribute to the therapeutic effects of second-generation antipsychotics (SGAs). Certain SGAs have been reported to be superior to first-generation antipsychotics (FGAs) in the treatment of negative symptoms, but this effect is confounded by the observation that FGAs may cause secondary negative symptoms such as EPS.

Studies of treatment with antidepressants, mainly serotonin specific reuptake inhibitors (SSRIs), have yielded inconsistent findings, with a recent detailed meta-analysis supporting the addition of an SSRI as potentially helpful. However, current treatment guidelines conclude that the evidence for augmenting antipsychotic medication with an antidepressant in the treatment of negative symptoms of schizophrenia is not currently robust enough to be recommended for clinical practice.

FURTHER READING

For a review of nonpharmacological approaches to negative symptoms, see: Turner DT, McGlanaghy E, Cuijpers P, et al. (2018) A meta-analysis of social skills training and related interventions for psychosis. Schizophrenia Bulletin 44(3):475–491. doi: 10.1093/schbul/sbx146

Social skills training and cognitive behavioural therapy (CBT) have demonstrated efficacy in ameliorating negative symptoms, may reduce functional impairments and enhance social competence in the areas of self-care, work, leisure and family relationships. In general, these approaches have been greatly underutilized in clinical practice until the emergence of more recovery-focused approaches, which emphasize more holistic management of mental disorders.

2. Piotr lives alone (with family members nearby) and attends a local rehabilitation day hospital. He has had numerous trials of first-generation antipsychotics over the past 20 years. Lately, he has been receiving treatment with the second-generation antipsychotics—risperidone and olanzapine.

Continued on following page

(Continued)

In addition to his negative symptoms, he experiences persistent beliefs that government agents are reading his mind and that he hears voices of 'politicians commenting on everything I do'. These symptoms wax and wane and he is occasionally distressed by them. The staff in the day hospital have noted that he has difficulties with organization and understanding the nuances of interpersonal cues and relationships.

4. What psychopathological condition is described here?
5. What is the prevalence of schizophrenia?
6. What are the main aetiological theories to explain the neuropathology of schizophrenia?
7. What do you know about the different classes of antipsychotics in terms of their side-effect profile?

Piotr is describing thought broadcasting and third-person auditory hallucinations giving a running commentary. These are both first-rank symptoms of schizophrenia (see Chapter 2). Furthermore, the day hospital staff have observed some neurocognitive deficits, including difficulties with executive functioning, such as the ability to organize and abstract.

It is well recognized that patients with schizophrenia have significant neurocognitive deficits when compared with the normal population. These include difficulties with verbal and working memory, attention and concentration, executive functioning and processing speed. These difficulties impact upon the level of autonomy in patients with schizophrenia in terms of self-care, vocational outcomes, family contact and social functioning.

Causes of schizophrenia

There are several aetiological theories for schizophrenia, all falling under the umbrella of the neurodevelopmental hypothesis. A higher rate of motor and cognitive problems is evident for years before the more florid symptoms of acute illness. The neurodevelopmental theory relates to the typical onset of florid symptoms during the time of dopamine receptor 'pruning'. Epidemiologically, it has been noted that those born after obstetric complications, in winter or early spring are at greater risk of the illness. Overactivation of the immune system from prenatal infection or postnatal stress may result in the overexpression of inflammatory cytokines and subsequent alterations in brain structure and function.

There is also a clear genetic component. The lifetime risk of schizophrenia in the general population is just below 1%, rises to 6.5% in the first-degree relatives of affected individuals and is higher than 40% in those with an affected monozygotic twin.

The dopamine hypothesis

The development and effectiveness of haloperidol (a first-generation antipsychotic of the butyrophenone family) in the 1950s led to the emergence of the dopamine hypothesis as the central neurobiological underpinning of schizophrenia. According to the dopamine hypothesis, central dopaminergic hyperactivity in the mesolimbic tract precipitates positive symptoms, while the disrupted dopamine activity in the mesocortical circuits may explain the negative symptomatology.

Haloperidol, along with other antipsychotics, act as D2 receptor antagonists, with various degrees of affinity to the receptor. In addition, 5-HT2A antagonism and/or 5-HT1A agonism may contribute to the therapeutic effects of the SGAs. These receptors in the prefrontal cortex are also thought to contribute to the pathology of the negative symptoms. Other dopamine tracts are implicated in the development of side-effects (Table 25.2).

First-generation antipsychotics

FGAs all act by dopamine antagonism. In general, high potency antipsychotics (e.g. haloperidol, fluphenazine) cause greater EPS than low potency agents (e.g. chlorpromazine, thioridazine). In

TABLE 25.2 ■ Dopamine Tracts

Dopamine Tract	Function	Dopamine Antagonist Effect
Nigrostriatal	Extrapyramidal system, movement	Movement disorders (acute dystonia, akathisia, parkinsonism and tardive dyskinesia)
Mesolimbic	Emotional functioning, motivational behaviour	Relief of psychosis
Mesocortical	Cognition, executive function	Relief of psychosis, akathisia, worsening of negative symptoms
Tuberoinfundibular	Regulates prolactin release	Hyperprolactinaemia

contrast, low potency agents cause more sedation and anticholinergic side-effects. In addition, these agents can cause significant prolongation of the QT interval on electrocardiogram, which can precipitate a ventricular arrhythmia called 'torsades de pointes'.

Second-generation antipsychotics

SGAs have a rapid dissociation at D2 receptors and a strong affinity for blocking 5-HT2A receptors, therefore demonstrating a sustained antipsychotic effect with a significantly lower risk of EPS. Moreover, they have been associated with improved compliance. They have multiple additional receptor binding affinities and some of their adverse effects can be explained by their action at histaminergic, cholinergic, alpha-adrenergic receptor blockade.

SGAs are also associated with a variety of side-effects. Olanzapine, clozapine and quetiapine are particularly associated with sedation. Clozapine and olanzapine have well recognized anticholinergic effects and are especially associated with adverse metabolic effects, including weight gain, hyperglycaemia and dyslipidaemia that have been the subject of litigation in the United States. It is recommended that those patients who are prescribed an atypical drug associated with weight gain, and especially those with cardiovascular disease, have regular metabolic monitoring that includes weight, glycaemic status and lipids measured regularly. Risperidone and amisulpride are implicated in hyperprolactinaemia and can cause unwanted side-effects of gynecomastia, galactorrhoea, abnormalities of the menstrual cycle, impotence and osteoporosis. SGAs are also associated with QT prolongation (Table 25.3).

Clozapine

Clozapine is currently licensed for treatment-resistant schizophrenia, which is defined by the lack of response to adequate trials of two or more conventional antipsychotics (one of which must be an SGA).

TABLE 25.3 ■ Example of Monitoring Protocol for Patients on Antipsychotics

	Baseline	4 weeks	8 weeks	12 weeks	Quarterly	Annually
Personal/family history	*					
Weight (BMI)	*	*	*	*	*	*
Waist circumference	*					*
BP	*			*	*	
Fasting BG	*			*		*
Fasting lipids	*			*		*
ECG	*					*

BMI, body mass index; BG, blood glucose; ECG, electrocardiogram

Clozapine was first used in the 1960s but was withdrawn from the market following recognition of its association with neutropenia and agranulocytosis. Around 2%–3% of patients treated with clozapine will develop neutropenia, and less than 1% will develop agranulocytosis. In many countries, the re-introduction of clozapine was supported by regular full blood count monitoring with emphasis upon the potential for neutropenia. This typically involves a weekly blood test that can be stretched to fortnightly and monthly testing over time as agranulocytosis becomes less likely with sustained use.

Later, in 1988, it was shown that clozapine was more effective than conventional antipsychotics, and it was dispensed in the United Kingdom, although with compulsory monitoring for neutropenia and agranulocytosis.

FURTHER READING

For a review of the effectiveness of antipsychotic agents, including clozapine, see: Siskind D, McCartney L, Goldschlager R, Kisely S. (2016) Clozapine v. first- and second-generation antipsychotics in treatment-refractory schizophrenia: systematic review and meta-analysis. British Journal of Psychiatry 209(5):385–392. doi:10.1192/bjp.bp.115.177261

Clozapine remains the only antipsychotic known to be efficacious in individuals with treatment-resistance and has superior efficacy in decreasing suicidal behaviour and violence.

Clozapine is a powerful drug in treatment-resistant illness. As a general rule patients who have failed two previous antipsychotic medication trials experience full symptom remission (one-third), partial symptom remission (one-third) and minimal response (one-third). Clozapine has a complex pharmacodynamic profile with multiple receptor actions that also bring a variety of adverse effects, such as sialorrhea (excessive salivation), sedation, weight gain, metabolic disturbance and seizures.

In Piotr's case, it would be appropriate to discuss a trial of clozapine at this point while raising the practical aspects of its prescription, including regular monitoring of his full blood count, the importance of adherence and other potential side-effects.

The risk of myocarditis ($<1\%$) and lowering of seizure threshold should be discussed along with the likelihood of weight gain, hypersalivation and sedation.

The pharmacology of clozapine differs substantially from other antipsychotics in that it binds weakly to D_1 and D_2 receptors. However, it has an affinity for D_4, $5HT_2$, $5HT_3$, α_1 and α_2 adrenergic, ACh M_1, and H_1 receptors. It has not been established which individual or combination of these receptors is responsible for the efficacy of clozapine. Clozapine is associated with an extremely low rate of EPS and it is not believed to cause tardive dyskinesia.

---

3. Despite your encouragement, Piotr is reluctant to take clozapine, as he is not keen on the idea of regular blood testing and states that 'none of your tablets ever seem to make any difference'. You note that he has longstanding orofacial grimacing and that his feet seem to be moving without his voluntary control. He is disorganized, with a blunted affect, and he appears more distressed by his systemized delusions that the government is monitoring him. There is no evidence of suicidal or homicidal thinking. Piotr clearly states that he is not prepared to make any further changes to his medications and no longer wishes to attend the day hospital. He agrees to see you on a six-monthly basis only. His family remain concerned and ask for a 'brain scan...in case you have misdiagnosed him'. Staff at the day hospital report that Piotr is smoking more heavily than normal, and he has been seen in the company of other service users who have had issues with substance misuse.

   8. What do you think these motor symptoms are and what do you understand about the mechanism of their development?

   9. How are they treated?

  10. How would you address possible substance misuse?

  11. What is known about the radiological findings in schizophrenia?

EPS include dystonia (continuous spasms and muscle contractions), akathisia (motor restlessness), parkinsonism (characteristic symptoms such as rigidity), bradykinesia (slowness of movement), tremor and tardive dyskinesia (irregular, jerky movements). These features differ in their timing with dystonic reactions typically occurring within hours of commencing an antipsychotic, parkinsonism within days or weeks, acute akathisia within hours to weeks and tardive dyskinesia, usually only after many months or years of treatment.

In parkinsonism, bradykinesia can be easily mistaken for either depression or negative symptoms of schizophrenia. Physical examination should aid in its identification as it is frequently accompanied by rigidity in parkinsonism.

FURTHER READING

For a review of combination treatment strategies in schizophrenia, see: Correll CU, Rubio JM, Inczedy-Farkas G, et al. (2017) Efficacy of 42 pharmacologic cotreatment strategies added to antipsychotic monotherapy in schizophrenia. JAMA Psychiatry 74(7):675–684. doi:10.1001/jamapsychiatry.2017.0624

Piotr appears to have tardive dyskinesia, which is caused by the super-sensitivity of dopamine receptors in the nigrostriatal pathway. Treatment of tardive dyskinesia (along with dystonia, akathisia and neuroleptic malignant syndrome) is covered in detail in Chapter 24. Briefly, there should be a withdrawal of any prescribed anticholinergic agent, lowering of the dose of an antipsychotic agent (which may temporarily worsen the dyskinesia) and consideration of substitution with a less 'potent' agent. In this case, clozapine is the most appropriate medication.

In terms of treatment-resistance if, as is the case with Piotr, clozapine is not a preferred option, combinations of antipsychotic agents are often used in clinical practice to broaden receptor binding affinity. However it should be noted that there is a limited evidence base for this approach.

FURTHER READING

For a review of family interventions in schizophrenia, see: Pharoah F, Mari J, Rathbone J, Wong W. (2010) Family intervention for schizophrenia. Cochrane Database of Systematic Reviews 12:CD000088. doi:10.1002/14651858.CD000088.pub2

At this point it would be prudent to reassess Piotr's diagnosis, rule out any comorbid substance abuse and assess any current stressors, such as 'expressed emotion (EE)' in the home. People with schizophrenia from families that express high levels of criticism, hostility or over-involvement (i.e. high EE), have more frequent relapses than people with similar problems from families that tend to be less expressive of emotions. There is consistent evidence that high EE (including controlling attitudes, hostility and criticism) has discernible pathophysiological effects and a significant correlation with relapse frequency. Typical interventions include reducing exposure to the high EE environment (e.g. with daytime placements in day facilities). There is some evidence that family-based psychoeducational interventions can reduce the level of EE and that this is associated with better medication compliance, fewer relapses and fewer periods of hospitalization.

Drug analysis

Substance misuse is common in individuals with schizophrenia. Although there is a marked variation between studies, as many as 50% of affected individuals abuse alcohol or other substances. In addition, around 70% are addicted to nicotine. Cigarette smoking appears to regulate the mesolimbic dopamine system and improves cognitive performance by reducing so-called 'hypofrontality'. As such, it may be a form of self-medication. Conversely, it is a postulated causal factor in the development of psychosis and may significantly decrease antipsychotic levels (clozapine).

FURTHER READING

For a review of testing for illicit drug use in mental health services, see: Abraham A, Luty J. (2010) Testing for illicit drug use in mental health services. Advances in Psychiatric Treatment 16(5):369–379. doi:10.1192/apt.bp.108.005835

As in Piotr's case, when there is an inconsistency between history (there are no clear precipitating causes for his deterioration) and clinical symptoms/signs, drug testing may be necessary. On-the-spot screening by urine testing is usually sufficient. Nonetheless, confirmatory laboratory tests may be indicated if there is a diagnostic dilemma, if the patient disputes a screening result, or if there are serious implications to a positive result (e.g. in child protection cases). Urine screening is inexpensive and simple to administer with instant results. However, its usefulness may be limited by adulteration, urine tampering and false-positives. A further complication is that long-term cannabis use can produce positive results in the urine up to 45 days after cessation. The interaction between substance abuse and psychosis is discussed in detail in Chapter 12.

Neuroimaging

Neuroimaging is indicated as part of the workup in individuals presenting with a first psychotic episode and may be considered in those with an established psychotic illness for whom their symptomatology changes dramatically. In both situations, the primary role of neuroimaging is to rule out organic factors such as an intracerebral tumour or stroke.

Despite the request, there is no diagnostic test for the presence of schizophrenia. However, there is an increasing body of research identifying the neurobiological underpinnings associated with psychotic illnesses.

Structural magnetic resonance imaging findings in patients with schizophrenia have revealed widespread reductions in grey matter (GM). GM reduction in the medial temporal lobe structures, thalamus, basal ganglia, amygdala, hippocampus, parahippocampal gyrus and neocortical temporal lobe regions is linked to lateral ventricular enlargement and third ventricle enlargement.

FURTHER READING

For a review of the findings from functional image studies in schizophrenia, see: Fitzsimmons J, Kubicki M, Shenton ME. (2013) Review of functional and anatomical brain connectivity findings in schizophrenia. Current Opinion in Psychiatry 26(2):172–187. doi:10.1097/YCO.0b013e32835d9e6a

Studies have investigated the disordered functional brain anatomy of both the positive and negative symptoms of schizophrenia. These indicate that hallucinations are associated with abnormal brain activity in primary and secondary sensory areas. Disordered activation in nonsensory regions appears to contribute to the emotional impact of hallucinations as a factor underlying an inability to distinguish ongoing mental processing from memories. Brain activation studies support the view that auditory or verbal hallucinations are associated with an impaired ability of internal speech plans to modulate neural activation in sensory language areas. Negative symptoms of schizophrenia are associated with impaired function in frontal brain areas with resting blood flow and metabolism in the frontal cortex reduced in schizophrenia. Brain activation studies indicate impairment of working memory functioning and are linked to impaired functional connections between the frontal and temporal cortex.

---

4. Piotr's family meet with you to discuss further management options. They are concerned that his condition will deteriorate without more regular contact with the services. After meeting with the mental health advocacy services, they understand the limitations of medication and are interested in other models of care. They are particularly interested in the possibility of CBT. The meeting with the advocacy service has made them more optimistic in general, especially as the advocate told them that all service users could 'recover' from mental illness.

    12.   What nonpharmacological treatment options are available for the management of schizophrenia?

    13.   What is the prognosis in severe and enduring mental illness?

    14.   How would you respond to the family's observation about 'recovery?'

Psycho-social interventions

There are a variety of augmented models of routine care that may help to alleviate symptoms of chronic illness, improve engagement with services and improve social and occupational dysfunction. These interventions work in synergy with pharmacological approaches and are traditionally provided by rehabilitation and recovery teams in the Irish setting, as outlined in Table 25.4.

Prognosis

The prognosis for individuals with schizophrenia varies considerably. Overall, the life expectancy of persons with severe and enduring mental illness (e.g. schizophrenia) is 12–15 years shorter than for the general population. This effect is principally mediated by lifestyle issues and reflected in cardiovascular disease, respiratory illnesses and cancer statistics. In addition, the lifetime risk of suicide is significantly raised at 5%–10%.

Prognostic factors that can be assessed in the first episode are outlined in Chapter 4. The historical observation that one-third of affected individuals recover, one-third remit/relapse and one-third deteriorate appears to under-represent those with a favourable prognosis as demonstrated in more recent studies. The course of the first two years appears to predict long-term outcomes. Therefore, perhaps logically early intervention at medical, social and psychological levels is associated with long-term benefits (see Chapter 4).

TABLE 25.4 ■ Psycho-social Interventions

Intervention	Description	Evidence
Assertive community treatment/intensive case management	Multidisciplinary team intervention to maintain and improve contact	Reduced hospitalization and enhanced quality of life
Skills training	Provided as part of an integrated care plan	Skills for improved community functioning, improved interpersonal relationships and quality of life
Family-based services	Patients with ongoing family contact	Increased family involvement, reduced hospitalizations
CBT	Targets symptoms and coping strategies	Some evidence for a reduction in positive and negative symptoms
Substance abuse interventions	Targets comorbid alcohol or substance abuse	Fewer relapses, improved treatment adherence

CBT, cognitive behavioural therapy

Recovery

Response to intervention in schizophrenia is often referred to in terms of remission and recovery. For 'remission' the Diagnostic and Statistical Manual of Mental Disorders requires that there should be a 'complete return to full functioning', while other definitions require specific symptoms to be controlled and not interfering with functioning.

Further complexity has risen with service user-defined concepts of recovery. The 'recovery model' (which the mental health advocate in this case has referred to) incorporates a wide range of factors, which may be at odds with clinician defined criteria. The model has been described as a 'journey' (analogous with the recovery of those with addictions), that emphasizes user-empowerment, hope and optimism, personal responsibility, autonomy, self-management and person-centred treatments. The recovery model focuses on collaborative treatment approaches, finding productive roles for users, peer support and reducing stigma. The model is viewed by many as an antidote to the lack of optimism that many perceive with the medical model, which has significant limitations in terms of effectiveness for many people with a severe and enduring illness. The recovery approach is increasingly incorporated into the development of mental health services around the globe.

FURTHER READING

For a discussion of the recovery model in schizophrenia, see: Warner R. (2009) Recovery from schizophrenia and the recovery model. Current Opinion in Psychiatry 22(4):374–380. doi:10.1097/YCO.0b013e32832c920b

---

The recovery approach considers 'illness' and 'wellness' as independent variables and services have increasingly incorporated these values. It is apparent that, although schizophrenia remains a serious illness with a higher morbidity and mortality, most individuals with the condition can live a meaningful and satisfying life in the presence of treatment-resistant symptoms.

CHAPTER 26

Mark

School Refusal

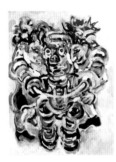

1. Understand the difference between school refusal, school phobia, truancy and condoned absence from school.
2. Appreciate the importance of detailed history taking from multiple sources (parents, school, general practitioner), especially when looking at a family history of psychiatric problems.
3. Appreciate the importance of working with the family, school, educational psychologist and educational welfare officer.
4. Understand the considerations for performing an age-appropriate mental health assessment.
5. Recognize how to assess social media use in a young person and how to probe for problematic experiences.
6. Understand what is meant by bullying and how to respond to it.

---

1. It is mid-October, and you are the nonconsultant hospital doctor on call in the child and adolescent mental health service. The receptionist informs you that a fax has come in from a local general practitioner marked urgent and for the attention of the duty doctor. You read the referral, and it describes a 12-year-old boy, Mark, who is refusing to attend school. His general practitioner described an 'anxious appearing young man, attended with his mother, refusing to attend school, expressing thoughts of killing himself'. Regarding background, the general practitioner reported only a family history of generalized anxiety disorder without further details.
   1. What are the child and adolescent mental health service referral criteria and how will you triage this referral?

The health, safety and environment (HSE) child and adolescent mental health service (CAMHS) standard operating procedure states that children up to the age of 18 with moderate to severe mental health disorders that were unsuccessfully treated in primary care are appropriate to refer to CAMHS. This includes children with suicidal thoughts or behaviour. Current exclusion criteria include children with moderate or severe intellectual disability, pure developmental disorders and children in need of educational assessment and intervention as there are alternate specialized services for the assessment and management of these difficulties.

In this case, the referral indicates that Mark is objectively anxious and has been thinking about suicide. However, there are very few details, and more information would be required to triage the referral properly. A comprehensive collateral history at this stage will inform whether the child should be seen on an emergency, high priority or routine basis.

---

2. You contact Mark's mother, Mary, whose phone number was also on the general practitioner's referral. You tell Mary that you have received the referral and would like to get some more information.

Mary is very concerned with Mark's behaviour over the last few weeks. She reports that 'he has been spending more time in his room and has been avoiding going to school. This is new behaviour for him. He previously seemed to enjoy school. He has always been bright and received positive reports from his teachers. He has not explained this change other than saying that he hates school and does not want to go anymore. On a few occasions, he has refused to put on his uniform, which led to arguments with Mark crying and having a tantrum. He has missed school on four occasions over the last three weeks, including being home from school today.

Mary spoke to Mark's teacher last week who reassured her that Mark was just finding the transition to secondary school difficult. She said that this was common, and Mark would be fine after some more time.

When you raise the subject of Mark's suicidal thoughts, Mary begins to cry. 'What am I supposed to do?' she asks. 'He says he will kill himself if I make him go to school'.

Mary adds that Mark's two older brothers did very well in the same school and never had any such difficulties. They are both now in college and getting on 'great'. She worries that there is something wrong with Mark. 'He needs help, doctor', she says. 'I don't want anything to happen to him. He needs to be seen now!'

She denies ever having suspected Mark of doing anything to physically harm himself in the past.

2. Mary has become distressed on the phone. What are the implications of this for you?
3. Would you see Mark as an emergency (today), high priority (within a month) or as a routine referral (on the general waiting list, currently standing at four months)?
4. What is school refusal and what are the differential diagnoses?

There are several things for a doctor to take into consideration when a patient or family member becomes distressed on the phone, including the following:

1. It can be an indication of the severity of the situation and how much of an impact it is having on the family.
2. The details of the case aside, the distress should be addressed at the time in so far as is possible. The doctor might spend a little more time talking with Mary, acknowledging the difficulty she is experiencing, and being clear about a plan for handling the referral.
3. You are aware of the general practitioner's letter that there is a family history of anxiety. Mark's mother becoming upset might make you think about the level of distress within the home. What kind of atmosphere is Mark living in now?

Considering Mary's distress, Mark's comments about ending his life, his recent change in behaviour and self-isolation in his bedroom, you decide to see Mark as soon as possible. Mary is happy to bring Mark to the CAMHS office later this afternoon. You ask that both parents attend with Mark so that you can get a better impression of the family unit.

The definition of school refusal is 'child-motivated refusal to attend school or difficulties remaining in school for an entire day'. Common factors in its development include the following:

- Social and peer-related difficulties
- Learning and curriculum difficulties
- Difficulties with the physical environment.

The differential diagnosis includes the following:

- Truancy: Occurs when the child is absent from school without the knowledge and agreement of parents. Often associated with antisocial behaviours, oppositional defiant disorder or conduct disorder.
- School phobia: Occurs when the child has a specific fear of someone or something at school.
- Condoned absence: Occurs when the child is absent from school with the knowledge and agreement of his parents. Parents may believe that school is harming the child in some way, or they want a child at home to help with housework or just for company.
- Generalized anxiety, social anxiety or separation anxiety.

---

3. Mark arrives with his mother. You first meet them both together and explain to them what to expect before asking questions. When establishing who comprises Mark's family, Mary tells you that Mark's father, Patrick, was too busy with work to attend this appointment, to which Mark makes a grunting sound.

After this, you notice that Mark is quiet throughout this meeting and mostly stares at the floor and plays with the zip on his coat.

Mary is tearful as she speaks and tells about how her 'little boy' has changed and how she is worried about him. In particular, she is concerned about how missing school might affect his future. 'He has missed so many days already this year', she says. 'He had a sore throat in the first week and a tummy bug the week after. Now he just doesn't want to go to school at all'.

She describes Mark's older brothers as being sportier than Mark, and that his eldest brother played football for Limerick. She says that Mark has always been more introverted than his siblings and she has worried about this. He was attached to her as a preschool child, always wanting to be with her and getting very upset when she had to leave him, particularly when dropping him to crèche. He did, however, seem to enjoy primary school and 'made very nice friends', some of whom are now in the same secondary school as Mark.

She denies there is anything particularly stressful at home. Her husband works long hours in his accountancy practice and she works part-time in a clothes boutique in the local shopping centre.

5. What do you think is significant in Mary's account?
6. What is separation anxiety disorder and how does it present?
7. What is attachment and how does it relate to school refusal and anxiety disorders?

Mark's father was too busy to attend. You believe it is difficult to assess the significance of this as the appointment was arranged urgently. It may have been entirely unavoidable, but it is worth noting to see if a pattern emerges over time.

There seems to be a consistent theme of comparing Mark to his siblings and an expectation that he conform to both their interests and achievements.

Mary highlights that Mark was 'very attached' to her as a child, that he had difficulty separating from her in preschool years and that she has always worried about him. It is worth thinking about the kind of attachment Mark had with his mother and how that might impact his mental health today.

Worries in children are common and are a normal part of child development. Children with anxiety disorders have more intense worries. Approximately 1 in 10 children and adolescents will fulfil the diagnostic criteria for an anxiety disorder throughout their childhood. Comorbidity with other anxiety disorders and depression is common. Childhood anxiety can have an unremitting course and persist into adulthood.

Separation anxiety presents as inappropriate fear in a child when separated from their main attachment figure, usually a parent. It often presents around times of change, such as starting in crèche, playschool, Montessori or moving from primary school to secondary school.

Attachment is a measure of the bond or relationship between a carer (e.g. a parent) and the person being cared for (e.g. the child). Good, secure attachment develops from appropriate stimulation, warmth and control from the parent to the child. Insecure attachment, lack of appropriate stimulation and inappropriate parenting styles predispose children to psychological difficulties.

Severe attachment problems can manifest as disturbed and developmentally inappropriate social relatedness across most contexts.

For example, attachment issues relating to over-concerned mothers and under-interested fathers can sometimes lead to separation anxiety and subsequently, school refusal in children (Table 26.1).

---

4. You ask to speak to Mark alone and Mary consents. You begin by asking Mark a little about himself, what his interests are and how he feels about school. Mark is initially quite nervous. However, he gradually opens up about his interests, which are quite varied.

He describes his ambitions to be a 'YouTuber'. He tells you he has 233 subscribers and 10,000 views on his channel. You make a note about social media use to remind yourself to come back to this topic later.

Moving onto school, Mark explains he 'hates it', 'doesn't fit in' and 'doesn't want to go back'. He reports he has no struggles academically and finds his homework manageable. He has no friends in school, and he reports that all his friends are online. He feels he is bullied and picked on, and when he goes to retrieve his books from his locker, he is often pushed and shoved around. When you ask whether he has told his parents about this, Mark says that he has not, stating his mother would get too worked up about it and start crying, and his father would just tell him to stand up for himself.

8. What would happen if Mary did not consent to you speaking with him on his own?
9. Should you have a chaperone with you speaking to children on their own?
10. How would you adapt your interview style when talking with Mark?

Particularly, in older children, it can be beneficial to speak to a child without a parent present. If a good rapport can be established, children may disclose more to a professional when alone as there are often topics they find it difficult to speak about in front of their parents.

Mary is Mark's mother and, as Mark is under 18 years, can refuse to allow you to speak to him alone. Some parents may not feel comfortable having their child assessed without their presence because they expect the experience to be difficult and wish to advocate for their child. Usually, parents want what is best for their child and having a conversation with a parent in such circumstances, explaining the rationale for seeing the child alone and reassuring the parent about any concerns, can often lead to consent being granted. If the parent does not change their mind, the interview can proceed with the parent present.

In certain cases, it is prudent to have a chaperone or a second professional present to assess children either on their own or with their parents, but it is not always necessary.

The content and the tone of questions must be adapted to the developmental stage of the child. Like all psychiatric consultations, warmth, empathy, kindness and genuineness contribute to good

---

TABLE 26.1 ■ **Types of Attachment Including Associated Caregiver and Child Behaviours**

Attachment Type	Caregiver Behaviours	Child Behaviours
Secure	React quickly and positively to the child's needs	Distressed when the caregiver leaves
		Happy when the caregiver returns
	Responsive to the child's needs	Seek comfort from a caregiver when scared or sad
Insecure–avoidant	Unresponsive, uncaring	No distress when caregiver leaves
	Dismissive	Does not acknowledge the return of caregiver
		Does not seek or contact a caregiver
Insecure–ambivalent	Responds to child inconsistently	Distress when caregiver leaves
		Not comforted by the return of caregiver
Insecure–disorganized	Abusive or neglectful	No attaching behaviours
	Responds in frightening ways	Often appear dazed, confused or apprehensive in the presence of a caregiver

therapeutic interactions. Asking open questions first but leading on then to the appropriate use of closed questions to redirect or prompt the child is useful.

---

5. Mark describes feeling frustrated, particularly with his parents, whom he says do not understand him and do not really want to know him. He feels they want him to be like his brothers. He gets on reasonably well with both brothers, but they do not have much in common. They are both older, they live away from home, and he reports that when they return home 'all the family talks about is sport'.

You ask him about his online friends. He talks to them mainly through online games like 'Fortnite', typically about the game they are playing or about how they do not like school. He mentions several social media apps, only some of which you are familiar with. He says that he uses these only to communicate with his friends and does not tend to 'follow' people. He denies ever being bullied online or ever receiving communications that might have been inappropriate.

You try to quantify the amount of time he spends gaming, on social media and electronic devices in general, but this proves difficult as he is vague, saying things like 'not that much' or 'it's different every day'. He says he cannot put precise times on it. He did say that he is online until at least midnight on school nights, and later at weekends.

Mark does not feel particularly 'happy', but also denies his mood is typically low, except when he thinks about going into school. He feels his energy is low, but he can enjoy things, particularly playing games online. His sleep has been poor, finding it takes him at least an hour to get to sleep after switching his phone off at night. At this time, his thoughts would be racing, often with negative thoughts about school. Once he gets to sleep, he rarely wakes during the night and is extremely tired when called for school in the morning. He finds it difficult to eat breakfast, but his appetite is fine for dinner in the evenings. He is having some difficulty concentrating on schoolwork but does not think his grades have slipped.

Besides feeling low when he thinks about school, he also feels anxious. The thought of going in and seeing 'those guys' makes him feel 'on edge' and 'nervous'. He has tried not to think about them on the way into school but finds this difficult. He has noticed that his muscles would be tense at these times. He agrees this may be affecting his appetite for breakfast as his stomach does not feel right. When he gets home, if the day has not been too bad, he can relax. He does not tend to worry about anything else. There are no other situations such as crowds or public places that make him anxious. He does not particularly like it when a teacher asks him a question in front of the class, or if put on the spot for his opinion in front of a group of his peers, but he has not noticed any physical symptoms at this time, such as sweating, being short of breath or feeling his heart is pounding.

When you ask him about the thoughts of harming himself, he gets annoyed. He said that he told his mother on one occasion that he would kill himself if she made him go to school. He said he did not mean it, but that he only said it so that he could stay at home. He denied having had any thoughts of hurting himself or of ending his life.

11. What is the relevance here of social media use? What would you consider excessive use with regards to social media, computer games and electronic devices?

12. What do you think the preferred diagnosis is?

Social media use can be associated with positive effects by promoting socialization and executive functioning but also has considerable potential for negative effects that include exploitation, harassment, bullying and reduction of self-esteem and self-worth. Teachers and parents report bullying within social media as common. The difficulties lie in the pervasiveness of social media and smartphones and the associated difficultly in moderating its use.

Clear evidence-based guidelines are lacking in the area of harm reduction with regard to social media, but many guidelines suggest a maximum of three hours per day of screen-time (this includes all smartphone, console use, computer use) that is purely recreational or social.

FURTHER READING

For a review of the concept of school refusal, see: Elliot JG, Place M. (2017) Practitioner review: school refusal: developments in conceptualization and treatment since 2000. Journal of Child Psychology and Psychiatry 60(1):4–15. doi:10.1111/jcpp.12848

Problematic use is associated with the symptoms of emotional dysregulation when use is interrupted or curtailed, salience (total preoccupation with social media), tolerance (consuming more and more social media), irritability, anxiety when social media use is restricted), conflict (such as interpersonal problems as a direct result of social media usage) and relapse (e.g. returning to excessive social media use after a period of abstinence).

---

6. You meet with Mark's mother alone. You ask her about Mark's relationship with his father, and you get a sense they have struggled over the last few months as they seem to have very little in common. Mary corroborates most of what Mark says about his sleep and appetite. She was aware that Mark uses his mobile phone a lot and is quick to inform you she never approved of him getting one. She is happy to remove the phone immediately, but you caution that such an approach may make things worse in the short term.

You explain that the consultation time is coming to an end and you will not have time to cover everything from the history today. You ask her to complete a child development questionnaire.

Finally, you invite Mark back in. You get written consent from both Mark and Mary to contact the school to request a school report and to speak with Mark's homeroom teacher or principal. You ask Mark to keep a sleep diary. You inform the family that you are concerned about the amount of Mark's screen-time. Mark is annoyed with this but agrees to come to an arrangement with his parents about appropriate limits, including switching off all screens one hour before bedtime and to leave his phone off overnight.

You give Mark's parents a copy of a sleep diary, a school attendance diary and written information from the Department of Education on school refusal. You advise the parents that on the days that Mark does not attend school, he should do schoolwork at home and not have access to his phone or his Xbox. You ask them to return in two weeks.

You discuss the case at the multidisciplinary team meeting. You give a summary of the case and explain some parts of the history are incomplete because you spent a lot of time building rapport and trying to understand the family dynamic. The occupational therapist gives you advice on dealing with school anxiety/refusal and encourages the use of the attendance diary. She suggests getting his locker location changed to somewhere more appropriate and discussing your concerns about bullying with the principal but explains that it is better to empower the parents to take responsibility for this. The clinical psychologist is interested in the developmental history and role of attachment issues. She is happy to see Mark for cognitive behavioural therapy for anxiety when you have completed the formulation.

You contact the school principal after you have reviewed the school reports. He informs you that Mark is new to the school but based on previous standardized tests and individual teacher's assessments, there is unlikely to be an underlying learning or educational issue. He was unaware of the bullying issue but reports that the school has a policy for managing bullying and will intervene quickly to address any issues. He states Mark has struggled to adapt to the new school and his teachers report he does not seem to have many friends. He reports that no educational psychology assessment has been performed and this particular case is unlikely to meet the threshold for a report under the National Educational Psychological Service, but he will make the referral.

13. What is 'bullying' as defined by the Department of Education and the Department of Health?

Bullying is defined in the anti-bullying procedures for primary and post-primary schools as 'unwanted negative behaviour, verbal, psychological or physical conducted by an individual or group against another person (or persons), and which is repeated over time'.

FURTHER READING

For a discussion of bullying in schools, see: Menesini E, Salmivalli C. (2017) Bullying in schools: the state of knowledge and effective interventions. Psychology, Health & Medicine 22 (Suppl1):240–253. doi:10.1080/13548506.2017.1279740

The HSE Dignity at work policy describes workplace bullying as repeated inappropriate behaviour, direct or indirect, whether verbal, physical or otherwise, conducted by one or more persons against another or others, at the place of work and/or in the course of employment, which could reasonably be regarded as undermining the individual's right to dignity at work.

---

7. You meet the family again two weeks later, and this time both parents attend. They report that things are a lot better now that many issues are out in the open. You review the child development questionnaire and note normal milestone development. You do not find evidence of an insecure or disorganized attachment nor the presence of separation anxiety in earlier years.

When you speak to Mark alone, you ask him about his friends and whether he has a boyfriend or a girlfriend. He says that he has friends online but fewer friends this year in school or at home.

Regarding school he has attended 8/10 school days, missing the two previous Mondays. His father has taken over giving him a lift to school in the morning and accompanies him to the front gate of the school. He is sleeping more regular hours and has accepted the curtailment of screen-time. He says the principal put his locker on the same floor as his common room and he does not have to go into the 'locker room' anymore. There was a talk about bullying in the school, and for the time being, people are leaving him to his own devices. He still does not like school, but it is more manageable now.

14. What are the potential long-term effects of school refusal?
15. What are the treatment options?

Effects of school refusal include the following:

- Impacts education
- Reduces future opportunities
- Affects social development
- May undermine self-esteem.

Legally, parents are responsible for making sure their children are educated. An educational welfare officer is tasked with the job of ensuring that children attend school.

Treatment depends on the severity of the symptoms and how entrenched the refusal to attend school is:

- Education for the patient, the family and the school about the condition.
- The patient is encouraged to attend school, on a gradual or partial basis working toward complete attendance.
- Severe cases may require a change of school or home-schooling.
- Precipitants such as bullying and social anxiety must be addressed.
- Educational Psychologist service from the school or Department of Health should be involved early on.
- Education welfare officer from Child Protection Services should be involved in cases that meet the threshold for an excessive number of absences.
- Cognitive behavioural therapy (CBT)-style therapy can be helpful.
- Intense CBT and other behavioural approaches can be implemented for difficult cases.

   Occasionally, low dosage serotonin specific reuptake inhibitors can be helpful for patients with comorbid anxiety.

Page numbers followed by "b", "f" and "t" indicate boxes, figures and tables respectively.